# OBSTETRICS AND GYNECOLOGY RECALL

# RECALL SERIES EDITOR

**LORNE H. BLACKBOURNE, M.D.**
General Surgeon
Major, Medical Corps
United States Army
Fort Eustis, Virginia

# OBSTETRICS AND GYNECOLOGY RECALL

### EDITOR

**F. JOHN BOURGEOIS, M.D., F.A.C.O.G., F.A.C.P.**
Associate Professor
Department of Obstetrics and Gynecology
University of Virginia
Charlottesville, Virginia

### ASSOCIATE EDITORS

**PAOLA A. MULLIN, M.D.**
Resident
Department of Obstetrics and Gynecology
University of Virginia
Charlottesville, Virginia

**DANIEL S. VELJOVICH, M.D.**
Resident
Department of Obstetrics and Gynecology
University of Virginia
Charlottesville, Virginia

## Williams & Wilkins
### A WAVERLY COMPANY

BALTIMORE • PHILADELPHIA • LONDON • PARIS • BANGKOK
BUENOS AIRES • HONG KONG • MUNICH • SYDNEY • TOKYO • WROCLAW

Editor: Elizabeth Nieginski
Managing Editor: Darrin Kiessling
Manager, Development Editing: Julie Scardiglia
Marketing Manager: Rebecca Himmelheber
Development Editor: Carol Loyd
Production Coordinator: Cindy Park
Design Coordinator: Mario Fernandez
Typesetter: Port City Press, Inc.
Printer: Vicks Lithograph & Printing
Digitized Illustrations: Port City Press, Inc.
Binder: Vicks Lithograph & Printing

Copyright © 1997 Williams & Wilkins

351 West Camden Street
Baltimore, Maryland 21201-2436 USA

Rose Tree Corporate Center
1400 North Providence Road
Building II, Suite 5025
Media, Pennsylvania 19063-2043 USA

Accurate indications, adverse reactions and dosage schedules for drugs are provided
in this book, but it is possible that they may change. The reader is urged to review
the package information data of the manufacturers of the medications mentioned.

Printed in the United States of America

**Library of Congress Cataloging-in-Publication Data**

Bourgeois, F. John.
   Obstetrics and gynecology recall / F. John Bourgeois.
      p.   cm.—(Recall series)
   Includes index.
   ISBN 0-683-18214-5
   1. Obstetrics—Examinations, questions, etc.   2. Gynecology—Examinations,
questions, etc.  I. Title.  II. Series.
   [DNLM:  1. Obstetrics—examination questions.  2. Genital Diseases,
Female—examination questions.  WQ 18.2 B772o 1997]
   RG111.B68  1997
   618′.076—dc21
   DNLM/DLC
   for Library of Congress                          97–10753
                                            CIP

*The publishers have made every effort to trace the copyright holders for borrowed
material. If they have inadvertently overlooked any, they will be pleased to make
the necessary arrangements at the first opportunity.*

To purchase additional copies of this book, call our customer service department at
**(800) 638-0672** or fax orders to **(800) 447-8438.** For other book services, including
chapter reprints and large quantity sales, ask for the Special Sales department.

Canadian customers should call **(800) 665-1148**, or fax **(800) 665-0103.** For all
other calls originating outside of the United States, please call **(410) 528-4223** or
fax us at **(410) 528-8550.**

**Visit Williams & Wilkins on the Internet:** **http://www.wwilkins.com** or contact
our customer service department at **custserv@wwilkins.com**. Williams & Wilkins
customer service representatives are available from 8:30 am to 6:00 pm, EST, Monday
through Friday, for telephone access.

98 99 00
2 3 4 5 6 7 8 9 10

# Dedication

This book recognizes Annie Bourgeois, who valued veracity and education, and did not care to compromise either. It is further an acknowledgment of the scholarship of W. Norman Thornton, Jr., M.D., who understands that the framework of knowledge and understanding does not require large volumes of words, but does require prioritization. I hope it reflects the philosophy of Joe Covelli, M.D., who understood that in clinical medicine compassion without accuracy doesn't do much good. However, it is dedicated to you.

# Contents

# Contributors

Gina Adrales, M.D.
Terry Allen, M.D.
Jessica Biesecker, M.D.
Susan Bliss, M.D.
Megan Bray, M.D.
Amy Erdman, M.D.
Maria Gluch, M.D.
Kathie Hullfish, M.D.
Amir Jazaeri, M.D.
Elizabeth Kane, M.D.
Sunita Kulshrestha, M.D.
Kelly MacMillan, M.D.
Helen Malone, M.D.
Tanya Paul, M.D.
John Schnorr, M.D.
Amy Timmons, M.D.
Charrell Washington, M.D.

# Preface

It's no accident that it's called "Recall." The questions and answers contained in this book review the fundamentals of obstetrics and gynecology, absent lengthy explanations and literature citations. *Obstetrics and Gynecology Recall* is designed to complement, not replace, more weighty sources. It is intended as a touchstone for testing students' mastery of already-gained knowledge—a good use for this book during both the clerkship and while preparing for the inevitable final exam.

But that's not all. What if you are just beginning your clerkship, and you are assigned a patient with a condition that you have barely heard of? Your guidebook to the essentials is *Obstetrics and Gynecology Recall*. By evening rounds you can be conversant regarding the condition, and well-prepared to consult a more comprehensive reference—a good way to generate knowledge and a great way to guarantee good evaluations.

Whether you need a rapid way to begin learning the fundamentals, or require a concise review of the key elements of obstetrics and gynecology to efficiently test your knowledge base, *Obstetrics and Gynecology Recall* is the place to start *and* to finish.

# Section 1

Obstetrics

# 1

# Obstetric Glossary

**Abortion**

Pregnancy termination prior to 20 weeks' gestation with fetus weighing less than 500 grams
    Complete—all products of conception are evacuated
    Incomplete—some products of conception remain in the uterus
    Inevitable—vaginal bleeding with an open cervix
    Threatened—vaginal bleeding with a closed cervix

**Abruption**

Complete or partial separation of the placenta prior to the delivery of the fetus

**AFP**

Alpha-fetoprotein; produced primarily by the fetal liver, used as a screening test for congenital birth defects and chromosomal anomalies

**Amniocentesis**

Removal of amniotic fluid, usually by transabdominal aspiration; used either for therapeutic or diagnostic purposes

**Amniotic fluid**

During the first trimester, an ultrafiltrate of maternal plasma
Later in gestation, transudation of fetal plasma across the fetal skin
At 12 to 24 weeks, fetal urine begins to contribute.
Other sources include the fetal gastrointestinal and respiratory tracts, as well as transudate across the umbilical cord.

**Apgar score**

Assessment of the newborn, primarily at 1, 5, and 10 minutes by evaluating tone, heart rate, irritability, color, and respirations

**β-HCG**

Beta subunit of human chorionic gonadotropin
Produced by the syncytiotrophoblast
Maintains the corpus luteum in early pregnancy
Used to detect pregnancy

**Biophysical profile**

Intrauterine evaluation of the fetus using nonstress test (NST), fetal breathing movements, fetal movement, fetal tone, and amniotic fluid index (AFI)

**Bishop score**

A scoring system used to assess the likelihood of success of induction of labor using factors such as dilatation, effacement, station, consistency, and position of the cervix

**Breech**

Complete (5%–10%)—flexed thighs and knees, feet above the buttocks
Frank (50%–75%)—flexed thighs, extended knees
Footling or incomplete (20%)—leg(s) extended below the umbilicus

**Chadwick's sign**

A clinical sign consisting of a bluish discoloration to the cervix and vaginal walls that may suggest pregnancy

**Chloasma**

"Mask of pregnancy"; brownish patches of facial skin that may occur during pregnancy or with oral contraceptive use (also known as melasma)

**Chorioamnionitis**

Acute or chronic infection/inflammation of the fetal membranes

**CVS**

Chorionic villi sampling—placental tissue is removed between 9 and 12 weeks by either transabdominal or transvaginal means and used for genetic evaluation

**Coombs**

Used to detect maternal red blood cell antibodies

| | |
|---|---|
| **Corpus luteum** | Physiologic ovarian cyst; maintains progesterone production during early pregnancy until the placenta begins to function |
| **CST** | Contraction stress test |
| **Crown rump length** | In early pregnancy, used to estimate gestational age; add 6.5 weeks to the measurement obtained on ultrasound to estimate gestational age |
| **DES** | Diethylstilbestrol; fetal exposure to this drug may result in genital-tract anomalies, including incompetent cervix, cervical adenosis, increased risk for clear-cell adenocarcinoma of the cervix, and other uterine structural anomalies in women. Used archaically to prevent abortion |
| **DIC** | Disseminated intravascular coagulopathy |
| **"Double setup"** | Pelvic exam performed in the operating room with the means to perform an emergent cesarean section if there is significant bleeding or fetal distress; previously performed in women with suspected placenta previa |
| **Eclampsia** | Seizures during pregnancy; the most severe manifestation of pregnancy-induced hypertension |
| **EDC** | Estimated date of confinement ("due date"); 280 days from the first day of the last menstrual period |
| **FHR** | Fetal heart rate (normal is between 120 and 160 bpm, fetal bradycardia is < 120 bpm, and fetal tachycardia is > 160 bpm) |
| **FHT** | Fetal heart tone—refers to auditory detection of FHR |

**Episiotomy**

Surgical procedure performed at the time of vaginal delivery in an attempt to minimize stretching of the perineum
In this country, the most common form is a midline episiotomy extending from the posterior aspect of the vaginal introitus through the superficial perineal muscles and down through the vaginal mucosa.

**FSE**

Fetal scalp electrode—used to monitor fetal heart rate after rupture of the fetal membranes has occurred

**Forceps**

Mechanism to assist vaginal deliveries by shortening the second stage of labor
Indications include maternal exhaustion, fetal distress, and fetal malposition.
Several different types (e.g., Keilland, Piper, Tucker-McLean) are available, depending on the indication.

**GDM**

Gestational diabetes mellitus

**GTD**

Gestational trophoblastic disease

**Gravida**

The number of times a woman has been pregnant or a pregnant woman

**hCG**

Human chorionic gonadotropin

**HELLP**

Subset of preeclampsia characterized by Hemolysis, Elevated Liver enzymes, and Low Platelets

**hPL**

Human placental lactogen or human placental somatomammotropin

**Hydrops**

Anasarca of the fetus associated with ascites, generalized edema, pleural effusions, etc; most commonly ascribed to anemia as a consequence of hemolysis

| | |
|---|---|
| **Hyperemesis gravidarum** | Occurs in approximately 5/1000 pregnancies<br>Associated with nausea and vomiting causing dehydration, electrolyte imbalance and weight loss<br>Etiologic factors include psychosocial, thyroid disease, and trophoblastic disease. |
| **IUGR** | Intrauterine growth restriction<br>Asymmetric—Head growth remains near normal.<br>Symmetric—The entire fetus is small. |
| **IVF** | In vitro fertilization |
| **Kell antigen** | Major red blood cell antigen, may cause hydrops if present |
| **Labor** | Uterine contractions leading to cervical dilatation and effacement |
| **Leopold maneuvers** | Examination of maternal abdomen that allows fetal weight, position, and lie to be estimated |
| **Lie** | Relation of fetal spine to maternal spine; vertical or longitudinal is normal. |
| **Macrosomia** | Fetal weight greater than 4,000 grams; complicates approximately 5% of births<br>Risk factors include maternal obesity, postdate pregnancy, maternal diabetes including GDM, and multiparity. |
| **Magnesium sulfate** | Used in the treatment of preterm labor and eclamptic seizures |
| **Mastitis** | Infection of the breast, most commonly secondary to infections with *S. aureus* or *Streptococcus* as a result of breast-feeding<br>Feeding from the affected breast may be continued, in contrast to a breast abscess, in which feeding must be discontinued until treated. |

**Meconium**

Infant's first bowel movement, composed of sloughed cells from intestinal mucosa

May occur in utero as a result of stress and may lead to respiratory compromise if aspiration occurs

**Molar pregnancy**

Please refer to the chapter on gestational trophoblastic disease (see Chapter 41).

**MSAFP**

Maternal serum alpha-fetoprotein

**Nifedipine**

Calcium channel blocker used to treat preterm labor

**Nitabuch's layer**

Layer between the uterus and the invading trophoblasts; absence will lead to abnormal placental implantation (i.e., accreta, increta, and percreta)

**NST**

Nonstress test

**NSVD**

Normal spontaneous vaginal delivery

**Nuchal cord**

Umbilical cord around the fetal neck; may lead to distress during labor and delivery

Frequent cause of variable decelerations during childbirth

Often innocuous

**Oxytocin**

Hormone released by the pituitary that stimulates labor onset; synthetic form is pitocin and is used in the induction of labor.

**Pfannenstiel**

Low transverse abdominal incisions

**Placenta**

Accreta—attachment of the placenta in the uterine musculature (myometrium) secondary to absence of Nitabuch's layer

Battledore—umbilical cord attachment to the edge of the placenta

Circumvallate—associated with preterm labor and bleeding; caused by inappropriate placentation

Increta—invasion of the placenta into the myometrium

Percreta—penetration of the placenta
 through the myometrium to the serosa
Previa—placenta covering various
 degrees of cervical os
Vasa previa—placental vessels crossing
 the cervical os
Velamentous—umbilical cord vessel
 attachment to the placenta by thin
 membranes; may lead to vasa previa

**Postdatism**

Gestational age greater than 42 weeks

**Postpartum hemorrhage**

Greater than 500 cc blood loss at the
 time of vaginal delivery.
Most common causes include uterine
 atony (inability to contract), retained
 products of conception (POC),
 obstetrical lacerations, abnormal
 placental implantation, and bleeding
 dyscrasia.

**Preeclampsia**

Pregnancy-induced hypertension; please
 refer to Chapter 15, Hypertensive
 Disorders in Pregnancy.

**Preterm**

Gestational age less than 37 weeks

**PROM**

Rupture of fetal membranes prior to the
 onset of labor

**PPROM**

Preterm rupture of fetal membranes
 (i.e., prior to 37 weeks' gestation)

**PUPPPs**

Pruritic urticaria, pustules, and plaques
 of pregnancy

**Pseudocyesis**

The belief that one is pregnant without
 being pregnant

**Puerperium**

The period of time surrounding birth

**Rh**

Major blood group antigen of
 importance during pregnancy
Incompatibility between mother (-) and
 fetus (+) may lead to hemolytic
 disease of the newborn.

**RhoGAM**    Rh immune globulin given to gravidas who are Rh negative if there is suspicion of fetal–maternal bleeding; for example, is given if there is bleeding during any trimester, after delivery, and prophylactically at 28 weeks

**Scanzòni**    Maneuver describing rotation of the fetal head through an arc of 180° to facilitate delivery from OP to OA

**Sheehan syndrome**    Pituitary ablation as a result of hypotension after delivery
May result in amenorrhea, inability to breast-feed, etc.

**Shoulder dystocia**    Inability to deliver the fetus through the maternal pelvic outlet because of either macrosomic infant or relatively contracted pelvis

***Streptococcus* group B**    Found in approximately 30% to 40% of healthy women; may be a risk factor for preterm labor or premature rupture of membranes

**Terbutaline**    Betamimetic medication used in the treatment of preterm labor

**Tocolysis**    Therapy initiated to stop preterm labor

**TOL**    Trial of labor

**Triple screen**    Offered between 8 and 18 weeks' gestation
Involves three tests performed on maternal serum AFP, estriol, and hCG
Used to detect birth defects of chromosomal anomalies

**VBAC**    Vaginal birth after cesarean

**White's classification**    Used to classify diabetes in pregnancy; please refer to the chapter on gestational diabetes.

**Wood's maneuver**        Used during a shoulder dystocia to rotate the anterior shoulder counterclockwise to an oblique position in an attempt to facilitate delivery

**Zavanelli**        Replacement of the fetal head through the vagina followed by a cesarean section; used in rare cases of **severe** shoulder dystocia

# 2

# Maternal Physiology

**What are hPL and hCG?**

hPL = Human placental lactogen hormone
hCG = Human chorionic gonadotropin hormone

**Where are they produced?**

hPL and hCG are produced in the syncytiotrophoblasts of the placenta.

**What are their functions?**

hPL antagonizes effects of insulin and enhances lipolysis to ensure adequate blood glucose for the fetus; hCG stimulates the corpus luteum to produce progesterone and estradiol until the placenta is capable of autonomous steroidogenesis.

**What changes occur in the skin during pregnancy?**

Striae gravidarum ("stretch marks"); vascular spiders (telangiectasias) and palmar erythema caused by increased estrogen levels; hirsutism and acne secondary to increased progesterone levels; hyperpigmentation of nipples, areolae, axillae, umbilicus, midline abdomen ("linea nigra"); and melasma or chloasma of the face ("mask of pregnancy") due to increased levels of melanocyte-stimulating hormone

**What changes occur in the breast during pregnancy?**

Enlargement, increased cystic consistency, dilatation of superficial venous patterns, darkening of areolae, sebaceous gland hypertrophy, colostrum production in late pregnancy

**What is the Chadwick sign?**

Bluish discoloration of the upper vaginal vault and cervix secondary to normal cyanosis during early pregnancy

**Other vaginal changes in pregnancy?**

Increased vascularity and distensibility

**What is the Hegar sign?**

Softening of the lower uterine segment; often occurs in early pregnancy

**How is this sign appreciated during examination?**

Cervix is distinctly separate from the lower uterus; a soft isthmus is located between the cervix and uterus.

**What is the leukorrhea of pregnancy?**

Increased vaginal discharge of pregnancy secondary to increased vaginal capillary permeability and desquamation of vaginal epithelial cells

**What is ectropion?**

Increased eversion of cervical columnar epithelium onto the exocervix; can be especially prominent during pregnancy

**What percentage of cardiac output is devoted to uterine blood flow in pregnancy?**

20% (approximately 500 ml/min) at term

**In the nonpregnant state?**

Less than 1%

**What percentages of uterine blood flow are devoted to perfusing the different parts of the uterus?**

5% perfuses the myometrium.
10%–15% perfuses the endometrium.
80%–85% perfuses the placenta.

**What is the blood flow to the kidneys, breasts, and skin in pregnancy?**

Renal: 400 ml/min
Breasts: 200 ml/min
Skin: 400 ml/min

**What changes in blood volume, red cell mass (RCM), and plasma mass occur in pregnancy?**

Blood volume increases by 30%–50%.
RCM increases by 35%.
Plasma volume increases by 50%.

**What is a consequence of the increase in plasma volume in pregnancy?**

Physiologic "anemia" of pregnancy due to the relatively greater increase in plasma volume compared to RCM; hematocrit decreases approximately 5%, but the RBC count does not decrease.

**When does this effect peak during pregnancy?**

Near the late second/early third trimester

**What causes true anemia in pregnancy?**

Iron deficiency, folate deficiency, hemoglobinopathies

**What changes in heart rate, stroke volume, and cardiac output occur during pregnancy?**

Heart rate: increases 5%–15%, maximizing at term
Stroke volume: increases 20%–35%, maximizing during the second trimester
Cardiac output: increases 35%–45%, maximizing at 20–24 weeks' gestation; further increases of up to 40% during the second stage of labor

**What are the consequences of these changes?**

Rotation and elevation of the heart on the longitudinal axis, which manifests as slight left axis deviation on EKG and the appearance of cardiomegaly on chest x-ray

**What heart murmurs are normal in pregnancy?**

Late systolic or ejection murmurs

**What effect does pregnancy have on blood pressure?**

Blood pressure: falls from the first trimester to the middle of the second trimester; increases to prepregnancy levels by term
Systolic pressure: decreases approximately 4 mm Hg
Diastolic pressure: decreases approximately 10–15 mm Hg

**What is the baseline blood pressure in pregnancy?**

Early first-trimester blood pressures

**What are the consequences of vena cava compression caused by the enlarging uterus in pregnancy?**

Decreased cardiac output (secondary to decreased venous return) can cause nausea, dizziness, and syncope ("supine hypotensive syndrome") if not compensated for by increased peripheral resistance.
Increased venous pressure proximal to the area of compression can lead to worsening varicose veins in the legs and vulva, increased lower extremity edema, and decreased venous flow, which contributes to the increased risk of thrombosis in pregnancy.

**What changes in respiratory rate, tidal volume, total lung capacity, and vital capacity occur during pregnancy?**

Respiratory rate: unchanged or slightly increased

Tidal volume: increased up to 40%

Total lung capacity: decreased from about 4200 to 4000 ml secondary to increased pressure from the enlarging uterus on the diaphragm (residual volume is decreased from 1000 to 800 ml)

Vital capacity: unchanged

**Why is vital capacity unchanged during pregnancy?**

Increased tidal volume is negated by decreased expiratory reserve volume.

**What blood gas changes occur in pregnancy?**

Increased pH and decreased $PCO_2$ secondary to hyperventilation (increased minute ventilation secondary to 40% increase in tidal volume at term)

Decreased serum $HCO_3$ due to increased renal excretion to compensate for mild respiratory alkalosis

Net pH between 7.40 and 7.45

**How do WBC and platelet counts change in pregnancy?**

WBC counts: increase slightly in pregnancy (10,000 to 14,000/mm³); minimal left shift

Platelet counts: decrease slightly in later pregnancy, which may be related to increased platelet aggregation

**What is the significance of thrombocytopenia during pregnancy?**

It is not physiologic and should be investigated.

**What are normal WBC count values during labor?**

WBC count can reach 25,000–30,000/mm³ without infection (average during labor and early puerperium is 14,000–16,000/mm³).

**How is the coagulation system affected by pregnancy?**

Pregnancy is a hypercoagulable state.

Coagulation factors I, II, VII, VIII, IX, and X are increased as a result of increased hepatic synthesis.

Tissue thromboplastin (III) is synthesized by the placenta.

**What are the consequences of the coagulation system changes during pregnancy?**

Increased risk of thromboembolism (especially in the late third trimester and puerperium); pulmonary embolism ranks second in causes of maternal mortality after hemorrhage.

**How does progesterone affect smooth muscle in pregnancy?**

Inhibits smooth muscle peristalsis in GI, urinary, and biliary tracts

**What are the consequences of smooth muscle inhibition?**

GI tract: delayed gastric emptying, reflux esophagitis, and constipation
Urinary tract: ureteral dilatation, urinary stasis, and predisposition to pyelonephritis
Biliary tract: stasis plus changes in serum bile salt concentrations; may predispose to cholelithiasis and cholecystitis

**What are the effects of pregnancy related to appendicitis?**

Diagnosis may be delayed (and mortality is thus higher) because of the altered position of the appendix in the upper RLQ secondary to enlarging uterus.

**What are the effects of pregnancy related to pancreatitis?**

Increased frequency of cholelithiasis and perhaps hyperlipidemia lead to increased frequency of pancreatitis in pregnant women.

**How are renal blood flow and glomerular filtration rate (GFR) altered in pregnancy?**

Both increase approximately 40%–50%.

**What effects do these changes have on serum creatinine, BUN, and uric acid concentrations?**

Serum concentrations decrease because of increased excretion secondary to the increased GFR.

**What accounts for the increased incidence of pyelonephritis in pregnancy?**

Progesterone-mediated laxity of ureteral smooth muscle leads to inhibition of peristalsis in the ureter.
Pressure of the enlarging uterus on the ureter (right greater than left due to the tendency of the pregnant uterus to lie to the right) leads to ureteral dilatation and urostasis.

High incidence of cystitis in pregnancy predisposes to upper urinary tract infection (UTI).

**What is the major risk associated with pyelonephritis in pregnancy?**

Preterm labor

**What are the common UTI organisms in pregnancy?**

Gram negatives: *Escherichia coli* (70%–80%), *Klebsiella pneumoniae* (5%–10%), *Proteus* species (5%–10%)
Gram positives: Group B streptococci (3%–5%), enterococci (3%–5%), staphylococci (1%–3%)

**Does pregnancy affect thyroid function?**

No, but results of thyroid function tests can be affected.

**How are thyroid function tests affected in pregnancy?**

Thyroid-binding globulin (TBG): increased secondary to estrogen-stimulated hepatic synthesis; reflected in low thyroid uptake [triiodothyronine ($T_3$) resin uptake] values
Total thyroxine ($T_4$) and total $T_3$: elevated, because a significant percentage of each bind TBG
Free $T_4$ and free $T_3$: normal
Thyroid-stimulating hormone (TSH): normal

**What lab values suggest true hyperthyroidism and hypothyroidism in pregnancy?**

True hyperthyroidism: elevated free $T_4$
True hypothyroidism: elevated TSH

**Can $T_3$, $T_4$, or TSH diffuse across the placental membrane?**

Yes; transfer is negligible.

**What about thyroid-stimulating immunoglobin and propylthiouracil?**

Yes

# 3
## Female Anatomy

**What are the layers of the abdominal wall?**

From external to internal: skin, subcutaneous fat, superficial fascia (Scarpa's), anterior rectus sheath, muscle, posterior rectus sheath, preperitoneal fat, and peritoneum

**What is the arcuate line?**

Also known as the linea semicircularis
Superior to the arcuate line, the posterior aponeurosis of the internal oblique and aponeurosis of the transversalis lie posterior to the rectus abdominis.
Inferior to the arcuate line, these aponeuroses lie anterior to the rectus abdominis.

**Which bones compose the bony pelvis?**

Ilium, ischium, pubis, sacrum, and coccyx
The pubis, ilium, and ischium join to form the innominate bone (Figures 3-1 and 3-2).

Figure 3–1

Figure 3–2

**What are the four female pelvic configurations?**

Gynecoid
Android
Anthropoid
Platypelloid

**What is a gynecoid pelvis?**

"Typical" female pelvis shape found in approximately 50% of women
The anteroposterior and the transverse diameters are relatively equal, with straight pelvic sidewalls.
The ischial spines are not usually prominent.
The pubic arch is wide.

**What is an android pelvis?**

"Typical" male pelvis shape found in one-third of white women and one-sixth of nonwhite women
Convergent sidewalls, prominent ischial spines, and a narrow pubic arch

**What is an anthropoid pelvis?**

This pelvic shape is found in 25% of white women and in approximately 50% of nonwhite women.
The anteroposterior diameter is greater than the transverse diameter, giving this pelvis a "heart" shape.

**What is a platypelloid pelvis?**

Rarest pelvic type, found in 3% of women
The transverse diameter is greater than the anteroposterior diameter, with wide sidewalls.

**What is the pelvic inlet?**

Its boundaries are the sacral promontory posteriorly, the pubic ramus and symphysis pubis anteriorly, and the linea terminalis laterally.

**What is the obstetric conjugate?**

The shortest anteroposterior diameter between the sacral promontory and the symphysis pubis
Can only be measured radiographically
Normal measurement for the obstetric conjugate is > 10 centimeters (cm).

**What is the true conjugate?**

The anteroposterior diameter between the promontory of the sacrum and the superior margin of the symphysis pubis

**What is the diagonal conjugate?**

The distance between the sacral promontory and the inferior margin of the symphysis pubis; measured clinically

**What is the midpelvis?**

Measured at the level of the ischial spines
The interspinous diameter (the transverse of the midpelvis) should be at least 10 cm.

**What are the organs of the external female genitalia?**

Mons pubis, labia majora, labia minora, clitoris, vestibule, urethral opening, vagina, perineum, and perineal body

**What is the composition of the labia majora?**

Embryologically homologous to the male scrotum
Point of termination for the round ligaments
Composed primarily of subcutaneous fat with a prominent venous plexus and sebaceous glands

**What is the composition of the labia minora?**

Primarily composed of connective tissue and smooth muscle with dense nerve innervation
Fuse superiorly to form the frenulum and prepuce of the clitoris

**What is the composition of the clitoris?**

Homologous to the penis
Composed of a glans and two crura
Glans contains two corpora cavernosa, which are generously supplied with nerve fibers.

**What are the Bartholin glands?**

Homologous to the bulbourethral (Cowper's) gland in the male

Located beneath the vestibule on either side of the vagina, and open at the lateral border of the vagina

**What and where is the urethral opening?**

Located on the anterior edge of the vestibule and surrounded by Skene's or the paraurethral ducts, which are homologous to the prostate in the male

**What is the composition of the perineum?**

The area between the mons pubis, the buttocks, and the thighs laterally

Support for the perineum is provided by the pelvic and urogenital diaphragms.

The urogenital diaphragm is the area between the pubis symphysis and the ischial tuberosities.

The muscles of the perineum are the bulbocavernous, ischiocavernous, "sphincter" of the urethra, superficial and deep transverse perineal muscles, and the external sphincter of the anus (Figure 3-3).

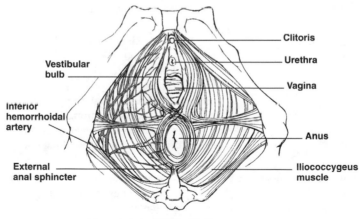

Figure 3–3

**What is the blood supply to the perineum?**

The internal pudendal artery

**What is the innervation to the perineum?**

Primarily from the pudendal nerve, which consists of the labial branch off the ilioinguinal, the perineal branch from the femoral cutaneous, and a branch from the genitofemoral nerve

| | |
|---|---|
| **What is the lymphatic drainage of the perineum?** | Through the inguinal nodes |
| **What structures comprise the pelvic diaphragm?** | The levator ani and coccygeal muscles |
| **What is the composition of the vagina?** | The vagina is a muscular organ that extends from the vulva to the uterine cervix.<br>Anterior to the vagina lies the bladder, which is separated from the vagina by the vesicovaginal septum.<br>Posterior to the vagina, the rectovaginal septum separates the vagina and the rectum.<br>The upper portion of the vagina is separated by the cervix into the anterior and posterior and lateral fornices.<br>The lateral fornices lie 1.0–1.5 cm from the point at which the uterine artery crosses the ureter.<br>The epithelium of the vagina is rugated stratified squamous epithelium. |
| **What is the blood supply to the vagina?** | Upper third: cervicovaginal branch of the uterine artery<br>Middle third: inferior vesical arteries<br>Lower third: internal pudendal artery and middle rectal artery<br>Venous drainage: through an interconnected venous plexus that drains into the internal pudendal vein |
| **What is the innervation to the vagina?** | No specific innervation; occasional free nerve endings are found in the papillas.<br>Parasympathetic innervation is supplied by S2–S4. |
| **What is the lymphatic drainage of the vagina?** | Lower third: through the inguinal nodes<br>Upper two-thirds: through the internal and external iliac nodes |
| **What are the organs of the female internal genitalia?** | The uterus and its supporting structures, the fallopian tubes and ovaries |

**What is the relationship of the uterus to the other pelvic organs?**

Sits between the bladder and the rectum
The posterior wall of the uterus is
   covered by peritoneum; the peritoneal
   reflection forms the pouch of Douglas
   between the uterus and the rectum.
Anteriorly, the vesicouterine peritoneum
   covers the uterus.
The bladder is in direct contact with the
   uterus (Figure 3–4).

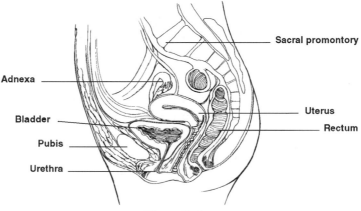

Figure 3–4

**What are the parts of the uterus?**

Uterine cervix, isthmus, corpus, and
fundus (Figure 3–5)

Figure 3–5

**What is the uterine cervix?**

Extends from the isthmus (constricted)
   portion of the uterus into the vagina
Portio: portion of the cervix visible from
   the vagina

Internal os: opening of the cervix into the isthmus
External os: opening of the cervix into the vagina
Cervical canal:
   Area between the internal and external os
   Measures approximately 4 cm
   Lined by columnar epithelium, which forms the endocervical glands

**What is the blood supply to the uterine cervix?**

Cervical branch of the uterine artery, which enters the cervix after coursing through the cardinal ligament

**What is the innervation to the uterine cervix?**

Autonomic nerves that course with the pudendal artery; the sympathetic nerves from T12 to L3

**What is the lymphatic drainage from the uterine cervix?**

Through the external and internal iliacs to the common iliacs
The para-aortic nodes may also be involved.

**What is the uterine corpus?**

The "body" of the uterus
Composed of serosal, muscular, and mucosal layers
Mucosal layer is the endometrium, which is composed of a ciliated columnar surface epithelium; glands; and blood vessels known as the spiral arteries.
The muscular layer is called the myometrium.
   Composed of smooth muscle and connective tissue
   The smooth muscle of the myometrium is arranged in a complex fashion.

**What are the ligaments of the uterus?**

The broad, round, and uterosacral ligaments extend from both sides of the uterus.
The cardinal (Mackenrodt's) ligaments or the transverse ligaments of the cervix extend from either side of the cervix (Figures 3-6 and 3-7).

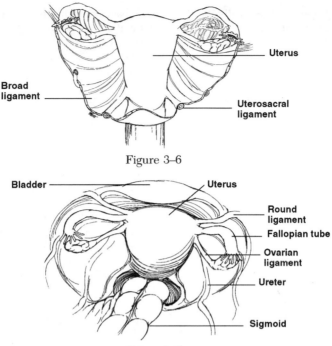

Figure 3–6

Figure 3–7

| **What are the broad ligaments?** | Composed of a reflection of the peritoneum |
|---|---|

**What are the broad ligaments?**

Composed of a reflection of the peritoneum

Extend from the lateral margin of the uterus to the pelvic sidewall

Comprise the mesosalpinx medially, and laterally form the infundibulopelvic ligament

The uterine vessels and the ureters are contained within the base of the broad ligaments.

**What are the round ligaments?**

Dense bands of connective tissue that extend from the lateral uterine fundus to the upper portion of the labia majora

Homologous to the gubernaculum in the male

**What are the uterosacral ligaments?**

Dense bands of connective tissue that extend from the inferior and posterior portion of the uterus and attach to the fascia over the sacrum

**What are the cardinal ligaments?**

Dense bands of connective tissue located at the base of the broad ligament
Provide most of the support to the uterus

**What is the blood supply to the uterus?**

Primarily the uterine and ovarian arteries
Uterine artery:
Usually arises as a branch of the internal iliac artery (hypogastric)
Courses along the base of the broad ligament toward the lateral uterine wall
Divides into the cervicovaginal and uterine branches; uterine branch further divides into the fundal, ovarian, and tubal arteries
Also provides multiple perforating branches, called radial arteries, into the uterus
Crosses over the ureter ("water under the bridge") approximately 2 cm lateral to the cervix
Ovarian arteries branch directly off the aorta and anastomose with the uterine arteries.
Further anastomoses in the pelvis include that between the inferior mesenteric artery and the internal iliac (hypogastric) and internal pudendal arteries; that between the middle sacral artery and the lumbar sacral artery; and that between the deep circumflex artery (off the external iliac) and branches of the internal iliac.
Venous drainage of the uterus is through the uterine vein and the pampiniform plexus.

**Why is the collateral circulation to the pelvic viscera important?**

In profuse uterine or pelvic hemorrhage, the uterine or even the internal iliac (hypogastric) artery can be ligated to decrease bleeding by decreasing the pulse pressure. The collateral circulation ensures that the pelvic viscera are adequately supplied with blood.

**What is the lymphatic drainage of the uterus?**

Through the internal and external iliac nodes

The fundus of the uterus may drain to the para-aortic lymph nodes.

**What is the composition of the fallopian tubes?**

Eight- to 14-cm muscular tubes that extend laterally from the cornua of the uterus

Segments: interstitial, isthmic, ampullary, and infundibular

Similar to the uterus, composed of serosal, muscular, and mucosal layers

Muscular layer contains an external longitudinal layer and an internal circular layer of muscle.

The mucosa is composed of columnar epithelium.

The epithelial layer contains ciliated cells, which promote ova transport toward the uterus.

**What is the blood supply to the fallopian tubes?**

Primarily from the uterine and ovarian arteries, as well as from the previously mentioned anastomoses

The venous drainage is through the pampiniform plexus and the ovarian veins.

**What is the lymphatic drainage of the fallopian tubes?**

Through the aortic nodes

**What is the relationship of the ovaries to other pelvic structures?**

The ovaries are lateral to the uterus and are normally located in the ovarian fossae, which lie in the pelvic sidewall at the bifurcation of the common iliac artery.

The ovary is attached to the broad ligament by the mesovarium.

The suspensory ligament (infundibulopelvic ligament) is the lateral continuation of the broad ligament and contains the ovarian artery, vein, and nerves.

The ovarian ligament connects the ovary with the lateral wall of the uterus; this ligament runs within the broad ligament (mesovarium ligament).

**What is the composition of the ovary?**

Consists of cortex and medulla
Cortex (outer layer):
    Contains the ova in various stages of maturity
    Outermost layer of the cortex is the tunica albuginea.
Medulla (central region) of the ovary contains connective tissue and the blood supply to the ovary.

**What is the blood supply to the ovary?**

Through branches from the uterine artery, ovarian vessels, and numerous anastomoses
The venous drainage is through the pampiniform plexus to the ovarian veins.
    The right ovarian vein drains into the inferior vena cava.
    The left ovarian vein drains into the left renal vein.

**What is the lymphatic drainage of the ovaries?**

Primarily through the aortic nodes
Rarely, they may drain through the iliac node group.

**What is the innervation to the ovaries?**

Sympathetic and parasympathetic nerves that course along the ovarian and infundibulopelvic ligaments

**What are the branches of the internal iliac (hypogastric) artery?**

Anterior (visceral):
    Uterine
    Superior vesical
    Middle vesical
    Inferior vesical
    Middle hemorrhoidal
    Inferior hemorrhoidal
    Vaginal
Anterior (parietal):
    Obturator
    Inferior gluteal
    Internal pudendal
Posterior:
    Iliolumbar
    Lateral sacral
    Superior gluteal (Figure 3–8)

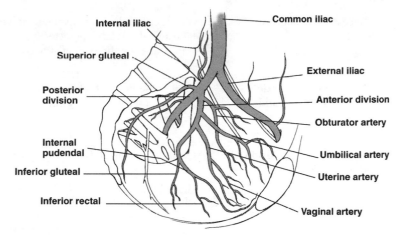

Figure 3–8

**What is the innervation of the pelvis?**

The hypogastric plexus supplies the sympathetic innervation; parasympathetic innervation is by S2–S4.

As stated earlier, the perineum is also innervated by L1 (ilioinguinal), S1–S3 (femoral cutaneous), and L1–L2 (genitofemoral).

**What is the relationship of the bladder to the other pelvic organs?**

Anteriorly, the bladder rests against the lower abdominal wall and the pubic bones.

Posteriorly, the bladder abuts the vagina and cervix.

**What is the composition of the bladder?**

Consists of a dome and base

The muscle of the dome of the bladder becomes thin with distention of the bladder.

The base consists of the trigone and the detrusor of the bladder; these muscles vary less with distention.

**What is the blood supply to the bladder?**

Superior and inferior vesical arteries and the middle hemorrhoidal artery

The superior vesical artery arises from the anterior branch of the internal iliac (hypogastric) artery; the inferior branch arises from the anterior branch of the internal iliac, the internal pudendal, or the vaginal artery.

**What is the innervation to the bladder?**

Sympathetic and parasympathetic nerves
The external urethral sphincter is innervated by the pudendal nerve.

**What is the lymphatic drainage of the bladder?**

Through the internal iliac nodes
The distal urethra drains to the inguinal nodes.

**What is the composition of the ureters?**

Measure approximately 25 cm from the renal pelvis to the trigone of the bladder
Segments: abdominal and pelvic
Composed of an inner longitudinal layer of muscle and an outer circular layer. Besides the muscular layer, the ureter has an outer serosal layer and an inner mucosal layer.

**What is the course of the ureters?**

With regard to the abdominal ureter, both the right and left ureters follow a similar course.
They run retroperitoneally down the anterior surface of the psoas major, then follow the common iliac artery and cross the iliac vessels before entering the pelvis.
The right ureter crosses the common iliac artery at the bifurcation, whereas the left ureter crosses 1–2 cm above the bifurcation.
Both then follow the lateral pelvic wall and down the medial leaf of the broad ligament where it crosses under the uterine artery.
Both then continue medially and enter the cardinal ligaments. At this point, the ureter is approximately 1.5 cm lateral to the cervix.
Both continue medially to enter the bladder at the trigone of the bladder.

**What is the blood supply to the ureters?**

Several anastomoses from many vessels, including the renal, common iliac, internal iliac (hypogastric), ovarian, uterine, vaginal, vesical, and superior gluteal arteries

**What are the most common points of injury to the ureter during gynecologic surgery?**

The pelvic brim and the point at which the ureter crosses under the uterine artery and at the trigone of the bladder

**How can the ureters be differentiated from vessels during surgery?**

Two ways: watch for ureteral peristalsis, and identify Auerbach's plexus.
Auerbach's plexus is the area of anastomoses of the vessels supplying the ureter.
Visualized on the anterior surface of the ureter

**What is the relationship of the rectum to the other pelvic organs?**

The rectum is the continuation of the sigmoid colon and begins at the point on the sigmoid colon where the mesentery ends (usually at the curvature of the sacrum).
The rectum does not have teniae coli or appendices epiploicae.
The distal third of the rectum is below the peritoneal reflection and lies posterior to the vagina.
The rectum continues into the anal canal.

**What is the blood supply to the rectum?**

Superior hemorrhoidal artery, which is a branch of the inferior mesenteric, and the middle and inferior hemorrhoidal arteries

**What is the innervation to the rectum?**

The sympathetic innervation follows the vasculature.
The parasympathetic innervation is from S2–S4.

**What is the lymphatic drainage from the rectum?**

Rectum: through the iliac nodes
Anus: through the inguinal nodes

**During what kind of gynecologic surgery is the rectum most commonly injured?**

Vaginal surgery, primarily vaginal hysterectomy, because the rectum lies only millimeters from the posterior vaginal wall

**What are the most common points of injury to nerves during gynecologic surgery?**

During radical gynecologic surgery, such as a radical hysterectomy, or during iliac and obturator node dissection, the genitofemoral or obturator nerves can be severed.

Injury to the obturator nerve interferes with adduction of the thigh and hip and with sensory function on the medial aspect of the thigh.

Injury to the genitofemoral nerve leads to anesthesia in the perineum.

During inguinal lymph node dissection, the anterior branches of the femoral nerve can be injured, which can interfere with sensory function on the anterior aspect of the thigh.

During abdominal surgery with the placement of a self-retaining retractor, the femoral nerve may be injured.

May cause temporary or permanent injury

Prohibits flexion of the hip; patient is not able to lift leg off the bed.

If there is improper placement of a patient's leg in stirrups during surgery, the peroneal nerve may be injured.

Causes sensory and motor loss over the lateral lower leg

The patient will have footdrop.

# 4

# Prenatal Care

**What are the goals of prenatal care?**

Ensure mother's health.
Ensure delivery of a healthy infant.
Anticipate problems.
Diagnose problems early.

**What should the initial visit consist of?**

Confirmation of pregnancy with urine or blood test
History
Physical examination
Laboratory screening

**What medical history is especially relevant?**

Venereal diseases, diabetes mellitus, hypertension, heart disease, autoimmune disorders, kidney disease, urinary tract infections, seizure or other neurologic disorder, psychiatric disorders, hepatitis, phlebitis, varicose veins, thyroid dysfunction, trauma, blood transfusions, pulmonary disease (tuberculosis or asthma), breast disease, and any previous surgery

**What social history is particularly pertinent?**

Cigarette use
Alcohol use
Illegal drug use
Domestic violence

**What family history is pertinent?**

Family history (both sides) of inherited disorders, birth defects, or mental retardation, including thalassemias, neural tube defects, Down syndrome, Tay-Sachs disease, sickle cell disease, hemophilia, muscular dystrophy, cystic fibrosis, and hereditary (Huntington) chorea

**How is menstrual history obtained?**

Pertinent questions include:
When was the last menstrual period?
Are the patient's periods regular?
What is the usual interval between periods?

Did the last period conform to the usual pattern in terms of timing, volume, and appearance?
Is the patient taking oral contraceptive pills?
Is the patient nursing?

**What obstetric history is pertinent?**

Pertinent questions include:
What were the patient's previous pregnancy outcomes?
Is there a history of infertility, which might suggest an anatomic or hormonal abnormality?
Were previous deliveries by cesarean section and how was the section done?
If deliveries were vaginal, how were they done?

**What gynecologic history is pertinent?**

Pertinent questions include:
Has the patient had any sexually transmitted diseases, including gonorrhea, chlamydia, herpes, warts, syphilis, hepatitis B, and human immunodeficiency virus (HIV) infection?
Has the patient had gynecologic surgery?
Does the patient have any known uterine or other gynecologic anomalies?
Has the patient had previous first-trimester spontaneous abortions?

**What are the normal findings from physical examination particular to pregnancy (depending on gestational age), and noteworthy abnormalities?**

Vital signs: Blood pressure decreases during second trimester; pulse increases.
Head, eyes, ears, nose, and throat: None
Neck: Diffuse mild enlargement of the thyroid
Skin:
  Increased pigmentation of the face (chloasma), abdomen (linea nigra), and vulva
  Stretch marks on the abdomen, thighs, or breasts
Lungs: Elevation of the diaphragm late in pregnancy

Heart:
> Soft systolic murmur due to increased
> maternal cardiac output
>
> Heart rate is increased.
>
> S2 is loud.

Breasts: Increased nodularity

Abdomen:
> Fetal heart tones at 14 weeks using
> Doppler
>
> Uterus grows out of pelvis at 14
> weeks; at 20 weeks, uterus is at the
> umbilicus; after 20 weeks, the EGA
> equals the distance in centimeters
> from the pubic symphysis to the
> uterine fundus.

Upper abdomen tympany is heard late
in pregnancy because of displacement
of the small bowel and distention of
the stomach.

**What are the normal findings from pelvic examination particular to pregnancy (depending on gestational age), and noteworthy abnormalities?**

Vulva and perineum:
> Hyperpigmentation, varicose veins, or
> hemorrhoids
>
> Herpes or condyloma are abnormal
> and noteworthy.

Vagina:
> Increased secretions
>
> Trichomoniasis or bacterial vaginosis
> are abnormal and noteworthy.

Cervix:
> Softer and pigmented
>
> Cervical mucus is more copious, often
> appearing thick and yellow.

Bimanual: Uterine size is enlarged.

**How is the shape of the pelvis assessed?**

The diagonal conjugate is the distance
from the pubic symphysis to the sacral
promontory, which marks the pelvic
inlet.

Check the ischial spines to determine if
they are prominent, because they mark
the midpelvis.

Assess the pelvic sidewalls to determine if
they are parallel or convergent.

Assess the shape of the sacrum.

**What laboratory evaluations are recommended?**

Complete blood count to screen for
anemia

Hepatitis B surface antigen test

Type and screen for maternal Rh status
and antibodies to Rh or other blood
antigens

Rubella titer

HIV, because the risk of transmission to
the fetus can be reduced

Rapid plasma reagin (RPR) to screen for
syphilis

Urine culture: Initial test for
asymptomatic bacteriuria because
pregnant women are more susceptible
to urinary tract infections, leading to
pyelonephritis

Cervical cultures for gonorrhea and
chlamydia

Pap smear

Triple screen

Glucose screen to detect gestational
diabetes mellitus

Ultrasound to screen for fetal
abnormalities is recommended by
some experts.

**What laboratory screens
should be performed after
the initial visit, and when
should they be performed?**

Triple screen at 15 to 20 weeks
Glucose tolerance test at 24 to 28 weeks
Ultrasound at 20 weeks

**What is a triple screen?**

Blood test that measures maternal serum
α-fetoprotein (MSAFP), human
chorionic gonadotropin (hCG), and
estriol (E3)

**What is it used to
determine?**

The combination of measurements of
MSAFP, hCG, and E3 with gestational
age and maternal age and weight assist
in determining increased risk of neural
tube defects or certain chromosomal
anomalies, such as trisomy 21 and
trisomy 18.

**Abnormal results?**

Trisomy 21: Elevated hCG and low
MSAFP and E3

Trisomy 18: Low levels of all three

Neural tube defects (spina bifida,
myelomeningocele): Elevated MSAFP

| | |
|---|---|
| **Follow-up after abnormal result?** | Detailed ultrasound and possibly amniocentesis |
| **What is a 1-hour glucose screening test?** | One hour after the patient drinks a 50-g oral glucose load, blood is drawn for glucose measurement. |
| **Normal value?** | < 135 mg/dl |
| **Follow-up after abnormal result?** | Three-hour glucose tolerance test |
| **What is a 3-hour glucose tolerance test?** | Patient prepares by consuming a high-carbohydrate diet for 3 days before the test.<br>After the patient drinks a 100-g oral glucose load, blood is drawn for glucose measurement at time 0, and at 1, 2, and 3 hours. |
| **Normal values?** | Fasting < 105 mg/dl<br>After 1 hour < 190 mg/dl<br>After 2 hours < 165 mg/dl<br>After 3 hours < 145 mg/dl |
| **Abnormal values?** | An abnormal fasting value alone or two other abnormal values indicate gestational diabetes. |
| **What is examined during an ultrasound?** | Fetal growth by measuring biparietal diameter, head circumference, femur length, humerus length, and abdominal circumference<br>Intracranial contents<br>Spine (neural tube defects)<br>Fetal organs, including diaphragm, kidneys, liver, and a four-chamber view of the heart<br>Placenta (location and grade)<br>Amniotic fluid volume |
| **What warning signs should the patient be aware of?** | Vaginal bleeding:<br>In the first trimester, bleeding can indicate pending miscarriage.<br>In the second or third trimester, bleeding may indicate placenta previa, placental abruption, or labor. |

Swelling of face or fingers, severe
headache, or blurry vision may
indicate preeclampsia.
Dysuria, chills, or fever may indicate
pyelonephritis or other infection.
Fluid leaking from the vagina could
indicate premature rupture of the
membranes.
Decreased fetal movement may indicate
fetal compromise.

**When should return visits
be scheduled and what
should each visit include?**

Every 4 weeks until 28 weeks
Screening: Urinary tract infection,
proteinuria, hypertension, preterm
labor, gestational diabetes, and fetal
well-being
Every 2 weeks until 36 weeks
Screening:
All of the above plus fetal growth
At 36 weeks, screening for chlamydia
and gonorrhea
Every week until 41 weeks
Screening: All of the above
After 41 weeks, twice weekly until
delivery
Screening: Fetal well-being by
evaluation of amniotic fluid index and
nonstress test

**How is maternal condition
evaluated at each visit?**

Blood pressure: Actual and any change
or trend
Weight: Actual and trend
Symptoms: Headache, vision, pain,
nausea, vomiting, bleeding, dysuria
Vaginal examination if indicated

**How is fetal condition
evaluated at each visit?**

Fundal height (to assess growth): Actual
and trend
Fetal heart rate
Presenting part
Fetal activity
Amniotic fluid
Nonstress test at 41 weeks and later

**What is the recommended
total weight gain during
pregnancy?**

Approximately 12 kg
For underweight women, slightly more;
for overweight women, less

**What is the recommended weight gain throughout pregnancy?**

1 kg in the first trimester; 0.5 kg per week after 20 weeks

**How is the weight gain accounted for during pregnancy?**

9 kg is accounted for by the fetus, placenta, amniotic fluid, uterine hypertrophy, increase in maternal blood volume, breast enlargement, and maternal extracellular and extravascular fluid. The remainder of the weight gain is fat.

**Can lack of weight gain be harmful in pregnancy?**

Severe underweight (near-starvation) is required to establish clear differences in pregnancy outcome.
Starvation affects fetal birth weight, but does not cause central nervous system damage.

**What are the recommended daily allowances in pregnancy?**

Calories:
Increase daily caloric intake by approximately 300 calories per day depending on prepregnancy nutritional status.
Birth weight is influenced more significantly by the number of calories, not the form of calories.
Protein: Preferably from animal sources, such as meat, milk, eggs, cheese, poultry, and fish, to provide appropriate amino acids
Iron:
300 mg of iron is transferred to the fetus, and 800 mg is incorporated into maternal hemoglobin mass.
6 mg per day requirement in the second half of pregnancy
Very few women have sufficient iron stores, and diet seldom contains enough iron to meet the demand.
To ensure adequate iron intake, supplementation is recommended.
Another important aspect is the availability of the ingested iron; calcium and magnesium compounds can inhibit iron absorption.
Calcium:
30 g of calcium (or 2.5% of total

maternal calcium) is needed for the fetus.

Most maternal calcium is in bone and can be easily mobilized to meet the needs of the fetus.

In addition, absorption by the intestine increases during pregnancy.

Iodine:

Increased fetal requirement and theoretical increased maternal renal losses

Use of iodized salt meets this requirement.

Copper:

Pregnancy affects copper metabolism because it increases serum ceruloplasmin and plasma copper.

However, copper deficiency in pregnancy has not been documented.

**What elements do not need supplementation in pregnancy?**

Chromium, manganese, potassium, sodium, fluorine, zinc, phosphorus, and magnesium

**Which substances are potentially toxic in pregnancy?**

Iron; zinc; selenium; and vitamins A, $B_6$, C, and D

**What vitamins are important in pregnancy?**

Folic acid:

Maternal folate requirements are slightly increased during pregnancy; thus, patients are more prone to folate deficiency, which rarely leads to hypersegmented neutrophils or megaloblastic anemia.

Neural tube defects: Centers for Disease Control and Prevention recommends 0.4 mg daily for all women of childbearing age to prevent neural tube defects.

Vitamin $B_{12}$:

Deficiency is usually seen only in strict vegetarians.

In breast-fed infants of vegetarians, $B_{12}$ deficiency may be pronounced.

Excessive vitamin C ingestion can lead to deficiency of $B_{12}$.

Vitamin C: Recommended requirement in pregnancy is 20% higher than for nonpregnant woman.

**What are the current recommendations for exercise during pregnancy?**

Women who exercise regularly may continue their prepregnant level of exercise, unless they have a hypertensive disorder of pregnancy, multifetal gestation, intrauterine growth restriction, or heart disease.

Women who did not previously exercise should slowly begin a low-impact exercise program.

Fetal reactivity is maintained even during vigorous exercise.

**Employment?**

Continue prepregnancy employment.

**Travel?**

No harmful effect on an otherwise healthy woman

Greatest risk is not being near an appropriate facility if a problem should arise.

Seat belts should be worn properly with three-point restraints; lap belt should be placed under abdomen and shoulder belt between breasts.

**Coitus?**

If abortion or preterm labor threatens or if placenta previa has been diagnosed, coitus should be avoided.

**Smoking?**

Cessation should be emphasized because of increased risk of low birth weight.

**Alcohol?**

Should be avoided because prolonged exposure to alcohol can lead to fetal alcohol syndrome

**Caffeine?**

In 1980, the Food and Drug Administration advised pregnant women to limit caffeine intake, although it has not been shown to be teratogenic.

**Illicit drugs?**

Chronic use of cocaine is harmful to the fetus, causing intrauterine distress, low birth weight, placental abruption, and complications of drug withdrawal after birth.

**Medications?**

In general, any drug that exerts a systemic effect on the mother crosses the placenta.
The advantages to be gained by taking any medication must clearly outweigh any risks.

**Provide an explanation and preventive measures (if applicable) for the following concerns expressed by pregnant women.**

**Bowel habits?**

May become irregular owing to relaxation of smooth muscle and compression of the lower bowel by the enlarging uterus
Hemorrhoids are common because of impaired venous return.
Appropriate diet prevents this problem.

**Nausea and vomiting?**

The cause is not clear.
Small feedings at more frequent intervals help.

**Backache?**

Mild backache can usually be alleviated with comfort measures and by avoiding strain.

**Round ligament pain?**

Usually occurs during the second trimester as the uterus grows and stretches the round ligaments
Rest alleviates this pain.

**Varicose veins?**

Congenital predisposition to varicose veins
Can become more pronounced as pregnancy progresses
Management: Elevation and support stockings

**Heartburn?**

Caused by reflux due to upward displacement and compression of the stomach by the uterus, decreased gastrointestinal motility, and relaxation of the lower esophageal sphincter due to progesterone

Small, frequent meals help prevent heartburn.

**Fatigue?**

Common during the first trimester

**Leukorrhea?**

Increased vaginal discharge is due to increased mucus formation by cervical glands in response to hyperestrogenemia.

Patients who complain of vaginal discharge must be evaluated for trichomoniasis, vaginitis, or bacterial vaginosis.

# 5     Labor and Delivery

**What is labor?**

Regular uterine contractions that cause progressive effacement and dilatation of the cervix and lead to expulsion of the fetus and placenta from the uterus

**What are Braxton Hicks contractions?**

"False labor"; contractions that occur with variable frequency and do not cause progressive cervical dilatation and effacement

**What is cervical dilatation?**

The cervix being dilated or stretched beyond the normal dimensions

**How is it measured?**

In centimeters; measured at the width of the internal os of the cervix

**What is effacement?**

Shortening of the cervix and thinning of the cervical walls caused by the pressure of the fetus's head as it descends into the birth canal during labor

**How is effacement expressed?**

In terms of percentage of total effacement [i.e., 0% effacement (normal) to 100% effacement (completely thinned cervix)]

**What is engagement?**

Descent of the biparietal diameter of the fetal vertex below the level of the pelvic inlet

**What is station?**

Marks the descent of the fetal presenting part through the maternal pelvis

**How is station measured?**

In centimeters relative to the level of the maternal ischial spines
    0 station: presenting part at the ischial spines
    +1, +2, +3: above the ischial spines
    -1, -2, -3: below the ischial spines to the perineum

## UNCOMPLICATED LABOR

**What are the stages of labor?**

First stage: from the onset of contractions causing progressive cervical dilatation to complete dilatation of the cervix
Second stage: from complete cervical dilatation to the birth of the fetus
Third stage: from the birth of the fetus to the delivery of the placenta

## FIRST STAGE OF LABOR

**What are the two phases of the first stage of labor?**

Latent: cervical effacement and early dilatation
Active: slope of cervical dilatation changes; usually begins when the cervix is 3–4 cm dilated and contractions are regular

**How long does the latent phase of labor last?**

Primigravidas: up to 20 hours
Multiparas: up to 14 hours

**What is the normal progress of cervical dilatation during the active phase of labor?**

Primigravidas: at least 1.2 cm/hr
Multiparas: at least 1.5 cm/hr

**What conditions may slow progress in the active phase of labor?**

Uterine dysfunction, fetal malposition, cephalopelvic disproportion (CPD)

**How should the mother be positioned during the first stage of labor?**

Mother may ambulate (provided that intermittent monitoring is performed) or recline in the lateral recumbent position.

**By what method and how often should the fetus be monitored in uncomplicated pregnancies?**

Intermittent by auscultation

**In complicated pregnancies?**

Continuous fetal heart rate (FHR) monitoring

| | |
|---|---|
| **When should vaginal examinations be performed in the first stage?** | On initial presentation of patient with contractions<br>Latent phase: sparingly if membranes have ruptured<br>Active phase: approximately every 2 hours<br>If the patient reports the urge to push or FHR decelerates |

## SECOND STAGE OF LABOR

| | |
|---|---|
| **How long should the second stage of labor last?** | Primigravidas: 30 minutes to 2 hours; with epidural analgesia, approximately 3 hours<br>Multiparas: 45 minutes (average) |
| **What are the seven cardinal movements of labor?** | Engagement (usually occurs before the onset of true labor), descent, flexion, internal rotation, extension, external rotation, and expulsion |
| **What forces bring about descent?** | Combined forces of uterine contractions, maternal bearing-down efforts, and gravity |
| **When does descent occur?** | A variable degree of fetal descent occurs before the onset of labor and during the first and second stages. |
| **When does the fastest rate of descent occur?** | During the second stage of labor |
| **How long does it last?** | Until the fetus is delivered |
| **What is flexion?** | Flexion of fetal neck toward chest |
| **When does flexion begin?** | Partial flexion exists before labor as a result of the natural muscle tone of the fetus. |
| **What causes flexion?** | During descent, resistance from the cervix, the walls of the pelvis, and the pelvic floor results in further flexion of the cervical spine, causing the fetus's chin to approach its chest. |

| | |
|---|---|
| **What determines presentation of the fetus?** | The relationship of the fetal occiput to the maternal pelvis |
| **What are the types of presentations?** | Left and anterior (LOA), transverse (LOT), or posterior (LOP)<br>Right and anterior (ROA), transverse (ROT), or posterior (ROA) |
| **What is internal rotation?** | Turning of the fetal head as the fetus descends through the pelvis. |
| **When does it occur?** | As the head descends through the pelvic cavity and meets the muscular sling of the pelvic floor |
| **Why does it occur?** | The presenting part of the fetus naturally seeks the most favorable position as it descends through the pelvis. |
| **What type of presentation is most favorable at the pelvic brim?** | Transverse |
| **What type of presentation is most favorable at the outlet?** | Because of the shape of the pelvic arch, the sagittal suture of the fetal head in the anteroposterior (AP) position relative to the pelvis |
| **What is extension?** | Extension of the fetal neck to negotiate under the pubic symphisis |
| **What forces bring about extension?** | Combined forces of descent, flexion, and internal rotation |
| **What is the purpose of extension?** | Because the vaginal outlet is directed upward and forward, extension must occur before the head can pass through. |
| **What happens at crowning?** | As the head continues to descend, the perineum bulges, followed by crowning; crowning occurs when the largest diameter of the fetal vertex is encircled by the vulvar ring. |
| **What is the station at crowning?** | +5 |

**After crowning?**

The vertex then extends as the occiput, nose, mouth, and chin pass over the perineum.

**What is external rotation?**

Return of the delivered head to its position at the time of engagement and its alignment with the fetal back and shoulders

**What is expulsion?**

Delivery of the anterior shoulder under the symphysis pubis, followed by delivery of the posterior shoulder and then the body

**How should the mother be positioned during the second stage of labor?**

In any comfortable position except supine

**When should the mother be directed to bear down?**

With each contraction

**Why is this direction important for patients receiving regional anesthesia?**

Reflex sensations may be impaired.

**How often should the fetus be monitored during the second stage of labor?**

Continuously or after each contraction

**Why?**

FHR decelerations secondary to head or cord compression may occur during this stage.

**How often should vaginal examinations be performed during the second stage?**

Every 30 minutes with particular attention to descent, extent of internal rotation, and development of molding or caput

**What are the goals of assisted vaginal delivery?**

Minimize maternal and fetal trauma.

**What are the steps of an assisted vaginal delivery?**

The patient is usually placed in the lithotomy position; the skin over the perineum and upper thighs is cleansed with antiseptic solution; appropriate sterile leggings and drapes may also be applied.

As the perineum bulges with the fetal vertex, an episiotomy is performed if necessary.

The fetal vertex delivers by extension; the Ritgen maneuver may facilitate delivery of the head.

The airway (oral cavity first, followed by nares) is cleared of blood and amniotic fluid using a suction bulb or suction catheter.

The operator checks for a nuchal cord (an umbilical cord that encircles the neck).

The shoulders then descend and rotate into the AP position relative to the maternal pelvis; delivery of the anterior shoulder is assisted by gentle traction on the head; delivery of the posterior shoulder is assisted by gentle elevation of the head.

The rest of the body is delivered without difficulty; the cord is clamped and cut.

**What is the Ritgen maneuver?**

The operator inserts a hand and applies upward pressure on the fetal chin and with the other hand applies gentle downward pressure on the fetal occiput to allow controlled delivery of the fetal head.

**What is the procedure for a nuchal cord?**

A nuchal cord can often be reduced over the head. If the cord is too tight, it can be clamped and cut on the perineum.

## THIRD STAGE OF LABOR

**How long does the third stage of labor last?**

No more than 30 minutes

**What are the stages of placental delivery?**

Separation of the placenta from the uterine wall
Expulsion from the vagina

**When does the placenta separate from the uterine wall?**

Within 5 to 10 minutes of the end of the second stage

**What are the signs of placental separation?**

The uterus becomes firm and globular.
A gush of blood flows from the vagina.
The umbilical cord lengthens outside the vulva.
The uterine fundus rises in the abdomen.

**What is the Brandt-Andrews maneuver?**

Exertion of traction on the umbilical cord with one hand while the uterus is lifted out of the pelvis by suprapubic pressure on the uterus with the other hand; pressure on uterus is stopped as the placenta passes through the introitus.

**Why must the operator be careful in performing this maneuver?**

The membranes can tear and be left behind as the placenta is lifted away from the introitus.

**Why is the placenta examined after delivery?**

To ascertain its complete removal from the uterine cavity

**How can the placenta present at the time of its delivery?**

Duncan (**D**ull = Duncan): rough maternal edge presentation
Schultze (**S**hiny = Schultze): fetal membrane presentation

**How is uterine hemostasis achieved after delivery of the placenta?**

Vasoconstriction by myometria contraction

**How can uterine contractions after delivery of the placenta be stimulated?**

Agents such as oxytocin, methylergonovine, prostaglandin; massage

**What types of lacerations may require repair?**

First-degree laceration involves the vaginal mucosa or perineal skin.
Second-degree laceration extends into the submucosal tissue of the vagina or perineum with or without involvement of the muscles of the perineal body.
Third-degree laceration involves the anal sphincter.
Fourth-degree laceration involves the rectal mucosa.

## OPERATIVE DELIVERY

### CESAREAN SECTION

| | |
|---|---|
| **What is a cesarean section (C/S)?** | Delivery of the fetus through incisions in the anterior abdominal wall and the uterus |
| **What are the indications for a C/S?** | Maternal/fetal<br>  Dystocia<br>Maternal<br>  Maternal disease<br>    Eclampsia/severe preeclampsia<br>    Diabetes mellitus<br>    Cervical cancer<br>  Previous uterine surgery<br>    Previous classic cesarean section<br>    Previous uterine rupture<br>    Myomectomy<br>  Obstruction in birth canal<br>  Fibroids<br>  Ovarian tumors<br>Fetal<br>  Fetal distress<br>  Cord prolapse<br>  Fetal malpresentation<br>    Breech<br>    Transverse<br>    Brow<br>Placental<br>  Placenta previa<br>  Abruptio placentae |
| **What are the three types of C/S?** | Low transverse, classic, and low vertical |
| **C/S classifications refer to which incision: abdominal or uterine?** | Uterine |
| **What is the most common type of C/S?** | Low transverse |
| **What is a low transverse C/S?** | The incision is made transversely in the lower uterine segment. |

| | |
|---|---|
| **Advantage?** | Decreased risk of scar rapture in subsequent pregnancies and generally less bleeding and adhesion formation |
| **What is a classic C/S?** | A vertical incision is made into the upper contractile portion of the uterus. |
| **Indications?** | Preterm breech fetus<br>Fetus in a transverse lie with the back down<br>Restricted access to the lower uterine segment secondary to fibroids or dense adhesions<br>When a hysterectomy is to follow the delivery of the fetus<br>Presence of an invasive cervical cancer<br>Postmortem C/S to rescue a live fetus from a deceased mother |
| **What is a low vertical C/S?** | A vertical incision is made in the lower uterine segment that can extend into the vagina or into the contractile portion of the uterus. |
| **Indications?** | Preterm breech |
| **What are the maternal morbidities for C/S?** | Risk of maternal death is four to six times greater than for a vaginal delivery.<br>Complications: hemorrhage; injury to surrounding structures such as the bowel, bladder, blood vessels, nerves and ureters; postoperative complications<br>Postoperative complications: thromboembolic events; pain; prolonged hospitalization; postoperative infection involving the uterus, wound, bladder, lung, and IV site |
| **How are subsequent pregnancies managed?** | Decision to repeat C/S depends in part on the indications for the primary surgery.<br>Repeat C/S if any of the previously mentioned indications are present.<br>Previous classic C/S mandates a repeat C/S.<br>Patients with previous transverse C/S may labor in subsequent pregnancies unless contraindications exist. |

## OBSTETRIC FORCEPS DELIVERY

**What are forceps?**

An instrument used to provide traction, rotation, or both to the fetal head when the unaided expulsive efforts of the mother are insufficient to accomplish safe delivery

**What do forceps used for traction (Simpson's and Tucker) look like?**

They have a pelvic curve that corresponds to the axis of the birth canal.

**What do forceps used for fetal rotation (Kielland's) look like?**

They do not have a pelvic curve.

**What are the indications for a forceps delivery?**

Maternal
    Exhaustion: inability to expel the fetal
       head
    Medical conditions
       Cardiac disease (e.g., mitral
         stenosis)
       Pulmonary disease
Fetal
    Failure of the fetal head to rotate
       completely
    Control of the fetal head during a
       vaginal breech delivery
    Fetal heart rate decelerations with
       complete cervical dilatation and
       adequate station

**How are forceps deliveries classified?**

According to the station and position of the presenting part at the time the forceps are applied

**Classifications?**

Outlet forceps: applied when the scalp is
    visible at the introitus without
    separating the labia
Low forceps: applied when the vertex is
    at +2 station
Mid-forceps: applied when the head is
    engaged but the leading part is above
    +2 station or when the sagittal suture
    is not in the AP plane of the mother

| | |
|---|---|
| **Under what circumstances should forceps be applied to the unengaged fetal head?** | Under **no** circumstances |
| **What are the requirements for a forceps delivery?** | The fetal vertex **must** be engaged.<br>The position of the fetal vertex must be certain.<br>Membranes must be ruptured.<br>Uterine contractions must be present.<br>The cervix must be fully dilated.<br>The bladder should be emptied.<br>Adequate anesthesia is optimal. |
| **What are the complications of a forceps delivery?** | Maternal<br>  Trauma to soft tissues<br>  Bleeding from lacerations<br>Fetal<br>  Bruising or lacerations to the face<br>  Injury to the fetal scalp or cranium |

## VACUUM-ASSISTED DELIVERY

| | |
|---|---|
| **What is a vacuum?** | An instrument that uses a suction cup applied to the fetal head to exert traction to aid the mother's expulsive efforts |
| **What are the indications for a vacuum-assisted delivery?** | Same as those for a forceps delivery, except for:<br>Face or breech delivery<br>Assisting fetal rotation<br>Vacuum can also be used in multiparas in whom a small rim of cervix remains and the rim will displace easily over the fetal head. |
| **What is an advantage of a vacuum-assisted delivery compared to a forceps delivery?** | May require a smaller episiotomy than that for a forceps delivery |
| **What are the contraindications to a vacuum-assisted delivery?** | Preterm deliveries because of risk of fetal head and scalp injury from the suction cup |

| | |
|---|---|
| **What are the complications of a vacuum-assisted delivery?** | Vaginal laceration due to entrapment of vaginal mucosa between the suction cup and the fetal head<br>Fetal scalp injuries<br>Serious fetal eye injury if used in a face presentation |

## COMPLICATIONS AND ABNORMALITIES OF LABOR AND DELIVERY

| | |
|---|---|
| **What is dystocia?** | Literally, "difficult labor" |
| **What are the causes of dystocia?** | Ineffective uterine expulsive forces<br>Abnormal presentation, position, or fetal structure<br>Disproportion between the size of the fetus and the maternal pelvis<br>Obstruction of the birth canal |
| **What are the three Ps?** | Power: strength of the uterine contractions<br>Passage: maternal pelvis<br>Passenger: fetal size relative to the maternal pelvis |
| **Significance?** | Any abnormal progression during labor is likely caused by an abnormality in one of the three Ps. |

### ABNORMALITIES OF THE UTERINE EXPULSIVE FORCES

| | |
|---|---|
| **When is the latent phase of labor considered prolonged?** | Primigravida: latent phase exceeds 20 hours<br>Multipara: exceeds 14 hours |
| **Causes?** | Hypertonic uterine contractions that do not lead to effective contractions and cervical dilatation<br>Hypotonic uterine contractions<br>Premature or excessive use of sedatives or analgesics |
| **What are the management options for a prolonged latent phase?** | Hypertonic uterine activity: therapeutic rest with morphine sulfate or an equivalent drug<br>Hypotonic contractions: IV oxytocin in a continuous infusion beginning with 0.5 mU to 1.0 mU per minute and increased incrementally; artificial rupture of membranes (AROM) |

**Why is AROM controversial?**

Added risk of intrauterine infection when performed in the latent phase and labor does not improve

**What abnormalities can occur during the active phase of labor?**

Protraction disorder: failure of the cervix to dilate greater than 1.2 cm/hr in a primigravida and 1.5 cm/hr in a multipara after the cervix has reached an accelerated slope of dilatation (usually at 3–4 cm)

Arrest of dilatation: period of 2 or more hours without progress in cervical dilatation, usually at 3–4 cm

Arrest of descent: period of more than 1 hour without a change in station of the fetal presenting part with adequate contractions

**What is failure to progress?**

Failure of either cervical dilatation or descent of the fetal vertex during labor despite adequate uterine contractions

**Etiologies?**

CPD, uterine anomalies, uterine fibroids, cervical mass; often no definable etiology

**How is adequacy of labor measured?**

With an intrauterine pressure catheter (IUPC)

**What measurement is considered adequate?**

Greater than 200 Montevideo Units (MVU) in a 10-minute period

**What are the management options for a prolonged active phase?**

Oxytocin infusion
IUPC to assess adequacy of labor
Fetal scalp electrode

**When is a C/S necessary for failure to progress?**

No cervical change occurs for 3–4 hours despite adequate labor; the size of the fetus, adequacy of the pelvis, and the well-being of the fetus should also be assessed.

Second stage of labor exceeds 2 hours (3 hours if epidural analgesia is used), provided maternal expulsive effort has been sufficient; some patients can be delivered by forceps.

| | |
|---|---|
| **What other factors should be considered when assessing the need for a C/S?** | Physician must balance the morbidity incurred by the mother from C/S against the benefit to the infant from avoiding prolonged labor and possible difficult delivery. |

## ABNORMAL PRESENTATIONS AND POSITIONS

| | |
|---|---|
| **What are the abnormal fetal presentations and positions?** | Presentations other than vertex, positions other than occiput anterior (OA) and longitudinal |
| **What is a breech presentation?** | Presentation of the fetal buttocks or lower extremities into the maternal pelvis |
| **What are the types of breech presentation?** | Complete (5%–10%): flexed thighs and flexed knees, feet above the buttocks<br>Frank (50%–75%): flexed thighs and extended knees<br>Footling or incomplete (20%): leg(s) extended |
| **What is the effect of a breech presentation on the progress of labor?** | Only a small effect on rate of dilatation and descent; however, likelihood of dysfunctional labor is greater |
| **What are the criteria for a trial of labor?** | Estimated fetal weight > 1500 or < 3800 g<br>Frank breech presentation<br>Nonextended fetal head (may be determined by ultrasound)<br>Adequate maternal pelvis<br>Absence of fetal anomaly that may impair vaginal delivery<br>Evidence of fetal distress<br>Ability to perform a rapid C/S |
| **Why is vaginal delivery contraindicated for a footling breech presentation?** | 20% prolapse of the cord; entrapment of the aftercoming head on the cervix may occur because the fetal trunk does not adequately dilate the cervix. |
| **When should a C/S be performed?** | When the above criteria for a trial of labor are not met<br>In some institutions: if a dysfunctional labor pattern develops |

| | |
|---|---|
| **What is the perinatal morbidity for a breech?** | Ranges from 9% to 25% in breech fetuses (three to five times higher than in a vertex infant at term) |
| **What factors contribute to increased risk of morbidity and mortality in breech presentations?** | Factors that may have caused the breech presentation, such as prematurity and congenital anomalies |
| **What is a face presentation?** | Fetus with the face presenting at the introitus |
| **Cause?** | Complete extension of the fetal head results in a larger diameter of the fetal presenting part; does not include the normal extension of the fetal vertex that occurs as one of the cardinal movements of labor |
| **How is a face presentation managed?** | Mentum posterior: vaginal delivery of a term infant is impossible<br>Spontaneous rotation of the fetus to mentum anterior occurs in most cases.<br>Rotation with forceps should **not** be attempted.<br>C/S if spontaneous rotation does not occur; sometimes required if it does occur |
| **What is a brow presentation?** | Fetus with the brow presenting at the introitus |
| **Cause?** | Incomplete extension of the fetal head results in a presentation midway between a vertex and a face presentation. |
| **Effects on dilatation and descent?** | Dilatation: usually none<br>Descent: may be prolonged because this presentation provides a larger diameter to maneuver the maternal pelvis |
| **How is a brow presentation managed?** | May convert spontaneously to a vertex or face<br>Observation to determine whether spontaneous conversion will occur<br>C/S if conversion does not occur<br>Vaginal delivery if the fetus is unusually small or the maternal pelvis large |

| | |
|---|---|
| **What is an occiput transverse position?** | Failure of the head to rotate to an OA or OP position |
| **Causes?** | CPD<br>Altered pelvic architecture<br>Relaxed pelvic floor that does not encourage rotation |
| **Why does arrest of descent occur with this presentation?** | The OT position leads to a larger diameter of the presenting part. |
| **How is a persistent OT position managed?** | Normal-size pelvis or small fetus: oxytocin augmentation if arrest is secondary to inadequate contractions<br>Large pelvis or smaller fetus: no labor management necessary<br>Manual or forceps rotation<br>C/S if rotation fails or CPD exists |
| **What is an OP position?** | The occiput is in the posterior instead of the normal anterior position. |
| **How is an OP position managed?** | No fetal distress: observation with expectant management<br>Delivery of the fetal head may occur spontaneously.<br>Difficult delivery of head or maternal exhaustion: forceps delivery |
| **What is a transverse lie?** | The fetal spine lies transverse to the maternal vertical axis. |
| **Causes?** | Fetal prematurity, pelvic deformity, abnormal placental location |
| **How is a transverse lie managed?** | Before labor and rupture of membranes: expectant management because of possibility of spontaneous resolution<br>Risk for cord prolapse if membranes rupture<br>C/S: term infant with a transverse lie<br>Low transverse C/S: if infant is "back up"<br>Classic C/S: if infant is "back down" |

## ABNORMALITIES OF FETAL STRUCTURE

| | |
|---|---|
| **What is fetal macrosomia?** | Fetal weight greater than 4000 g |
| **Above what percentage of normal fetal weight constitutes macrosomia?** | 90% for a term pregnancy |
| **Etiology of fetal macrosomia?** | Genetic determinants, maternal diabetes, maternal weight gain during the pregnancy, or post-term gestation |
| **What is a shoulder dystocia?** | Inability to dislodge the anterior shoulder from under the pubis symphysis |
| **Can traction on the fetal head help?** | No |
| **What is the risk of exerting traction on the fetal head in this condition?** | May damage the brachial plexus and cause Erb's palsy |
| **What is Erb's palsy?** | Results from stretching or tearing of the upper branches of the brachial plexus<br>Paralysis of the deltoid and flexor muscles<br>Paralysis is transient and resolves within 3 to 6 months after delivery. |
| **How is a shoulder dystocia managed?** | The following maneuvers in the following order:<br>McRoberts maneuver: flexing the maternal thighs to alter the angle between the sacrum and the spine<br>Downward pressure with the hand over the maternal suprapubic region to guide the anterior shoulder under the symphysis<br>Pushing the anterior shoulder into an oblique position<br>Pushing the posterior shoulder forward; may lead to rotation and delivery<br>Moving the posterior shoulder across the fetal chest to facilitate delivery; may lead to rotation of the fetus and delivery<br>Fracture of one or both of the fetal clavicles |

| | |
|---|---|
| **What if none of the above maneuvers work?** | The fetal head is manually replaced into the vagina and delivery is accomplished by C/S (Zavanelli maneuver); this technique is rarely performed, and is considered a last resort. |
| **What are other fetal anomalies that can affect delivery?** | Fetal hydrocephalus, fetal ascites, gastroschisis, omphalocele, spina bifida, sacral teratomas |
| **Management?** | Depends on prenatal diagnosis of the fetal anomaly and the severity of the defect |

## FETAL DISTRESS

| | |
|---|---|
| **What is the etiology of fetal distress?** | Hypoxia caused by the temporary interruption of blood flow that supplies the fetus with oxygen through the placental exchange of respiratory gases during a contraction |
| **What is the role of fetal health in fetal distress?** | In a normal fetus, sufficient oxygen exchange occurs during the interval between contractions; a fetus whose oxygen supply is marginal cannot tolerate the stress of contractions and becomes hypoxic. |
| **What are the results of hypoxia?** | Contraction-related FHR changes and fetal acidosis |
| **How is fetal acidosis assessed?** | Blood is sampled from the presenting part. |
| **How is baseline FHR determined?** | Determination of the rate in beats per minute (BPM) and the variability |
| **What is a normal FHR?** | Between 120 to 160 BPM |
| **What is short-term variability?** | Also known as beat-to-beat variability; reflects mechanical events of the cardiac cycle |
| **How is short-term variability calculated?** | The standard deviation calculated from the baseline interval between beats |

| | |
|---|---|
| **What is normal short-term variability?** | Fluctuates between 5 and 25 BPM |
| **What is long-term variability?** | Fluctuations of FHR that occurs in cycles, usually three to five cycles per minute |
| **What are the types of FHR decelerations?** | Early, late, and variable |
| **What is an early deceleration?** | A deceleration, the radii of which occur prior to the peak of contraction. |
| **Cause?** | Fetal head compression leads to an increase in intracranial pressure, which elicits a vagal response with subsequent decrease in FHR. |
| **Description?** | Onset, maximal fall, and recovery coincide with the onset, peak, and end of the uterine contraction; nadir of the deceleration coincides with the peak of the contraction. |
| **What is a late deceleration?** | A deceleration, the radii of which occur after the peak of contraction. |
| **What does it indicate?** | Uteroplacental insufficiency |
| **Description?** | Onset, maximum decrease, and recovery are shifted to the right in relation to the contraction. |
| **How is severity measured?** | By the magnitude of the decrease in FHR at the nadir of the deceleration |
| **Grades of severity?** | Mild: FHR drops < 15 BPM<br>Moderate: FHR drops 15–45 BPM<br>Severe: FHR drops > 45 BPM |
| **What are the management options for late decelerations?** | 1) Left or right lateral maternal position<br>2) Oxygen by face mask<br>3) Stop oxytocin infusion if uterine hyperstimulation is suspected of causing the decelerations.<br>4) A tocolytic drug may be necessary to stop uterine contractions.<br>5) Monitor maternal blood pressure to exclude maternal hypotension as the |

etiology (especially if an epidural has been administered).

Fetal blood sampling if late decelerations persist for > 30 minutes (some institutions)

**When is operative delivery for fetal distress indicated?**

①Fetal acidosis

⑦Persistent late decelerations in early labor

Deterioration of fetal status and vaginal delivery cannot be accomplished promptly

**What is a variable deceleration?**

A deceleration, the radii of which may occur before, during, or after the peak of contraction

**Cause?**

✷ Secondary to cord compression; causes a sudden increase in blood pressure in the central circulation of the fetus with a subsequent decrease in FHR

**Description?**

Onset and forms vary; may be nonrepetitive.

**How is severity measured?**

By the duration of the deceleration and the decrease in FHR

**Grades of severity?**

Mild: lasts < 30 sec, or > 80 BPM
Moderate: 30–60 sec
Late: > 60 sec, or < 70 BPM

**What are the management options for variable decelerations?**

①Change maternal position to the right or left side (may relieve fetal pressure on the cord).

⑦Temporarily stop oxytocin.

⑦Amnioinfusion to alleviate pressure on the cord

If deceleration occurs during the second stage of labor, delivery of the fetus with low or outlet forceps

C/S if progressive acidosis or deterioration of variability occurs and vaginal delivery is not imminent ✘

Persistent bradycardia: immediate delivery

| | |
|---|---|
| **What is an amnioinfusion?** | Instillation of sterile saline into the uterine cavity through a catheter |

## MECONIUM

| | |
|---|---|
| **What is meconium?** | Fetal colonic contents |
| **What is the significance of meconium before delivery?** | May indicate current or past fetal distress, but usually does not |
| **Classification?** | Light or heavy |
| **Outcome of light staining?** | **Not** necessarily associated with poor outcome |
| **Management of an infant with meconium-stained fluid?** | At delivery: fetus needs vigorous suction on the perineum.<br>Intubation may be necessary.<br>Check with laryngoscope for meconium below the vocal cords; indicates aspiration, which can lead to pneumonia.<br>Remove meconium from the oropharynx and trachea with suction through an endotracheal tube. |
| **What is terminal meconium?** | Usually occurs during the second stage of labor, after clear amniotic fluid has been noted earlier; usually heavy and thick |
| **Significance?** | Associated with some event late in labor causing fetal distress (e.g., umbilical cord compression or uterine hyperstimulation) |

# 6

# The Postpartum Period (Puerperium)

**What is the puerperium?**

Time period from delivery of the infant and placenta to 6 weeks postpartum, during which maternal reproductive organs and physiology return to the prepregnancy state

## ANATOMIC AND PHYSIOLOGIC CHANGES

**What are the anatomic and physiologic changes in the reproductive tract during the puerperium?**

Uterus: Weight decreases from about 1000 g at delivery to approximately 50 g 3 weeks postpartum

Cervix: Cervical opening contracts; cervix itself thickens; canal reforms. At 1 week postpartum, it is difficult to introduce a finger into the os.

Lochia:
> Days 1–3 after delivery, contains blood and appears red (lochia rubra)
> Days 3–4, becomes paler (lochia serosa)
> Day 10, is white or yellow-white (lochia alba)

Vagina: Rapidly regains tone but does not return to the prepregnancy state

Supportive tissues of the pelvic floor: Gradually regain tone

Menstruation: Resumes 6–8 weeks postpartum in nonnursing women; resumes in 70% of women by 10 weeks postpartum

Ovulation: May not occur for several months, especially in nursing women; contraceptive counseling still should be provided.

**What are the physiologic changes in the cardiovascular system?**

Peripheral vascular resistance: Markedly decreases immediately after delivery
Plasma volume: Rapidly decreases to prepregnancy level
Cardiac output: Returns to its prepregnancy state by 8–10 weeks
Hematocrit: Returns to prepregnancy level by 8 weeks

**What are the anatomic and physiologic changes in the urinary tract?**

Hydronephrosis: No evidence by 6–12 weeks in most patients; one study showed that 50% of patients continue to have mild urinary stasis at 12 weeks, suggesting long-standing changes secondary to pregnancy.
Glomerular filtration rate and creatinine clearance: Normal by 8 weeks

**What changes lead to lactation?**

Levels of placental hormones drop (especially estrogen).
Suckling leads to release of prolactin and oxytocin, which cause contraction of myoepithelial cells in the alveoli and milk ducts.

**When is colostrum secreted?**

Approximately 2 days postpartum

**When is mature milk secreted?**

Approximately 3–6 days postpartum

**What are the major components of mature milk?**

Proteins, lactose, water, and fat

**How do the nutrients in colostrum and milk compare?**

Colostrum contains more protein (globulin) and minerals than mature milk, but less sugar and fats.

**What are the psychological changes during the puerperium?**

Mild "maternity blues" occur in 50%–70% of women during the first week after delivery; not associated with hormonal changes.
Postpartum depression occurs in 10%–15% of women.
Postpartum psychosis occurs in 0.1%–0.3% of women.

| | |
|---|---|
| **What medications are effective for postpartum depression?** | Tricyclic antidepressants and serotonin uptake inhibitors |
| **What are the signs, symptoms, and duration of postpartum psychosis?** | Similar to those of acute psychosis; usually lasts 2–3 months. Several authors have not found an association between postpartum depression and prenatal depression, social class, parity, and marital status. |

## POSTPARTUM CARE OF THE MOTHER

| | |
|---|---|
| **How is uterine relaxation evaluated?** | The uterus should be firm, with its upper margin just below the umbilicus after delivery of the placenta. Palpation of the uterus through the abdominal wall at frequent intervals after delivery can detect uterine relaxation. |
| **What is standard care for the perineum?** | Application of an ice pack immediately postpartum to minimize swelling and discomfort "Sitz baths" to minimize discomfort and keep the area clean Evaluation for a hematoma if a woman complains of increasing pain |
| **When is RhoGAM indicated?** | When the mother is Rh- and the infant is Rh+ |
| **When and how much RhoGAM is given?** | 300 μg of RhoGAM within the first 72 hours after delivery |

## COMPLICATIONS OF THE POSTPARTUM PERIOD

### POSTPARTUM HEMORRHAGE

| | |
|---|---|
| **What is a postpartum hemorrhage?** | Vaginal delivery: Blood loss > 500 ml Cesarean section: Blood loss > 1000 ml |
| **When does it usually occur?** | In the immediate postpartum period, but can occur gradually over the first 24 hours |

**What is the term for hemorrhage after the first 24 hours?**

Late postpartum hemorrhage

**Usual cause?**

Subinvolution of the uterus or retention of placental fragments

**What is the incidence of postpartum hemorrhage?**

Occurs in approximately 8% of vaginal deliveries

**Etiologic factors?**

Uterine atony
Genital tract trauma
Retained placental tissue
Coagulation disorders
Ruptured uterus
Uterine inversion

**What is uterine atony?**

Inability of the uterus to contract; causes 75%–80% of postpartum hemorrhages

**Etiologic factors?**

Overdistention of the uterus secondary to multiple gestations, fetal macrosomia, or polyhydramnios
Grand multiparity (parity > 5)
Prolonged use of oxytocin for the induction or augmentation of labor
Use of magnesium sulfate for the treatment of preeclampsia
Uterine infection

**Treatment?**

Identification of at-risk patients
Adequate IV access
Manual exploration of the uterine cavity for evidence of retained placenta
Medications (use in the following order):
  1. Oxytocin 20 U in a liter of crystalloid given rapidly plus 10 U of oxytocin IV push
  2. Methylergonovine (Methergine) 0.2 mg IM
  3. 15-Methyl prostaglandin $F_{2\alpha}$ (Hemabate) 1 ampule IM
Evaluation for possible abnormal placentation or uterine rupture if above measures fail
**Last** resort: Surgery

**What are the surgical options for uterine atony?**

Patient has completed childbearing: Abdominal hysterectomy (definitive therapy for intractable postpartum hemorrhage secondary to uterine atony)

Patient has not completed childbearing: Ligation of the hypogastric or uterine arteries

**How are genital lacerations managed?**

Place first suture well above the apex of the laceration (or episiotomy) to incorporate any bleeding retracted arterioles.

Vaginal lacerations: Reapproximate the tissue without dead space; a running locked suture is the most hemostatic.

Cervical lacerations: These do not require suturing unless actively bleeding.

Expanding vaginal or vulvar hematomas: May require surgical evacuation of the clot; locate and ligate bleeding vessels.

**What kind of hematoma can develop from a large dissecting perineal hematoma?**

Retroperitoneal hematoma

**What is the management of retained placental fragments?**

Manual exploration of the uterus with manual removal of the placenta fragments

Curettage of the uterus (with adequate anesthesia) if hemorrhage continues

Hysterectomy or uterine repair (if possible) if evidence of abnormal placentation (placenta accreta) is present

**What is an inverted uterus?**

The uterine fundus inverts into the uterine cavity.

**Cause?**

Excessive traction applied during the delivery of the placenta

**Management?**

Rapid intervention to prevent cardiovascular shock

Immediate intravascular volume replacement

Without removing the placenta, replacement of the uterus by placing a cupped hand around the fundus and elevating it into the long axis of the vagina

General anesthesia (halothane) to allow uterine relaxation

Oxytocin after uterine replacement

**How are coagulopathies managed?**

Postpartum hemorrhage associated with a coagulopathy: Infusion of blood products or necessary factors to correct specific defect

Significant thrombocytopenia: May require platelet transfusions

Von Willebrand disease: Fresh frozen plasma or DDAVP (a synthetic vasopressin analog)

## POSTPARTUM FEVERS

**What are the most common causes of postpartum fevers?**

Endometritis
Pelvic thrombophlebitis
Breast engorgement
Mastitis
IV site phlebitis

**What is endometritis?**

Inflammation most commonly caused by polymicrobial infection

Primarily involves the endometrium (specifically the decidua and the myometrium)

The most common cause of postpartum fever

**Signs and symptoms?**

Body temperature > 38.0°C
Increasing fundal tenderness
Change in lochia: More profuse or foul smelling
Leukocytosis, which may be difficult to interpret due to physiologic leukocytosis often seen postpartum

**Etiologic factors?**

Gram-positive cocci (group A streptococci, group B streptococci)

Gram-positive anaerobic cocci (*Peptostreptococcus, Petpococcus, Streptococcus, Bacteroides*) in up to 90% of cultures

Gram-positive bacilli (*Clostridium* and
  *Listeria*)
Gram-negative cocci (*Neisseria*
  *gonorrhoeae*)
Gram-negative bacilli (*Escherichia*,
  *Klebsiella*, and *Proteus*)

**What are the risk factors
for postpartum
endometritis?**

Prolonged rupture of membranes,
cesarean section after labor and
ruptured membranes, retained fetal
membranes or placental fragments

**What is the management
for postpartum
endometritis?**

Initial close observation for patients
  without significant symptoms and
  body temperature < 38.0°C
Clindamycin plus gentamicin (most
  tested and effective treatment);
  second- or third-generation
  cephalosporins; ampicillin/sulbactam
  sodium; extended-spectrum penicillins

**What is the management
of the patient who remains
febrile after several days
of antibiotic treatment?**

Search for other sites of infection (e.g.,
hematoma, pelvic abscess, septic pelvic
thrombophlebitis, or a wound infection)

**What is pelvic
thrombophlebitis?**

Extension of endometritis along the
  veins that drain the uterus; sometimes
  involves the ovarian veins (often
  including veins of the placental site)
  because they drain the upper part of
  the uterus
Usually a right unilateral process
Tests (e.g., Doppler ultrasound and
  computed tomography scan) usually
  not diagnostic
Often a diagnosis of exclusion when a
  patient does not respond to antibiotics
  for suspected endometritis but
  responds to addition of heparin

**Management?**

Treatment of phlebitis with continued
  use of antibiotics
Heparin therapy to increase partial
  thromboplastin time to two times
  above normal

| | |
|---|---|
| **What is breast engorgement?** | Lymphatic obstruction resulting in bilaterally tender breasts, often with mild temperature elevation; onset usually over the first days after delivery |
| **Management?** | Binding breasts with an Ace bandage or tight-fitting bra and placement of ice packs on the breasts<br>Avoidance of nipple stimulation<br>Parlodel (bromocriptine) therapy no longer recommended because of increased risk of cerebrovascular accident |
| **What is mastitis?** | Unilateral or bilateral infection of the breast; usually caused by *Staphylococcus aureus* and *Streptococcus* species; transmitted to the mother from the child's oropharynx |
| **Management?** | Breast-feeding or pumping from the affected breast<br>Antibiotic therapy with dicloxicillin<br>Formation of breast abscess:<br>　　Discontinuation of breast-feeding from the affected breast; may require surgical drainage and intravenous antibiotic therapy |

# 7

# Spontaneous Abortion

**What is an abortion?**

Termination of a pregnancy before 20 weeks' gestational age
Can also be defined as the expulsion of fetal tissue < 500 g
Can be spontaneous or induced by medical or surgical means

**What is preterm birth?**

Expulsion of a fetus after 20 weeks' gestational age and before 37 completed weeks' gestation

**What is intrauterine fetal demise?**

Death of the fetus after 20 weeks' gestational age

**What is a stillbirth?**

Expulsion of a dead fetus after 20 weeks' gestational age

**What are the categories of abortion?**

Induced abortion: Pregnancy termination by medical or surgical means for therapeutic or elective reasons
Spontaneous abortion ("miscarriage"): Pregnancy loss before 20 weeks' gestational age
Complete abortion: Abortion with complete expulsion of all products of conception (POC)
Incomplete abortion: Abortion without complete expulsion of all POC; fetal or placental components remain in the uterus.
Threatened abortion: Bleeding from the uterus (as seen on visualization of cervical os) without cervical dilatation and with or without contractions before 20 weeks' gestational age; no expulsion of POC
Inevitable abortion: Bleeding from the uterus with cervical dilatation with or

without perceived contractions before 20 weeks' gestational age; no expulsion of POC

Missed abortion: Fetal death before 20 weeks' gestational age without expulsion of POC

Septic abortion: Induced or spontaneous abortion with uterine and systemic infection

Recurrent abortion: Three or more consecutive spontaneous abortions

**How is spontaneous abortion evaluated?**

Confirm pregnancy by history, physical examination, and possibly ultrasound or human chorionic gonadotropin (hCG) assay.

Establish location of the pregnancy (intrauterine vs. ectopic) by history, physical examination, ultrasound, and hCG trends.

Establish whether expulsion of POC is partial, complete, or absent by history and pelvic examination.

May rule out retained POC with ultrasound if patient passes tissue.

May confirm fetal loss by laboratory tests (static or declining hCG values) or ultrasound (lack of fetal cardiac activity or movement, or the absence of POC); histologic evaluation of passed tissue can also help in diagnosing spontaneous abortion.

**What are the common pathologic findings in spontaneous abortion?**

Hemorrhage into the decidua basalis

Necrotic changes in tissue adjacent to bleeding

Edematous, thickened villi

Blood (carneous) mole: Ovum encapsulated in clotted blood

Fetal maceration: Skull collapse, hemorrhagic abdominal distention, red appearance, skin softening and peeling, organ necrosis

**What are the differential diagnoses of spontaneous abortion?**

Bleeding and pain are common gynecologic complaints and, without a β-hCG, the differential diagnosis includes:

Ectopic pregnancy

Placental separation
Hydatidiform mole
Bleeding submucous fibroid
Bleeding pedunculated fibroid
Cancer (cervical or uterine)
Dysfunctional uterine bleeding

**What is the incidence of spontaneous abortion?**

Occurs in 15%–20% of clinically diagnosed pregnancies
One study found a 50%–75% spontaneous abortion rate in chemically diagnosed pregnancies (positive hCG assay in women followed with sequential hCG assays).
Subclinical spontaneous abortion (early losses not diagnosed for lack of symptoms) rate is about 10%.

**During what trimester do most spontaneous abortions occur?**

First trimester

**In approximately how many early pregnancies do the common signs and symptoms of spontaneous abortion (pain and vaginal bleeding) occur?**

Approximately one in four

**How many of these pregnancies will be spontaneously aborted?**

Fifty percent

**What is the incidence of recurrent abortion?**

Estimates vary from 0.5% to 1% of pregnant women.

**What is the risk of recurrence of spontaneous abortion?**

Women who have had two consecutive spontaneous abortions have a 25%–45% risk of recurrence.
Women who have had a single early spontaneous abortion have an 80%–90% chance of delivering a viable infant in their next pregnancy.

**At what gestational age do most abortions occur?**

Eighty percent of pregnancy losses occur before 14 weeks' gestational age.
Fifteen percent are lost before implantation (undetectable clinically).
Two percent are lost during implantation.

**What are the etiologic factors of spontaneous abortion?**

Genetic

Over 50% of first trimester losses demonstrate abnormal karyotypes (30% at 16–19 weeks).

Half of the abnormal karyotypes are aneuploid (abnormal chromosomal number, e.g., trisomy, monosomy, triploidy, tetraploidy).

Half are euploid (single gene mutation or polygenic with a normal number of chromosomes).

Fetal: Abnormal morphologic embryonic growth and development [e.g., blighted ovum, in which the embryo is degenerated or absent (anembryonic)]

Maternal endocrinologic or metabolic disorders: Diabetes mellitus, thyroid dysfunction

Maternal autoimmune disorders: Antiphospholipid syndrome, lupus erythematosus

Infection: Implicated organisms include *Mycoplasma hominis, Ureaplasma urealyticum, Treponema pallidum, Borrelia burgdorferi, Chlamydia trachomatis, Neisseria gonorrhoeae,* and *Listeria monocytogenes.*

Uterine abnormalities: Müllerian defects, fibroids, adhesions

Incompetent cervix: Reduced ability of cervix to support pregnancy in uterus

Progesterone deficiency: Failure of corpus luteum or placenta to synthesize normal levels of progesterone (luteal phase defect) to maintain pregnancy

Trauma: Penetrating or blunt wounds or surgical trauma (e.g., corpus luteum cystectomy or appendectomy)

Drugs: Substances that may play a role include tobacco, alcohol, caffeine, aminopterin, methotrexate, chloroquine, oral hypoglycemic agents, and anesthetic gases.

Radiation: Lethal dose of approximately 10 radiation absorbed dose (rad) during implantation

Severe malnutrition

**What laboratory values can be helpful in managing spontaneous abortion?**

hCG assay
  Confirms pregnant status
  Serial values can be followed when the diagnosis is uncertain (e.g., in early pregnancy, in which falling or stable values suggest abortion).
Blood type and screen
  Blood type should be determined in all patients with bleeding in pregnancy.
  Rh immunoglobulin should be given within 72 hours if patient is Rh-negative.
Complete blood count: Determines extent of hemorrhage (if any) and likelihood of infection
Progesterone levels: Some authorities recommend this assay. This test determines whether the progesterone level is adequate to support the pregnancy.

**How is ultrasound useful in the evaluation of spontaneous abortion?**

Ultrasound (usually transvaginal in early pregnancy) is helpful in differentiating intrauterine pregnancy from extrauterine (ectopic) pregnancy when evaluating first-trimester bleeding without prior evidence of an intrauterine pregnancy.

**For each of the following hCG values, give the findings that should be seen on transvaginal ultrasound:**
  **hCG > 1500 MIU?**          Gestational sac

  **hCG > 5000 MIU?**          Fetal pole

  **hCG > 17,000 MIU?**        Fetal heart motion

**What is the discriminatory zone?**

The hCG value above which the gestational sac should be seen in the uterus

**How should a patient with threatened abortion be managed when the β-hCG is below the threshold for visualization of a sac and no intrauterine pregnancy is seen?**

This clinical scenario (early pregnancy with inability to rule in an intrauterine pregnancy or rule out an ectopic pregnancy) is frequently encountered. The principal management is close follow-up, but the following measures are commonly accepted in stable patients (no pain or hemodynamic instability):

Serial β-hCG measurements to determine trend (intrauterine pregnancies generally have a doubling of β-hCG values every 48 hours, whereas ectopic pregnancies generally have an abnormally low increase in β-hCG values)

Serial ultrasound examinations to determine whether there is a gestational sac once the discriminatory zone is reached

Ectopic precautions: The patient should be told to return with heavy bleeding, abdominal or pelvic pain, dizziness, syncopal episodes, or any symptom that might suggest ectopic pregnancy.

Suction curettage remains an option for patients who do not desire the pregnancy and are either noncompliant or otherwise poor candidates for follow-up

**How is threatened abortion diagnosed?**

Bleeding or cramping in early pregnancy
Closed cervix

**How is threatened abortion treated?**

Intravenous fluids for stabilization if needed
No known proven "treatment" exists that prevents miscarriage, although pelvic rest (avoiding intercourse) may be beneficial.

**What is the follow-up if spontaneous abortion occurs after threatened abortion?**

Follow-up with repeat physical examinations is justified if the patient is stable and without pain.
Blood type and Rh screen followed by administration of Rh immunoglobulin to Rh-negative women

**On what is the diagnosis of inevitable abortion based?**

Bleeding or cramps with a dilated cervical os

**What is the treatment of inevitable abortion?**

Intravenous fluids for stabilization if needed

No treatment can prevent miscarriage once the cervix has dilated; therefore, options include (if bleeding is minimal and the patient is stable and compliant) dilation and curettage or spontaneous abortion at home with close follow-up to ensure that all POC has been passed.

Blood type and Rh screen followed by administration of Rh immunoglobulin to Rh-negative women

**What are the treatment options for women who do not want to pass tissue at home?**

Suction curettage or inpatient observation while aborting

**What are the risks of passing tissue at home?**

It is safe at the usual 6 to 8 weeks' gestational age and does not require hospitalization or intervention.

**On what is the diagnosis of incomplete abortion based?**

Continued bleeding after passage of tissue

**What is the treatment of incomplete abortion?**

Intravenous fluids for stabilization if needed

Removal of tissue protruding from os with ring forceps

Ultrasound to evaluate for intrauterine POC

D&C; treatment of choice to evacuate the uterine cavity definitively

Oxytocin or methylergonovine, or both, to stimulate uterine contractions to decrease blood loss

Blood type and Rh screen followed by administration of Rh immunoglobulin to Rh-negative women

Antibiotics after D&C

Histologic evaluation of any available tissue

**What is a side effect of methylergonovine?**

It is an ergot and can therefore exacerbate chronic hypertension.

**On what is the diagnosis of complete abortion based?**

Tissue is passed after bleeding and cramping.
Cramps and bleeding cease after tissue passage.

**What is the treatment of complete abortion?**

Histologic confirmation that tissue is POC and not a mole
hCG values may be followed if tissue is unavailable.
Blood type and Rh screen followed by administration of Rh immunoglobulin to Rh-negative women

**On what is the diagnosis of missed abortion based?**

Fetal demise is confirmed, signs and symptoms of spontaneous abortion are absent, and the cervix is closed.

**How can fetal demise be confirmed?**

Laboratory or ultrasonographic means can confirm fetal demise; usually both are used.
Laboratory: Static or abnormally slow increases in hCG values
Ultrasound: Absence of fetal cardiac activity in a fetus with prior cardiac activity or at a gestational age in which fetal cardiac activity should be demonstrated

**What is the treatment of missed abortion?**

Options include:
  Outpatient follow-up
  D&C
  Vaginal suppository or intra-amniotic prostaglandin administration to effect uterine contractions and delivery in the second trimester
Blood type and Rh screen followed by administration of Rh immunoglobulin to Rh-negative women

**Why do most authorities opt for intervention (D&C or prostaglandin administration) over observation?**

Intervention decreases the risk of infection or coagulopathy, depending on the estimated time since fetal death and estimated gestational age.

**What are the etiologic factors of coagulopathy after a missed abortion?**

Rarely develops after a missed abortion (after several weeks) as a result of trophoblastic tissue (thromboplastin) entering the maternal circulation and triggering the intrinsic coagulation pathway

**On what is the diagnosis of coagulopathy in a missed abortion based?**

Diagnosis is made with laboratory and clinical evidence of altered coagulation.

Platelet values
  Simple screening test
  Usually low in the coagulopathic patient
Low fibrinogen and increased fibrin degradation products also suggest coagulopathy.
Very rarely, full-blown disseminated intravascular coagulation can develop.

**On what is the diagnosis of septic abortion based?**

Evidence of localized infection:
  Suprapubic, uterine, pelvic, or cervical motion tenderness; foul-smelling cervicovaginal discharge; peritonitis)
  **and**
Systemic evidence of infection: Fever, shock, leukocytosis after an induced or spontaneous abortion

**What is the treatment for septic abortion?**

Intravenous antibiotic administration
Evacuation of the infected uterine contents
Hospitalization

**When is intensive care required for a patient with a septic abortion?**

If systemic sepsis occurs, to allow proper hemodynamic monitoring and respiratory care

**What factors should guide the choice of intravenous antibiotics?**

Initial antibiotic therapy should be broad spectrum and cover anaerobic and aerobic bacteria.
After results of culture, antibiotics should be chosen according to organism antibiotic sensitivities.

**When during the course of treatment of septic abortion should D&C be performed?**

Only after initiation of antibiotic therapy

**When is hysterectomy a treatment option for septic abortion?**

In cases unresponsive to antibiotics, particularly with abscess formation

**What questions should be asked when taking a history for recurrent abortion?**

Has the patient been exposed to environmental toxins or drugs?
Does the patient have known gynecologic or obstetric infection?
Does the patient have antiphospholipid syndrome-associated historical factors (thrombosis, autoimmune thrombocytopenia, or false-positive syphilis tests)?
Is the patient related to the father of the child?
Does the patient have a family history of recurrent pregnancy loss?

**What tests can be included in the work-up of recurrent abortion?**

Thyroid function evaluation
Hysterosalpingography
Parental karyotypes to determine parental chromosome abnormalities
Endometrial biopsy to determine the presence of a luteal phase defect (histologic dating of the endometrium lags behind menstrual dating by 3 days)
Antiphospholipid syndrome studies (Russell viper venom and anticardiolipin antibodies)

**What are potential treatments for recurrent pregnancy loss?**

Supplemental progesterone for luteal phase defect
Surgery to correct uterine abnormalities
Treatment of infection, if present
Empiric treatment of couple with doxycycline to eradicate *Mycoplasma* has been proposed.
Prednisone, aspirin, or both for antiphospholipid syndrome
Prenatal genetic studies if warranted by parental karyotypes

**What is the major threat to future reproductive potential when performing a D&C for septic abortion?**

Asherman syndrome (the development of extensive intrauterine synechiae)
Risk is increased if a D&C is performed in the presence of infection.

Can also result from overzealous uterine
curettage in the absence of infection

**Prevention?**

Treatment with antibiotics before the
D&C

**Treatment?**

Hysteroscopic lysis of adhesions

**What are the
complications of D&C for
inevitable, incomplete,
missed, or septic abortion?**

Uterine perforation: Can result from
dilation, curettage, forceps probing, or
an overly soft uterine wall that
permits easy instrument penetration
Bladder or bowel injury: Results from
uterine perforation and occasionally
the suction of bowel into the suction
curette
Fistula formation secondary to
perforation
Infection
Amenorrhea and infertility (Asherman
syndrome)

**Why is it important to
send tissue, if available,
for histologic
confirmation?**

Histologic evaluation can confirm:
Intrauterine pregnancy when chorionic
villi are present
Passage of POC
Ectopic pregnancy in the absence of
chorionic villi
Gestational trophoblastic disease

**For each of the following
structural or mechanical
causes of pregnancy loss
before 20 weeks'
gestational age that are
amenable to treatment,
give the diagnosis and
treatment.**

**Cervical incompetence
(premature cervical
dilatation)**

Diagnosis: Painless (no contractions)
dilatation of the cervix and passage of
POC
Treatment: Placement of a cervical
cerclage to reinforce the structural
integrity of the cervix; usually treated
in the second trimester

**Leiomyomas**

Diagnosis: Hysterosalpingogram, ultrasonography, or hysteroscopy
Treatment: Removal (myomectomy) at laparotomy, laparoscopy, or hysteroscopy; hysteroscopy is usually used now in treating submucosal fibroids in infertility patients.

**Müllerian anomalies, such as a "double uterus" (bicornuate, septate, or didelphic)**

Diagnosis: Hysterosalpingogram, hysteroscopy, and laparoscopy
Treatment: Surgery

**Uterine synechiae (intrauterine adhesions seen in Asherman syndrome)**

Diagnosis: Hysterosalpingogram, hysteroscopy, or both
Treatment: Hysteroscopic lysis of adhesions

**When are mechanical causes of early pregnancy loss usually treated?**

With the exception of premature cervical dilatation, which is a clinical diagnosis, extensive work-up and subsequent treatment of mechanical causes of early pregnancy loss is not undertaken until the patient has experienced three consecutive losses (recurrent pregnancy loss).

# 8

# Ectopic Pregnancy

**What is it?**

Extrauterine pregnancy
Most commonly occurs in the fallopian
tubes
Can also occur in the abdomen, ovary,
and cervix
Life-threatening condition for the
mother
Successful completion of the pregnancy
is not usually a consideration.

**Incidence?**

16.8/1000 pregnancies (~2%)
Has risen steadily since 1970

**What is its mortality rate?**

~3.5/10,000 cases (12% of all maternal
deaths)
Highest risk of mortality for interstitial
and abdominal gestations

**What are the major risk
factors?**

Salpingitis: Risk increases threefold;
chlamydial infection is more important
than *Neisseria gonorrhoeae.*
Intrauterine device (IUD): Conception
with an IUD in place (risk: 2%–3%)
results in sixfold increase in risk
compared to conception without an
IUD.
Other contraceptives:
Oral and subdermal progestin-only
contraceptives: Increased risk (if
pregnancy occurs at all)
Combination oral contraceptives:
Slightly increased risk (if pregnancy
occurs at all)
Barrier methods: No increased risk
Previous tubal pregnancy: 10%–25% will
have another tubal pregnancy.
Tubal sterilization: Failure is associated
with increased rates of ectopic
gestations (12% of pregnancies from
failure of Pomeroy technique; 60%–

70% of pregnancies from failure of
bipolar tubal cautery and fallopian
rings).

**What are the symptoms?**
Vary from asymptomatic to frank shock
Classic triad: **Abdominal pain**
(generalized in nature 50% of the
time), **abnormal uterine bleeding**,
and **history of amenorrhea**
Other: Dizziness or lightheadedness;
gastrointestinal symptoms (e.g.,
nausea, vomiting, and diarrhea)
Common for pain to worsen acutely
around the time of rupture

**What are the signs?**
Abdominal tenderness
Adnexal tenderness (unilateral or
bilateral)
Cervical motion tenderness in > 50% of
patients
A tender adnexal mass may be palpable
in approximately 50% of patients.
Fever: > 38.5°C (< 10% of patients)
Other: Depends on the presence and
extent of rupture and hemorrhage;
includes peritoneal signs, tachycardia,
tachypnea, and orthostatic changes

**What are the laboratory
findings?**
Complete blood count
Hematocrit—usually normal or slightly
decreased; more valuable when
measured serially to indicate blood
loss
White blood cell count—variable
(normal values in 50% of patients)
Serum β-human chorionic gonadotropin
(β-hCG):
Confirms pregnancy
Serial quantitative values show a
blunted rate of increase; in a
normal pregnancy, β-hCG doubles
every 2 days.
**Note:** Urine β-hCG values have a
high false-negative rate for
diagnosing ectopic pregnancies.

**What are the differential
diagnoses?**
Acute appendicitis
Adnexal torsion

Aborting intrauterine pregnancy
Corpus luteum cyst
Pelvic inflammatory disease
Degenerating fibroids (in pregnancy)
Endometriosis
Urinary tract infection
Gastroenteritis
Diverticulitis
Meckel's diverticulum

**What are other useful studies?**

Abdominal pelvic ultrasound
  Intrauterine and extrauterine
    pregnancies rarely occur
    simultaneously (1 in 40,000
    pregnancies); evidence of
    intrauterine pregnancy excludes an
    ectopic.
  Abdominal sonography can identify an
    intrauterine sac only when
    pregnancy is advanced enough for
    $\beta$-hCG levels to reach 5000–6000
    mIU/ml (~7 weeks after last
    menstrual period).
  Vaginal ultrasound: Detects an
    intrauterine sac at $\beta$-hCG levels
    between 1500 and 2000 mIU/ml (~6
    weeks after last menstrual period).
Culdocentesis
  Presence of nonclotting blood is
    diagnostic of free blood in the
    peritoneal cavity; supports diagnosis
    of ectopic pregnancy.
  Useful for surgical intervention along
    with other findings; not very
    sensitive or specific for ectopic
    pregnancy
Laparoscopy: Indicated to confirm
  doubtful diagnosis

**What are the treatment options?**

Laparoscopy, laparotomy, medical
treatment

**What does laparoscopic treatment entail?**

1. **Linear salpingostomy:** Linear
   incision over the antimesenteric
   aspect of fallopian tube; the ectopic is
   exposed and evacuated. Incision
   closes by secondary intention and
   tubes reepithelialize.

2. **Partial salpingectomy:** Performed when the tube is severely damaged or persistently bleeding; resection is minimal to save as much tube as possible for future reanastomosis.

**What are the indications for laparotomy?**

Profuse hemorrhage
Certain locations of the pregnancy (cornual, interstitial, abdominal, ovarian)
Inadequate visualization, exposure, or treatment of adnexa during laparoscopy

**What does medical management of ectopic pregnancy involve?**

Methotrexate

**What are the indications for medical management?**

Small unruptured ectopic (< 3 cm)
Plateaued or rising β-hCG titer after salpingostomy
Salpingectomy suggesting inadequate evacuation of the pregnancy

**What are the complications of an ectopic pregnancy?**

Persistent trophoblastic tissue (5%); requires subsequent surgery or methotrexate
Intra-abdominal hemorrhage
Rh sensitization secondary to fetomaternal hemorrhage: Rare; however, all Rh– patients should receive prophylactic dose of RhoGAM.

**What is the prognosis for patients treated for an unruptured ectopic pregnancy?**

Subsequent intrauterine pregnancy : ~70%
Recurrence of ectopic pregnancy: 8%
Infertility, probably secondary to tubal dysfunction and adhesion formation after treatment : 20%

# 9     Preterm Labor

**What is preterm labor?**

Contractions and progressive cervical change between 20 and 37 completed weeks' gestational age

**What is term labor?**

Labor after 37 completed weeks' gestational age

**What is a threatened abortion?**

Labor before 20 weeks' gestational age

**What is cervical incompetence?**

Also called premature cervical dilatation; cervical dilatation in the absence of contractions before term; should not be confused with preterm labor

**What is the incidence of preterm labor?**

Occurs in 5%–15% of all pregnancies; rates have remained unchanged for decades despite efforts to intervene.

**What is the percentage of neonatal deaths caused by preterm birth?**

Seventy-five percent of neonatal deaths not caused by congenital anomalies

**What are the risk factors for preterm labor?**

Preterm rupture of the membranes
Polyhydramnios
Multiple gestation
Maternal systemic disease
Low socioeconomic status
Nonwhite race
Maternal age: < 18 or > 40
Low prepregnancy weight
Multiple gestation (10% of all preterm births)
Fetal death
History of preterm births (17%–37% risk after one preterm birth)
Repeated second-trimester spontaneous abortion
Uterine infection/vaginal infection/ colonization [group B streptococcus (GBS), gonorrhea, *Chlamydia*, *Ureaplasma*, syphilis,

trichomoniasis, *Gardnerella*]
Uterine anomalies (unicornuate uterus,
   bicornuate uterus, uterine
   leiomyomata)
Cystitis
Pyelonephritis
Smoking
Cocaine use
Use of IUD
Lack of prenatal care
Fetal anomalies
Placental anomalies

**What is the percent of all preterm births caused by preterm labor?**

Approximately 30%

**What are other causes of preterm birth?**

Preterm premature rupture of the
   membranes (30%–35% of all preterm
   births)
Placental abruption
Placenta previa
Multiple gestation
Hypertensive disorders
Diabetes mellitus
Congenital malformations

**What constitutes "labor"?**

Regular uterine contractions with:
Contractions lasting at least 30 seconds
At least two contractions in a 10-minute
   period
Persistence of contraction pattern for at
   least 30 minutes
Progressive cervical change

**What questions should be asked in the history of the preterm labor patient?**

Does the patient have:
A history of preterm birth?
A history of cystitis or pyelonephritis?
A known multiple gestation?
A known placenta previa?
A known fetal anomaly?
A known uterine anomaly?
Good fetal movement?
Untreated infections?
Cigarette or cocaine use?
An accurate last menstrual period
   (LMP) or dating ultrasound?

**What conditions should be ruled out in preterm labor?**

Preterm premature rupture of the membranes
Placental abruption
Placenta previa
Fetal death
Infection
Multiple gestation
Fetal anomalies

**Why is gestational age important in preterm labor?**

It determines the real risks to the fetus in the extrauterine environment and guides aggressiveness of treatment.

**How is gestational age calculated?**

By determining the estimated date of confinement (EDC, "due date") using Naegele's rule:
$$EDC = (LMP + 7 \text{ days}) - 3 \text{ months}$$

**How is gestational age calculated when LMP is not precisely known and early ultrasonographic dating is not available?**

Use best estimate of the LMP and the earliest possible ultrasound to estimate gestational age.

**What form of preterm birth can be prevented?**

Iatrogenic preterm birth due to elective induction of labor or elective cesarean section when the maturity of the fetus is not precisely known

**What are preventive measures for preterm labor?**

Home uterine monitoring for women with a history of preterm labor
Prophylactic tocolytic agents for women at high risk for preterm labor
Reduced activity
Bed rest
Frequent cervical examinations to detect early cervical change

**What are general treatment options?**

Hydration
Bed rest
Tocolytic therapy
Glucocorticoid administration
Transfer of patient to a high-risk facility

**How do hydration and bed rest stop preterm labor?**

Hydration: Mechanism is unknown.
Bed rest: Little evidence supports its use.
Both continue to be used liberally because their use entails almost no risk and may benefit the patient.

**What are tocolytic drugs?**   Agents that decrease uterine contractions by a variety of mechanisms; used to stop the progression of labor when continued uterine contractions or labor could have negative consequences

**What are the short- and long-term goals of tocolysis?**   Short-term goal: Prevent delivery for at least 48 hours to allow administration of glucocorticoids to the mother (fetal lung benefits optimized at least 48 hours after institution of therapy)
Long-term goal: Allow fetus to gain lung maturity in utero to increase the chances of a good outcome after delivery

**Contraindications?**   Intrauterine fetal demise
Oligohydramnios
Intrauterine growth retardation
Fetal distress
Chorioamnionitis
Fatal congenital anomalies

**What are β-mimetic agents?**   β-Adrenergic agonists that act through smooth muscle relaxation

**Specific β-adrenergic agents used?**   Only ritodrine is FDA-approved for tocolysis, but terbutaline is commonly used.

**Side effects?**   Tachycardia
Palpitations
Tremors
Nervousness
Restlessness
Pulmonary edema
Decreased $K^+$
Insulin release
Increased glucose
Lactic acidosis

**Contraindications?**   Maternal heart disease
Hyperthyroidism
Uncontrolled hypertension
Pulmonary hypertension
Drug-dependent asthma
Possibly diabetes

**How do calcium channel blockers (nifedipine) act in tocolysis?**

They reduce smooth muscle activity and myometrial contractions by reducing cytoplasmic free calcium.

**Side effects?**

Minimal; animal experiments suggest fetal hypoxemia and decreased uteroplacental blood flow, but these effects are not found in humans.

**What are indomethacin (Indocin) and sulindac?**

Prostaglandin inhibitors that prevent prostaglandin-induced myometrial contractions by blocking prostaglandin synthetase activity; possibly more effective than ritodrine in delaying delivery and increasing birth weight

**What primary concerns limit the use of prostaglandin inhibitors as tocolytics?**

Premature closure of ductus arteriosus and fetal nephrotoxicity

**What is the mechanism of action of magnesium sulfate in tocolysis?**

Exerts stabilizing effects on smooth muscle by calcium antagonism

**Side effects?**

Decreased deep tendon reflexes, respiratory and cardiac depression, and drowsiness; not usually seen if renal function is normal and administration rates are acceptable (2 g/hour)

**Indications?**

First-line drug in obviously progressive labor, especially at an early gestational age
Second-line drug with failed oral tocolysis
When other tocolytics are contraindicated

**What is the therapy for magnesium toxicity?**

1 g calcium gluconate intravenously

**What are the beneficial effects of corticosteroids in preterm labor?**

Betamethasone or dexamethasone aids fetal lung maturity and decreases the incidence of neonatal respiratory distress syndrome (RDS), neonatal intraventricular hemorrhage, and neonatal mortality.

**At what gestational age should they be used?**

At 24–34 weeks' gestational age in women at risk for preterm delivery, before 30–32 weeks' gestation in women with preterm premature rupture of fetal membranes in the absence of clinical chorioamnionitis

**Neonatal risks?**

No evidence of increased neonatal infection risk or adrenal suppression

**Maternal risks?**

Generally low; include pulmonary edema (increased risk with tocolytics, fluid overload, or multiple gestation), slight increase in infection with preterm premature rupture of the membranes (controversial), and glucose/insulin control effects

**What common organism poses a threat to fetus and mother in preterm labor?**

Group B *Streptococcus* (GBS)

**Incidence of colonization?**

Fifteen percent to forty percent of pregnant women are colonized with GBS.
Fifty percent of these women colonize their infants during delivery.

**Maternal complications related to GBS?**

Chorioamnionitis, endomyometritis, cystitis, and pyelonephritis

**Prophylaxis and treatment?**

Culture of women in preterm labor and a penicillin (erythromycin or clindamycin in penicillin-allergic patients) until culture proves negative
Full course of antibiotics for women with positive GBS cultures to prevent maternal/sexual transmission of ODS, neonatal sepsis, chorioamnionitis, and postpartum endomyometritis

**Should patients at risk for delivery of a preterm neonate be transferred to high-risk centers before or after delivery?**

Historically, concern for potential delivery en route to perinatal centers prevented routine transfer of patients with risk of preterm delivery.
Current practice mandates transfer to a perinatal center of all stable women at risk of delivery if the fetus weighs less than 1500 g (~32–34 weeks).

**Should preterm neonates be delivered by cesarean section (C/S)?**

Cephalic presentation: Vaginal delivery has same outcome as C/S despite the theoretical risk of head trauma and intraventricular hemorrhage.
Breech: C/S is indicated because of the risk of head entrapment by the incompletely dilated cervix (infrequent but potentially devastating).

**What underlying fetal deficiency leads to neonatal respiratory distress syndrome (RDS)?**

Deficient surfactant biosynthesis in neonatal lung type II pneumocytes leads to RDS because of alveolar collapse from increased alveolar surface tension.

**Treatment?**

Surfactant administration for neonates at high risk for RDS

**What determines outcome in preterm neonates?**

Level of neonatal care
Gestational age
Birth weight
Presence of asphyxia
Presence of intracranial hemorrhage
Presence of periventricular leukomalacia
Presence of retinopathy of prematurity
Parental socioeconomic factors/education
Presence of necrotizing enterocolitis
Presence of congenital anomalies

**What are the generally accepted values for low–birth-weight neonates?**

$\geq$ 2500 g = "normal"
< 2500 g = low birth weight
$\leq$ 1500 g = very low birth weight
$\leq$ 1000 g = extremely low birth weight

**What is the difference in risk of neonatal death between normal and very low–birth-weight infants?**

Very low–birth-weight infants have a 200-fold increased risk of death compared with neonates weighing > 2500 g (Table 9-1).

**What is the incidence of RDS from 33 to 38 weeks' gestation?**

Decreases with increasing gestational age:
Thirty-one percent at 33 weeks' gestation
Thirteen percent at 34 weeks' gestation
Six percent from 35 to 38 weeks' gestation

**Table 9–1. Mortality rates by gestational age and birth weight**

| Gestational Age (wk) | Mortality Rate (%) | Birth Weight (g) | Mortality Rate (%) |
|---|---|---|---|
| 23 | 82 | 500–600 | 80–90 |
| 24 | 42 | 600–700 | 53–85 |
| 25 | 20 | 700–800 | 41–65 |
| 26–27 | 6 | 800–900 | 29–42 |
| 28–29 | 9 | 900–1000 | 17–25 |
| <26 | 44 | 1000–1250 | 13 |

Courtesy R. J. Boyle, MD, University of Virginia.

**What are the early and late problems associated with preterm birth?**

Early: Developmental delay, cerebral palsy, visual impairment, hearing loss, chronic lung disease, rehospitalization

Late: Mental retardation, learning disabilities, attention deficit disorder, language impairment, school problems

**What is the incidence of problems?**

Twenty-six percent of survivors weighing < 800 g have major handicaps.

Seventeen percent to twenty percent of survivors weighing 750–1000 g have major handicaps.

# 10

# Premature Rupture of the Membranes

**What is premature rupture of the membranes (PROM)?**

Disruption of the integrity of fetal membranes before the onset of labor

**What is preterm PROM?**

PROM before term (before 38 weeks' gestation)

**What is prolonged PROM?**

More than 24 hours elapse between rupture of membranes and the onset of labor (latent period).

**What is the incidence of PROM?**

Complicates 10% of all pregnancies
Associated with 30% of preterm births
Most common diagnosis on admission to neonatal intensive care units

**Does PROM occur more frequently at term or preterm?**

Ninety-four percent of all cases occur at term.
Five percent occur in pregnancies with fetuses weighing 1000–2500 g.
One percent of all cases occurs in fetuses weighing less than 1000 g (75% of these have prolonged PROM).

**How do term and preterm patients differ in their propensity to go into labor after PROM?**

Ninety percent of term patients will be in labor 24 hours after PROM.
Fifty percent of preterm patients will be in labor 24 hours after PROM.
Eighty-five percent of preterm patients will be in labor within 1 week after PROM.

**What are the causes of PROM?**

Not definitively known, but linked to:
Membrane infection
Hydramnios
Incompetent cervix
Abruptio placentae
Amniocentesis

**What organisms have been linked to PROM?**

*Ureaplasma urealyticum, Trichomonas vaginalis, Bacteroides* species, *Chlamydia trachomatis,* group B streptococcus (GBS), *Gardnerella vaginalis,* and others

**How do they cause PROM?**

Production of various factors that weaken fetal membranes and render them susceptible to rupture

It is unknown whether positive vaginal or amniotic fluid cultures are the result of (1) infection causing PROM through weakening of the membranes, or (2) PROM leading to colonization with microorganisms.

**What is a common symptom in PROM?**

Sudden "gush" of fluid or a steady "trickle" of fluid per vaginum that may or may not be associated with the passage of a small amount of blood or mucus. **Note:** Patients frequently confuse loss of urine, vaginal discharge, or bloody show with loss of amniotic fluid.

**How is PROM diagnosed?**

With a "sterile" speculum vaginal examination

**What are the three signs of PROM?**

1. Pooling of vaginal fluid in the posterior fornix
2. Positive nitrazine test
3. "Ferning" on a slide prepared with a thin layer of fluid obtained from the vaginal wall and allowed to dry

**How can false-positive diagnoses of membrane rupture be avoided?**

Nitrazine test: False positives can occur if discharge is obtained from the cervical os because the cervical mucus and amniotic fluid both have a pH higher than that of the vagina; blood, semen, or vaginitis can also raise pH.

Ferning: Cervical mucus can also cause "ferning" (a distinct arborization pattern seen under microscopy) in the absence of ruptured membranes.

Collection of fluid: Collect fluid *only* from the vaginal wall to avoid cervical mucus unless fluid can be seen flowing from the os into the posterior fornix with the Valsalva maneuver, cough, or fundal pressure.

**How is cervical dilatation evaluated in preterm PROM?**

No digital cervical examination if rupture of the membranes is confirmed or suspected in preterm patients due to the risk of introducing infection into the amnionic sac
Visualization with a "sterile" speculum for cervical assessment

**How is potential infection evaluated?**

Cultures for genital tract organisms, including GBS as well as gonorrhea and chlamydia
Amniocentesis in women with preterm PROM for Gram stain and culture to evaluate for infection
   Benefit: also allows evaluation of fetal lung maturity
   Risk: procedure carries some risk; questionable whether this practice results in improved pregnancy outcomes

**How is ultrasound useful in the evaluation of PROM?**

Evaluation of fetal biometry [in the absence of a known last menstrual period (LMP) or prior ultrasound] to determine gestational age of the fetus
Evaluation of amniotic fluid volume for oligohydramnios, which may help to confirm the rupture
Determination of fetal presentation (vertex, breech, or transverse) when vaginal examination is inappropriate and abdominal examination is inconclusive
Evaluation for a fetal anomaly if PROM occurs preterm

**What is a dye test?**

Injection of dye into the amniotic sac followed by evaluation of the presence of dye on a tampon placed intravaginally

**How can a dye test be used to evaluate PROM?**

To confirm diagnosis if equivocal
To determine if membranes have "sealed over" in a woman who has stopped leaking

**How is the fetus evaluated before initiating treatment in PROM?**

Rule out fetal stress (from cord compression in oligohydramnios or cord prolapse) with fetal heart monitoring in preterm or term PROM.

**Why is knowing the gestational age important in PROM?**

The risks to the fetus from preterm delivery vary with gestational age.

**How is gestational age determined?**

With the patient's LMP, or ultrasound if LMP is uncertain

**What are the risks of PROM to the fetus and the mother?**

Infection of the fetus (fetal/neonatal sepsis or death), the fetal membranes (chorioamnionitis), or the uterus (endomyometritis)

**Differences in risks between preterm and term PROM?**

Preterm PROM: The risks are primarily related to prematurity [respiratory distress syndrome (RDS), (IVH)] and secondarily related to infection.
Term PROM: No risk of prematurity; primary risk is infection.

**What is expectant management of PROM?**

Preterm patient: patient observation for evidence of chorioamnionitis without active attempts at tocolysis
Term patient: patient observation without active attempts at induction

**What is active management of PROM?**

Preterm patient: active attempts at halting the progression or preventing the onset of labor (to increase fetal maturation in utero) with or without the use of steroids or antibiotics
Term patient: active attempts at delivery of the infant (induction or augmentation of labor)

**What are the primary risks of expectant management versus active management in *preterm* PROM?**

Principal risks of preterm PROM are related to prematurity, not infection; delivery of the preterm fetus is undesirable.
Expectant management risk: chorioamnionitis
Active management risks: risks involved with tocolysis, risks of antibiotics, and risks of corticosteroids (i.e., long-term emergence of resistant organisms)

The debate of expectant management versus active interventions is ongoing, but the benefits of close observation for evidence of fetal or maternal infection and induction of labor if chorioamnionitis is diagnosed are established.

**What are the primary risks of expectant management versus active management in PROM at *term*?**

Principal risk is chorioamnionitis (with potential neonatal sepsis and maternal endomyometritis), not prematurity; delivery is desirable.

Expectant management risks: risks of awaiting the natural onset of labor (chorioamnionitis, a significant risk after 24 hours)

Active management risks: risks of labor induction (uterine hyperstimulation, fetal distress, and uterine rupture, all relatively small risks)

Because the risks of induction are relatively low and the morbidity of chorioamnionitis relatively high, most practitioners induce labor or augment labor 8–24 hours after membranes have ruptured.

**What maternal and fetal signs and symptoms suggest chorioamnionitis in PROM?**

Uterine tenderness on abdominal examination

Maternal white blood cell count ≥ 16,000

Maternal temperature ≥ 38°C

Maternal and fetal tachycardia

Flu-like symptoms, back pains, or a subtle change in vaginal discharge

Foul-smelling or purulent vaginal fluid on speculum examination

**Why is tocolysis in preterm PROM controversial?**

Tocolytics may mask an important sign of infection (uterine irritability with resultant contractions), versus tocolytics do not delay diagnosis because other reliable signs (fever ≥ 38°C, uterine tenderness, leukocytosis, purulent amnionic fluid, fetal or maternal tachycardia) can be used to diagnose chorioamnionitis.

Also, most studies have failed to show a benefit of tocolysis in preterm PROM.

**What role do antibiotics play in the treatment of PROM?**

A prophylactic penicillin may prevent chorioamnionitis and decrease the risk of neonatal infection in prolonged rupture of the membranes.

**Of preterm PROM?**

Antimicrobial therapy in the absence of chorioamnionitis is controversial unless a specific organism (i.e., gonorrhea, chlamydia, or GBS) is identified, although there is some evidence that the latent period may be prolonged.

**What about GBS?**

Antibiotics with GBS activity (IV penicillin, ampicillin, or erythromycin) should be given in both preterm and prolonged PROM until cultures prove negative.
If GBS is confirmed by culture, a full course of antibiotics should be given.

**What is the treatment of chorioamnionitis?**

In both term and preterm PROM: antibiotic therapy and prompt delivery of the fetus (labor induction) to prevent neonatal sepsis
Cesarean section: reserved for usual obstetric indications; consequences of postoperative uterine infection are severe during chorioamnionitis.

**What are the NIH recommendations for the use of corticosteroids in the treatment of PROM?**

Controversial because of the theoretical risk of immunocompromise and infection
Antenatal corticosteroid use for women with preterm PROM at less than 30–32 weeks of gestation in the absence of clinical chorioamnionitis

**Benefits of steroids in the treatment of PROM?**

Neonatal benefits; reduced incidences of IVH, RDS, and NEL (necrotizing enterocolitis)

**What are the risks of PROM associated with gestational age less than 25 weeks?**

Low odds of neonatal survival (< 25%) and a high risk of severe short- and long-term neonatal morbidity if fetus lives

**How is PROM managed in the nonviable gestation?**

Because of risks, termination of the pregnancy with intravaginal prostaglandin suppositories to induce labor should be considered.

**What are the complications of preterm PROM?**

*Fetus/Neonate:*
Neonatal sepsis
RDS
– IVH
Patent ductus arteriosus
Necrotizing enterocolitis
Pulmonary hypoplasia in fetuses < 24 weeks
Cord prolapse/intrauterine demise
*Mother:*
    Chorioamnionitis/endomyometritis
    Puerperal sepsis

# 11

# Intrauterine Growth Restriction (IUGR)

**What is intrauterine growth restriction (IUGR)?**

Intrauterine fetal growth less than expected

**What is a small for gestational age (SGA) infant?**

An infant below the 10th percentile in weight for its gestational age

**How many SGA infants are affected by IUGR?**

Thirty percent
The other 70% are merely constitutionally small and are not at risk for the increased morbidity and mortality of IUGR infants.

**What is the incidence of IUGR?**

Occurs in 3% to 7% of all pregnancies

**What are the potential risks to a fetus with IUGR?**

Sepsis
Hypoglycemia
Temperature instability
Asphyxia
Meconium aspiration
Metabolic derangements
Hematologic disorders
Malformations

**What are the classifications of IUGR?**

Symmetric and asymmetric

**What is symmetric IUGR?**

Overall decrease in infant size
Affects both head and body
Usually secondary to an early gestational insult

**What percentage of IUGR cases are symmetric?**

Twenty percent

**What is asymmetric IUGR?**

Decrease in subcutaneous fat and abdominal circumference (AC)

Relative sparing of head circumference (HC) and femur length (FL)

Usually secondary to an insult later in gestation

Verified as increased HC/AC ratio or FL/AC ratio

**What percentage of IUGR cases are asymmetric?**

Eighty percent

**What are the etiologic factors for symmetric IUGR?**

Congenital infection

Chromosomal anomalies

Congenital anomalies

Maternal drug use (including alcohol abuse)

**What are the etiologic factors for asymmetric IUGR?**

Maternal disease (hypertension, renal, cardiopulmonary)

Placental defects

Multiple gestation

**How does congenital infection affect fetal growth?**

By interfering with cellular development; generally, the earlier the infant is infected, the more severe the outcome.

**What percentage of IUGR cases are caused by congenital infection?**

Ten percent

**What organisms are most commonly involved in IUGR?**

TORCH infections: **T**oxoplasmosis, **O**ther = **S**yphilis, **R**ubella, **C**ytomegalovirus, **H**erpes

**How do chromosomal anomalies and congenital anomalies affect fetal growth?**

Overall decrease in cell number→symmetric IUGR

**What chromosomal anomalies are associated with IUGR?**

Trisomies 13, 18, and 21

**What congenital anomalies are associated with IUGR?**

Cardiac and renal anomalies with or without an associated chromosomal anomaly

**What percentage of IUGR cases are caused by chromosomal and congenital anomalies?**

Ten percent

**How does maternal drug use affect fetal growth?**

Smoking: leads to symmetric IUGR by affecting uteroplacental blood flow
Alcohol abuse: may cause dysmorphic features and IUGR (fetal alcohol syndrome)
Cocaine use: causes vasospasm and decreased uteroplacental blood flow

**How does maternal disease affect fetal growth?**

Maternal vascular disease (e.g., hypertension, diabetes, renal disease): decreased uteroplacental blood flow→decreased fetal oxygenation→ IUGR; IUGR is usually asymmetric because there is fetal circulatory shunting in favor of the brain.
Diseases that affect maternal oxygenation (e.g., hemoglobinopathies) also affect fetal growth.

**What placental defects lead to fetal IUGR?**

Decreased placental mass (decreases fetal oxygenation and transfer of nutrients)
Placental anomalies including placental abruption, circumvallate placenta, placental infarction, placenta accreta
Possibly abnormal placental implantation (may be a risk factor; placenta previa may limit oxygenation and nutrient transfer)

**How do multiple gestations lead to fetal IUGR?**

Decreased placental surface per fetus
Eighteen percent of twin gestations are associated with IUGR

**What tests are used to diagnose IUGR?**

Physical examination with measurement of maternal fundal height
Ultrasound evaluation of fetal size and interval growth

**How is fundal height measured?**

From the maternal pubis symphysis to the top of the uterine fundus

**How is fundal height measurement used in the diagnosis of IUGR?**

As a screening test

**What is fundal height lag?**

A fundal height that does not correlate with fetal gestational age

**When should fundal height lag raise suspicion of IUGR?**

A lag greater than 4 weeks

**What fetal indices are evaluated with ultrasound?**

Head circumference relative to abdominal circumference and femur length

Amniotic fluid volume (AFV)

Placental grade

Estimated fetal weight

Fetal gestational age: a MUST prior to assessing for IUGR; do not confuse a misdated fetus with a fetus with symmetric IUGR

Congenital anomalies: may indicate a chromosomal anomaly

**How are head and abdominal circumference used to assess for IUGR?**

Established head circumference to abdominal circumference ratios:

In normal fetuses: HC/AC > 1.0 before 32 weeks; HC/AC = 1.0 at 32 to 34 weeks; HC/AC < 1.0 after 34 weeks.

In fetuses with asymmetric IUGR: The head remains larger relative to the body; therefore, HC/AC is elevated.

In fetuses with symmetric IUGR: Both HC and AC are reduced; the ratio remains normal.

**When is femur length used to assess for IUGR?**

When fetal position prevents accurate measurement

Femur length is spared in asymmetrical IUGR, increasing the FL/AC ratio.

**How is AFV used to assess for IUGR?**

Decreased AFV may be an early sign of IUGR.

The absence of a "pocket" of amniotic fluid measuring ≥ 1 cm confirms a 96% risk of IUGR.

By convention, a 2-cm pocket is used to assess for IUGR.

**Why does decreased AFV occur in IUGR?**

Decreased renal blood flow secondary to shunting to other organs leads to decreased fetal urine output and, thus, decreased AFV.

**How is placental grading used to assess for IUGR?**

A placenta of a higher grade than expected for a gestational age may indicate decreased placental function and subsequent IUGR.

**What indices are evaluated in placental grading?**

Placental calcium deposits and indentations in the chorionic plate.

**What are the placental grades?**

Grade 0: no calcifications and no indentations in the chorionic plate
Grade 1: few calcifications throughout the placenta
Grade 2: calcifications along the uterine wall and indentations in the chorionic plate
Grade 3: significant calcium deposits and indentations in the chorionic plate that appear to outline individual cotyledons

**How is estimated fetal weight (EFW) determined with ultrasound?**

Established charts and formulas determine EFW using head circumference, abdominal circumference, and femur length.

**What are the most useful ultrasound criteria for determining IUGR?**

Decreased AFV, elevated HC/AC, and an EFW below the 10th percentile

**How are Doppler flow studies used to assess for IUGR?**

Doppler ultrasound can be used to evaluate uterine or umbilical artery flow.

**What are normal results of Doppler flow studies?**

Forward flow through the umbilical arteries throughout the cardiac cycle

**What are results of Doppler flow studies that may indicate IUGR?**

Decreased end diastolic flow with a corresponding increased systolic/diastolic ratio (S/D ratio > 2.6). Most reliable— no diastolic flow

**What is the general goal of monitoring fetuses with suspected IUGR?**

To balance the risks of delivering a premature infant against the risk of stillbirth

**What are the general considerations in management of the constitutionally small and asymmetric and symmetric IUGR fetuses?**

Constitutionally small fetuses: Majority of SGA infants are constitutionally small and do not require any intervention.

Symmetric IUGR: Due to possibility of early insult, therapy may not be available.

Asymmetric IUGR: It may be possible to alter the uterine environment or deliver the fetus early to minimize negative effects.

**What is the management plan for fetuses with IUGR?**

Serial examinations of the fetus

Maternal education about daily fetal activity

Ultrasound examinations every 3 to 4 weeks to evaluate the HC/AC ratio, EFW, possible congenital anomalies, AFV

Regular fetal monitoring:

Frequent nonstress tests (NST)

Contraction stress test (CST), biophysical profile (BPP), or Doppler flow studies if a fetus has a nonreactive NST (especially if the fetus had a previously reactive NST); CST is positive (fetal heart rate [FHR] decelerations in > 50% of contractions) in 40% of IUGR fetuses

Possible amniocentesis to time the delivery of the fetus

**What findings from amniocentesis indicate delivery?**

Evidence of fetal lung maturity (either an L/S ratio > 2 or the presence of phosphatidylglycerol)

**When should a preterm fetus with IUGR be delivered?**

Progressive growth lag, development of oligohydramnios or nonreassuring fetal monitoring exists; amniocentesis for evidence of fetal lung maturity can be helpful. Depends on degree of prematurity.

**What is the recommended management of progressive growth lag, development of oligohydramnios, or nonreassuring fetal monitoring when amniocentesis indicates fetal lung immaturity?**

Steroids to accelerate fetal lung maturity
Close fetal monitoring
Consideration of delivery if fetal condition worsens

**What is the intrapartum management of a fetus with IUGR?**

Continuous fetal heart rate monitoring
No late FHR decelerations during labor: normal delivery
Persistent FHR decelerations: possible cesarean section

**What are the etiologic factors of hypoglycemia in IUGR infants?**

Two factors:
1. Decreased glycogen stores secondary to malnutrition
2. Decreased sensitivity of gluconeogenesis pathway to hypoglycemia

**What are the etiologic factors of hypothermia in IUGR infants?**

Decreased body fat stores

**What are the etiologic factors of meconium aspiration in IUGR infants?**

Passage of meconium is common and its concern is high when amniotic volume is low.

**What metabolic derangements are common in IUGR infants?**

Hypocalcemia
Hypokalemia
Hyponatremia
Hyperphosphatemia

**What hematologic disorders are common in IUGR infants?**

Polycythemia secondary to fetal hypoxia and an increased production of red blood cells (RBCs) to compensate for the decreased oxygenation
Hyperbilirubinemia secondary to increased RBC breakdown

**What is the long-term follow-up for infants born with IUGR?**

By 2 years of age, most infants with IUGR have caught up to normal infants.

Neurologic complications: The extent of persistent neurologic damage in IUGR infants remains unclear.

Overall, the degree of long-term sequelae is related to the degree of growth retardation, prematurity, and gestational age at which the insult occurs (the earlier the insult, the greater the level of neurologic damage). Thirty-five percent of IUGR children have school performance problems.

# 12

# Hematologic Diseases in Pregnancy

**What normal hematologic changes occur in pregnancy?**

Fifty percent increase in maternal plasma volume (1,000 ml) plus 25% increase in red blood cell (RBC) mass→decrease in hematocrit.

Decrease in hematocrit is greatest in the second trimester.

Late pregnancy: Plasma expansion ceases while RBC mass continues to increase.

**How is the decreased hematocrit compensated for?**

Iron absorption from the duodenum increases.

**What defines anemia in pregnancy?**

A hematocrit less than 30 or a hemoglobin less than 10

**What are the etiologic factors of anemia in pregnancy?**

Most common: secondary to iron deficiency anemia

Other causes: nutritional deficiencies, acute blood loss, anemia from chronic disease, drug-induced hemolytic anemia, hemoglobinopathies, malignancy

## IRON DEFICIENCY ANEMIA

**What is the daily iron requirement in pregnancy?**

One gram of elemental iron needs to be absorbed into the bloodstream to maintain a steady state.

**What are the symptoms of iron deficiency anemia?**

Fatigue and lethargy; these symptoms are also common in pregnancy.

**What are the associated lab findings?**

Complete blood count (CBC): Hematocrit is decreased.

Peripheral blood smear: May show hypochromic microcytic cells; however, if the patient is also folate-deficient, normochromic normocytic cells may be seen

Other: decreased serum iron concentration, decreased saturation of transferrin, increased total iron binding capacity (also seen in 15% of pregnant women who are not iron deficient due to increase in proteins during pregnancy)

**What is the effect of iron deficiency anemia on a developing fetus?**

Causes no adverse effect on the fetus; the fetus maintains its iron stores by active transport mechanisms despite maternal deficiencies.

**What is the effect of pregnancy on anemia?**

A decrease in the hematocrit that is most marked in the second trimester

**What is the treatment?**

Supplemental iron (PO or IV or dietary)

**What is the dosage?**

180 mg of simple iron compounds, such as ferrous sulfate or ferrous gluconate, each day; doses in excess of this standard dose do not result in more rapid RBC production because excess iron is excreted in the stool.

**What are the instructions for maximum absorption?**

Ingest 30 minutes before a meal.

**What can increase or decrease absorption?**

Vitamin C ingestion increases iron absorption; simultaneous antacid ingestion decreases absorption.

**What are indicators of patient response to iron supplementation?**

A reticulocytosis indicating a hematologic response should be seen within 2 weeks of beginning iron therapy.

The hematocrit should increase by 1% to 2% each week.

## FOLATE DEFICIENCY

**What is folic acid?**

Folic acid (folate) is a water-soluble vitamin usually found in green vegetables, peanuts, and liver. It is a member of the B-complex group of vitamins. In humans, the only source of folate is from the diet.

**What are folic acid requirements in pregnancy?**

0.8 to 1 mg/day
Increased requirements with multiple gestations and patients with hemoglobinopathies

**What effects does folate supplementation around the time of conception and in early pregnancy have on fetal development?**

Supplemental folate (1 mg per day) around time of conception and in early pregnancy (organogenesis) may decrease the incidence of neural tube defects.

**What is the incidence of folate deficiency in pregnancy?**

Low serum folate levels occur in ~10% to 25% of pregnant women; second most common nutritional anemia in pregnancy

**What is the relationship between folate deficiency in pregnancy and megaloblastic anemia?**

Folate deficiency is the most common cause of megaloblastic anemia in pregnancy.
However, even without folate supplementation, less than 5% of patients with a folate deficiency will develop a megaloblastic anemia.

**What are the symptoms of folate deficiency?**

Fatigue and lethargy, which are related to the degree of anemia
Nausea, vomiting, anorexia, roughness of the skin, glossitis

**What are the lab findings?**

CBC: reveals normochromic macrocytic anemia or a normochromic normocytic anemia with hypersegmentation of neutrophils
Reticulocyte count: normal or low; elliptocytes may be seen.
WBC count: sometimes decreased
Platelet count: sometimes decreased
Concurrent iron deficiency may produce a mixed population of RBCs, detectable on smear, but not MCV.
Serum folate level: low (< 4)

**How is folate deficiency distinguished from vitamin $B_{12}$ deficiency?**

Unlike folate deficiency, vitamin $B_{12}$ deficiency may produce a peripheral neuropathy.

**What is the effect of folate deficiency on a developing fetus?**

Folate deficiency does not cause adverse effects on a developing fetus because the fetus preferentially obtains folate from the mother and maintains normal levels.

Although the incidence of congenital anomalies is not increased in folate-deficient mothers, folate supplementation around the time of conception may decrease the overall incidence of neural tube defects.

**What is the effect of pregnancy on folate requirements?**

Pregnancy increases the folate requirement by three- to fourfold.

Patients with multiple gestations, malabsorption syndromes, hemoglobinopathies, or those taking phenytoin are more likely to develop a folic acid deficiency.

**What is the treatment of folate deficiency?**

Folate supplementation with 1 to 3 mg folate daily

**What are the indicators of patient response to folate supplementation?**

Rapid increase in the reticulocyte count
After 1 week of treatment, the hematocrit may increase as much as 1% each day.

## SICKLE CELL DISEASE

**What is sickle cell disease?**

Most common hemoglobinopathy
Hemoglobin (Hb) S ("sickle") results from a single amino acid substitution of valine for glutamic acid in the beta chain of hemoglobin.
RBCs with Hb S:
Have reduced oxygen-carrying capacity and survival time (half-life of 5 to 10 days)
Have an increased chance of sickling

**How is sickle cell disease inherited?**

Autosomal recessive disease

**What is sickle cell trait?**

Sickle cell trait (Hb AS) is the heterozygous form of disease.

**What other hemoglobinopathies result in sickling?**

Hb C, Hb D, and Hb sickle cell-beta thalassemia

**What is sickle cell-Hb C disease?**

It is a double heterozygous condition in which patient carries one gene for Hb S and one gene for Hb C.

It causes milder hemolytic anemia and fewer painful crises than sickle cell-Hb S disease.

Pregnant women have an increased frequency of skeletal pain with respiratory and/or neurologic compromise in the third trimester, at term, and immediately postpartum.

Pregnant women have an increased tendency for complicated pregnancy; management during pregnancy is the same as that of sickle cell anemia.

**What is sickle cell-Hb D disease?**

Patients may be asymptomatic or may have a mild hemolytic anemia.
Pregnancy is usually uneventful.

**What is the incidence of sickle cell trait?**

Occurs in 1/12 of adult African Americans

**What percentage of Hb is Hb S in people with sickle cell trait?**

Twenty-five to thirty-five percent

**What is the incidence of sickle cell disease?**

Occurs in 1/625 of African-American children

**What percentage of Hb is Hb S in people with sickle cell disease?**

Ninety percent

**Diagnostic tests?**

Screening tests for the sickle cell gene (e.g., sickledex test)
Hb electrophoresis: diagnostic
Polymerase chain reaction and Southern blotting may be used for prenatal diagnosis.

**What laboratory findings are consistent with sickle cell disease?**

Hematocrit: Low
Bilirubin: Hyperbilirubinemia
(bilirubin = 1–7 in sickle cell disease;
15–20 in a crisis)

**What are the signs and symptoms?**

Patients with sickle cell trait are
asymptomatic.
Patients with sickle cell disease:
Have "crises," frequent painful vaso-
occlusive episodes in the
extremities, joints, and abdomen.
Have symptoms of anemia and
frequent infections.

**What is the pathophysiology of sickle cell crisis?**

Sickling of RBCs is triggered by hypoxia,
acidosis, and dehydration.
Sludging in small vessels results in
microinfarction of the affected organs.
Crises can lead to a rapid drop in
hematocrit, deoxygenation, and pain;
splenic sequestration may occur.

**What is the effect of sickle cell disease on a developing fetus?**

It has been hypothesized that sickling in
the uterine vessels may lead to
decreased fetal oxygenation.
Sickle cell trait has no adverse effect on
a developing fetus.
Sickle cell disease may complicate
pregnancy; associated with an
increased incidence of spontaneous
abortion, preterm birth, intrauterine
growth retardation, perinatal mortality,
stillbirth, pyelonephritis, and
preeclampsia.

**What is the effect of pregnancy on a person with sickle cell disease?**

Increased incidence of severe anemia,
vasooclusive episodes, and painful
crises

**What are the complications of the disease?**

Increased incidence of urinary tract
infections
Osteomyelitis, jaundice, cholelithiasis,
high-output cardiac failure secondary
to chronic anemia, infections, and
pulmonary and splenic infarctions

**What is the management?**    Pneumococcal vaccine to prevent
                               infection early in or prior to
                               pregnancy
                               Supplemental iron when iron deficiency
                               exists
                               Folic acid supplementation (1 mg/day)
                               Avoidance of crises with prevention of
                               infections and dehydration
                               Antenatal fetal surveillance with NSTs
                               Serial ultrasonography to assess fetal
                               growth
                               Monitoring for preeclampsia (e.g., blood
                               pressure checks)
                               Regular monitoring of reticulocyte
                               count, bilirubin, and hematocrit

**How is a crisis managed**    Search for an infection (up to one-third
**during pregnancy?**          of crises are associated with infection).
                               If no infection is found, search for other
                               possible causes of pain and/or anemia
                               such as ectopic pregnancy, placental
                               abruption, pyelonephritis, appendicitis,
                               and cholecystitis.
                               Manage pain with acetaminophen and
                               meperidine hydrochloride
                               (Demerol®); avoid morphine sulfate
                               because of its potential smooth muscle
                               constrictive properties.
                               Replace fluid and electrolytes because of
                               increased insensible fluid loss that
                               occurs during a crisis.
                               Prophylactic exchange transfusions and
                               simple transfusions significantly
                               decrease the incidence and severity of
                               painful crises. However, improvement
                               in perinatal outcome is controversial.
                               In labor, provide supplemental oxygen
                               and continuous fetal monitoring.

**How can sickle cell disease**    Through carrier screening in
**be prevented?**                  populations at risk and prenatal
                                   screening when both parents have
                                   the sickle cell trait
                                   When both parents have the trait, the
                                   risk of a child with disease is 25%.
                                   Prenatal diagnosis of this condition is
                                   possible.

## VON WILLEBRAND DISEASE

**What is von Willebrand disease?**

A lack of or abnormality in von Willebrand factor

**What is the function of von Willebrand factor?**

Von Willebrand factor is a glycoprotein complex that associates with and stabilizes factor VIII, enhances platelet aggregation, and contributes to the ability of platelets to attach to injured endothelium.

**What are the components of factor VIII?**

Factor VIII is a multimer composed of factor VIII-related cofactor, factor VIII-related antigen, and factor VIII-coagulant protein (VIIIc).

**What is the incidence of von Willebrand disease?**

Affects 1/10,000 individuals

**How is the disease inherited?**

As an autosomal dominant trait

**What are the symptoms?**

Easy bruising, easy bleeding, gingival bleeding, and epistaxis; abnormal menstrual bleeding

**How is the disease diagnosed?**

Bleeding time: prolonged
PTT: occasionally increased
Factor VIII levels: decreased
Platelet count: normal
Factor VIII cofactor: qualitatively or quantitatively deficient

**What is the function of factor VIII-related cofactor?**

Necessary for platelet adherence to the endothelium

**How does von Willebrand disease affect pregnancy?**

Patients have an increased incidence of postpartum hemorrhage related to concentration of factor VIIIc (problems arise if factor VIIIc value is < 50% of normal).

**What is the effect of pregnancy on women with von Willebrand disease?**

Clotting factors normally increase in pregnancy and thus bleeding time usually improves. Labor and delivery often proceed uneventfully because factor VIII levels usually increase to hemostatic levels beginning at 11 to 12 weeks.

**What is the management?**

Avoidance of episiotomies, deep injection of local anesthetic, and conduction anesthesia

Infusions of factor VIII–containing preparations if a patient has inadequate hemostasis

Transfusion with cryoprecipitate (rich in factor VIII) or fibrinogen if the concentration of factor VIIIc is below 50% at term

1-desamino-8-D-arginine vasopressin (ddavp) for patients with von Willebrand disease who have decreased levels of normal circulating factor (quantitative deficiency)

**What are the considerations for caesarean section?**

Factor VIIIc levels should be 80% of normal and the bleeding time should be in the normal range.

**Why does the risk of delayed postpartum hemorrhage exist?**

Postpartum, factor VIII levels fall to pre-pregnancy levels after 48 to 72 hours.

**What are the considerations for the newborn?**

Assume the newborn has von Willebrand disease; circumcisions should be performed only after exclusion of disease.

**What are the risks associated with cryoprecipitate infusion?**

Cryoprecipitate is pooled from several donors and therefore places the patient at a higher risk for transfusion-related infection.

## IMMUNE THROMBOCYTOPENIC PURPURA (ITP)

**What is ITP?**

An autoimmune disease in which the platelet count is < 150,000

**What is the pathophysiology?**

Production of antiplatelet antibodies→peripheral destruction and sequestration of platelets

**What are the symptoms?**

Epistaxis, gingival bleeding, ecchymoses
Tendency to bleed easily
    Severity of bleeding ranges from
      minimal to life-threatening.
    Abnormal skin and mucous membrane
      bleeding when the platelet count
      < 100,000 cells/mm$^3$
    Spontaneous bleeding when platelet
      count is < 20,000 cells/mm$^3$

**How is the disease diagnosed?**

Demonstration of an IgG platelet-
    associated antibody
CBC: reveals an isolated platelet
    deficiency (usually between 75,000
    and 150,000/mm$^3$)
Increased bleeding time if the platelet
    count is < 50,000
Coagulation tests: normal

**What other causes of thrombocytopenia must be ruled out?**

Hemolysis, elevated liver enzymes, and
low platelet count (HELLP) syndrome;
infection; DIC

**What is the effect of ITP on pregnancy?**

Increased incidence of spontaneous
    abortions
Increased incidence of hemorrhage at
    the time of delivery (most bleeding
    comes from genital tract injury;
    uterine bleeding is usually not
    increased).
Depression of fetal platelet count due to
    transplacental passage of circulating
    antiplatelet IgG

**What are the effects of ITP on the infant?**

Possible intracranial hemorrhage in
    severely thrombocytopenic infants
Thrombocytopenia in 70% of infants
    born to mothers with ITP; peaks 4 to
    6 weeks after delivery, is usually mild,
    and gradually corrects within 2 to 3
    months

**How does the maternal platelet count relate to fetal platelet count?**

There is no reliable relationship between
maternal platelet and fetal platelet
count.

| | |
|---|---|
| **What is the effect of pregnancy on persons with ITP?** | No known effect |
| **What is the management?** | Avoidance of trauma and salicylates (they impair platelet function)<br><br>Fetal blood sampling when mother has a known history of ITP; cesarean section if the fetal platelet count is < 50,000 cells/mm$^3$ (controversial)<br><br>Hospitalization and intravenous glucocorticoid therapy if the patient has a bleeding diathesis or if platelet count < 20,000 cells/mm$^3$<br><br>Platelet transfusions are of little help in pregnancy because the transfused platelets are destroyed 1 to 4 hours after infusion. |
| **What is the intrapartum management?** | Avoidance of fetal hypoxia, which can decrease the fetal platelet count<br><br>Avoidance of prolonged labor<br><br>Continuous fetal monitoring<br><br>Epidural anesthesia may be used if the platelet count is at least 100,000 cells/mm$^3$. |
| **What is the postpartum management?** | Breastfeeding is not recommended because of possible transmission of antiplatelet antibodies through breast milk. |
| **What is the rationale for using steroids for management of ITP in pregnancy?** | Steroids increase the platelet count by increasing platelet production; decrease antiplatelet antibody production, binding, and antibody-coated platelet destruction. |
| **What is the treatment?** | Corticosteroids (Prednisone®):<br>    Cornerstone of treatment<br>    80–100 mg/day initiated when the platelet count falls below 100,000 cells/mm$^3$<br>    Dose is then tapered to the minimum value that permits a stable platelet count.<br>    A favorable response is seen with a rise in the platelet count in 7 to 21 days. |

High-dose IV immunoglobulin if a
patient is refractory to steroids or in
need of acute treatment prior to
surgery
Splenectomy:
Produces remission in 70% to 80% of
patients
If performed prior to pregnancy, the
frequency and severity of
complications during pregnancy
decrease.
If performed during pregnancy for
failure to respond to steroids or
life-threatening hemorrhage, fetal
mortality rate may be as high as
30%.
Plasma exchange therapy for refractory
or complicated cases.

**What beneficial effects
does treatment have on
circulating antiplatelet
antibodies that cross the
placenta to the fetus?**

None; the drugs currently in use are
poorly transmitted across the placenta

# 13

# Post-term Pregnancy

**What is post-term pregnancy?**

Gestation of 42 weeks (294 days) or more

**What is the incidence?**

Occurs in 3% to 12% of all pregnancies

**Why is correct dating of pregnancy important in evaluating for post-term pregnancy?**

Incorrect determination of gestational age may lead to the misdiagnosis of a normal pregnancy as post-term.

**What are common errors that are made in dating a pregnancy?**

Inaccurate history of the last menstrual period (LMP)
Inaccurate estimation of ovulation (prolonged follicular phase)

**What are the etiologic factors?**

The cause of a post-term pregnancy can usually not be found.
Rare conditions that may predispose patients to prolonged gestation include:
  Anencephaly
  Fetal adrenal hypoplasia
  Absence of the fetal pituitary
  Placental sulfatase deficiency
  Extrauterine pregnancy
  Obesity: Women who are obese at conception may have as much as a 50% increase in the frequency of post-term pregnancy over that of the general population.
  Excessive weight gain during pregnancy: Weight gain has also been found to be an independent factor for post-term pregnancy that compounds the effect of pre-pregnancy obesity.

**What are the maternal complications?**

Consist mainly of maternal discomfort, anxiety, increased expense, and risk of antenatal testing
Increased induction and cesarean section rate, with the attendant risks

**For what complication are most cesarean deliveries performed in post-term pregnancies?**

Fetal distress

**What is the increase in the rate of cesarean deliveries?**

May be fourfold over nonpost-term pregnancies

**What is the increase in the rate of fetal complications?**

Two- to threefold increase in neonatal/perinatal morbidity rate

**Name the four main factors that contribute to neonatal/perinatal morbidity.**

Oligohydramnios, macrosmia, passage of meconium, dysmaturity

**What is oligohydramnios?**

Loss of amniotic fluid volume (AFV)
May lead to cord compression, which can cause both acute and chronic fetal hypoxia and sudden death
Peak AFV (mean = 1000 [ml]) occurs at 37 weeks; AFV declines after 37 weeks.
The mean volume at term is 800 ml; at 42 weeks, 250 ml.

**What is macrosomia?**

Fetal weight in excess of 4,000 g (8 lbs, 13 oz)
Fetuses grow at a rate of 224 g (or about 0.5 lb) per week for the last 4 weeks at term.
Occurs due to prolonged gestation with continued nutrition and resultant increased fetal growth.
Associated with an increased risk of shoulder dystocia or other birth trauma and a high cesarean section rate

**What is passage of meconium?**

It is thought to occur with maturation of innervation of the gastrointestinal tract or the presence of a fetal stressor.
Increased incidence with increasing gestational age:
    Rare prior to 32 weeks
    Occurs in 10% to 15% of normal term pregnancies
    Occurs in 25% to 30% of pregnancies at 42 weeks

The presence of meconium with oligohydramnios may result in meconium of increased viscosity, which increases the risk of aspiration pneumonia should aspiration occur.

**What is dysmaturity?**

Abnormal maturation in neonates associated with a characteristic appearance and increased morbidity and mortality rates

Classically described as a loss of vernix, peeling skin, loss of subcutaneous fat, long fingernails, thin abdominal girth, and an "old man" appearance, often with meconium staining of skin, nails, and placenta

Thought to result from placental insufficiency because area available for exchange of nutrients begins to decrease from a maximum of 11 $m^2$ at 37 weeks

**What is the difference between macrosomia and dysmaturity?**

Placental compromise does not occur in macrosomia; therefore, the fetus continues to grow.

**What is the antepartum management?**

Induction of labor between 42 and 44 weeks, regardless of cervical condition; most experts agree that at 42 weeks, if the patient is found to have a favorable cervix, induction should be recommended.

Trial of cervical ripening agents and/or antepartum testing if the cervix is unfavorable at 42 weeks

If at any time antepartum test results are abnormal, labor should be induced.

If the cervix ripens during this period, labor should be induced.

Some authorities begin screening earlier than 42 weeks.

**What does antepartum testing involve?**

Twice-weekly fetal surveillance by either nonstress test (NST) or contraction stress test (CST) combined with determination of AFV using the

Amniotic fluid index (AFI)

May also include several other tests (e.g., fetal kick counts, biophysical profile, placental grade, Doppler flow studies)

Fetal kick count is a simple screening tool that can be instituted early and done at home on a daily basis. The mother is instructed to lie on her left side for 1 hour three times a day after meals. If she notices decreased fetal movement (usually described as fewer than 4–5 kicks per hour), further evaluation is necessary.

AFI uses ultrasound to measure the vertical height of the largest amniotic fluid pocket in each of four quadrants. A value of 5 to 20 cm is considered adequate.

Biophysical profile measures five indices, including AFV, fetal tone, fetal body and respiratory movement, and NST.

Placental grade (0, 1, 2, or 3) is an assessment of placental maturity based on ultrasonographic changes in the chorionic plate, placental substance, and basal layer.

Grading cannot predict the likelihood of postmaturity syndrome, but correlates generally with gestational age, and may be of some value in the management of delivery when combined with placental thickness and other clinical variables.

Doppler flow studies of the umbilical artery have not been shown to add any useful information in evaluating post-term pregnancy in the absence of other complicating factors, such as hypertension.

**What are the risks associated with cervical ripening agents?**

Prostaglandin $E_2$ and dilapan laminaria risks include rupture of membranes, infection, bleeding, and allergic reaction including anaphylaxis.

**What is the intrapartum management?**

Close monitoring of fetal heart rate (FHR) and uterine contractions to monitor for variable decelerations that indicate umbilical cord compression

Amnioinfusion (i.e., infusion of saline into the amniotic sac of a patient with oligohydramnios)

Placement of a fetal scalp electrode and intrauterine pressure catheter after rupture of membranes to allow more accurate measurement of uterine contractions and FHR

Evaluation of amniotic fluid for meconium following membrane rupture; if present, evaluation of meconium viscosity

Presence of meconium: suctioning of the infant's oropharynx when the head is delivered and before the thorax is delivered to reduce the risk of aspiration pneumonia should aspiration occur

Consideration of macrosomia (especially with a prolonged second stage of labor) and shoulder dystocia in vaginal delivery

Avoidance of oxytocin overstimulation, because umbilical cord compression may occur secondary to decreased AFV

**What is the rationale for amnioinfusion for intrapartum management of a post-term pregnancy?**

May reduce cesarean section rate for fetal distress

May improve infant outcome by increasing AFV and thereby decreasing the risk of umbilical cord compression and meconium aspiration syndrome

# 14

# Multiple Gestation

**What is the incidence of multiple gestation?**

Occurs in 1.5% of all pregnancies

**List, define, and state the incidence of the two types of twin pregnancies.**

Dizygotic (also called fraternal) pregnancy results from the fertilization of two ova; comprises two-thirds of twin pregnancies.
Monozygotic (also called identical) pregnancy results from the fertilization of one ovum and then cleavage; comprises one-third of twin pregnancies.

**What factors influence the incidence of dizygotic twinning?**

Race (African Americans > whites)
Parity (increased incidence with increased parity)
Age (increases with maternal age up to 40 years)
Maternal size (increased incidence in larger women)
Family history
Fertility drugs including clomiphene citrate (Clomid®, 5%–10%) and menotropins (Pergonal®, 20%–40%)

**What factors influence the incidence of monozygotic twinning?**

No factors have been found; incidence is constant at 1/250. However, fertility drugs may increase the incidence.

**What types of placentas exist in twin pregnancies and how is the type determined?**

In dizygotic twins: The placental type is always dichorionic–diamniotic.
In monozygotic twins: Type of placenta depends on the timing of embryo cleavage.

**Table 14–1**

| Fertilization | 4 days | 8 days | 13 days |
|---|---|---|---|
| Dichorionic Diamniotic (30%) | Monochorionic Diamniotic (70%) | Monochorionic Monoamniotic (1%) | Conjoined twins (1/600) |

**How are twins usually diagnosed?**

Ninety-five percent of twin pregnancies are diagnosed prior to the onset of labor.
History:
  Use of fertility drugs
  Family history (if mother herself is a twin, incidence is 1/60)
  Rapid weight gain
Physical exam:
  Large uterine size for gestational age
  Identification of two fetal heart tones
  Visualization via ultrasound
Laboratory data:
  Possibly elevated MSAFP

**What are the complications?**

Increased mortality rate:
  Perinatal mortality rate is 6% to 12%, five to ten times higher than singletons
  Prematurity is the largest contributor to mortality.
  Twins with a monochorionic placenta have two to three times higher mortality rate than dichorionic twins because of:
  1. Twin–twin transfusion syndrome
  2. Cord accidents (occur in up to 50% of monoamniotic twins)
  3. Conjoined twins (occur in 1/50,000 live births)
Single fetal death in utero occurs in approximately 1% to 5% of twin pregnancies.
Preterm Delivery:
  It is the number one contributor to perinatal mortality.
  Fifty percent of twins deliver before 37 weeks.
  Ten percent of all preterm deliveries are multiple gestations.
Low birth weight: Fifty percent of twin infants have weights less than 2500 grams.
Prematurity
Intrauterine growth retardation (IUGR): may occur in up to 40% of twins

Discordant growth:
Estimated fetal weight (EFW)
difference is 25%.
Discordant growth causes IUGR of
one twin or macrosomia of the
other twin.
Twin–twin transfusion syndrome
(TTTS) results from the shunting
of blood through arteriovenous
communications within the
placenta.
1. Occurs in monochorionic
diamniotic twins, 5% to 10%
overall
2. Donor twin is small, anemic, and
may have oligohydramnios.
3. Recipient twin is large,
polycythemic, and may have
polyhydramnios.
4. Mortality rate is greater than
50%.
Pregnancy-induced hypertension:
Risk is twice as high as with
singleton pregnancy, or 12% to
16%.
It may be more severe with earlier
onset.
Malformations:
Risk is increased two to three times
compared to singletons.
Both twins are affected in less than
20% of cases.
Anomalies associated with twinning
include conjoined twins, TTTS.
Placenta previa/abruptio: slightly more
common
Cord accidents: Entanglement may
occur in 50% of monoamniotic
twins.
Operative delivery:
Malpresentation occurs in almost
20% of twin pregnancies.
Cord prolapse
Postpartum hemorrhage

**What is the mortality rate
for triplets?**

Fifteen to thirty percent

**At what average gestational age are triplets delivered?**

Thirty-three to thirty-five weeks

**What is the management?**

Early detection and frequent visits:
Ultrasound reduces missed diagnoses to less than 5%; visits should include education and screening for preterm labor.

Ultrasound:
To determine gestational age, evaluate anatomy, determine chorionicity

To assess serial growth and amniotic fluid volume (AFV) every 4 weeks

To confirm fetal presentations prior to delivery

Bed rest/Hospitalization:
May help prevent preterm delivery; controversial

Hospitalization is not cost-effective.

Prophylactic cerclage: useful in cases of incompetent cervix only

Tocolysis:
Its use prophylactically is not generally supported.

Use is similar to preterm labor in singleton pregnancies.

**How is the delivery of twins different from singleton deliveries?**

Average gestational age for twins is 37 weeks.

Delivery must be performed when cesarean section can be expedited.

Continuous fetal heart surveillance is mandatory.

Mode of delivery depends on presentation of twins:
Vertex–vertex presentation (45%): Vaginal delivery

Nonvertex presentation (20%): Cesarean section

Breech–vertex presentation carries risk of heads interlocking.

Vertex–nonvertex presentation (35%): Controversial

1. Deliver vertex twin vaginally.
2. Turn nonvertex twin to vertex; then deliver vaginally.

3. Vaginal breech delivery of second twin when:
   - Standard criteria are met for vaginal delivery
   - Second twin is of similar size
4. Breech extraction
5. Cesarean section of both twins

# 15

# Hypertensive Disorders in Pregnancy

**What are the three classifications of hypertensive disorders of pregnancy, and the conditions each includes?**

**Pregnancy-induced hypertension:**
Hypertension that develops as a consequence of pregnancy and regresses postpartum.
Hypertension without proteinuria or pathologic edema
**Preeclampsia:** Hypertension with proteinuria, pathologic edema, or both
Mild
Severe
**Eclampsia:** Hypertension with proteinuria and convulsions with or without pathologic edema
**Pregnancy-aggravated hypertension:**
Underlying hypertension worsened by pregnancy
Superimposed preeclampsia
Superimposed eclampsia
**Chronic hypertension:** Hypertension that antecedes pregnancy and persists postpartum

## PREGNANCY-INDUCED HYPERTENSION

### TRANSIENT HYPERTENSION

**What is transient hypertension?**

Development of hypertension as defined by blood pressure > 140/90 mm Hg that occurs in pregnancy or in the first 24 hours postpartum without edema or proteinuria
Blood pressure returns to normal within 10 days after delivery.

**How is transient hypertension managed?**

On an outpatient basis with close follow-up

## PREECLAMPSIA

**What is preeclampsia?**

An idiopathic disease exclusive to pregnancy, characterized by hypertension, proteinuria, and edema

Blood pressure > 140/90 mm Hg; this elevation must be present on two measurements at least 6 hours apart while patient is resting.

Proteinuria is defined as ≥ 300 mg or more of urinary protein per 24 hours, or ≥ 100 mg/dl.

**What are the two classifications of preeclampsia?**

Mild preeclampsia:
   Blood pressure ranges from 140/90 to 160/110 mm Hg.
   Proteinuria < 5 g/24 hrs
   Edema of face, hands, and feet
Severe preeclampsia
   Blood pressure > 160/110 mm Hg
   Proteinuria > 5 g per 24 hours
   Oliguria < 400 ml in 24 hours
   Cerebral or visual disturbances
   Epigastric pain or, more specifically, right upper quadrant (RUQ) pain that may indicate liver involvement
   Pulmonary edema
   Hepatocellular dysfunction
   Thrombocytopenia
   Intrauterine growth retardation (IUGR)
   Elevated serum creatinine
   Microangiopathic hemolysis

**What is the epidemiology of preeclampsia?**

Unique to human primates; does not occur in subhuman primates

Occurs in 6%–8% of pregnancies

Incidence is affected by parity.
   More common in nulliparous women (incidence of 14%–20% in primigravidas compared to 6%–7% in multiparas)
   Associated in multiparous women with multiple gestations, fetal hydrops, and coexisting vascular or renal disease such as diabetes mellitus, or when the paternity of current

pregnancy is different from that of
previous pregnancies

Affects women at either end of
reproductive age range

Onset typically after 20 weeks' gestation

Appears to be inherited and occurs
more commonly in families with
history of hypertension

More common in patients with essential
hypertension

Occurs more frequently in pregnancies
involving multiple gestations, in
polyhydramnios, and with the
occurrence of a hydatidiform mole

Second to embolism as most common
cause of maternal mortality in the
United States, accounting for 15% of
maternal deaths

Major cause of perinatal morbidity and
mortality in the United States

**What are the possible
etiologies of preeclampsia?**

They are unknown.
Possibilities include:
Immunologic phenomena
Genetic predisposition
Dietary deficiencies or excesses
(specifically calcium)
Vascular reactivity changes
Renin–angiotensin–aldosterone
system
Prostaglandins
Autonomic nervous system
Calcium
Endothelial cell function
Abnormal trophoblast invasion
Cardiovascular maladaptation
Coagulation abnormalities

**What is the
pathophysiology of
preeclampsia?**

The major feature is the generalized
occurrence of arteriolar constriction
leading to significantly elevated systemic
vascular resistance. Associated changes
include:
Uterine vascular changes: Endothelial
injury, ranging from swelling to
erosion in placental and nonplacental
sites

Hemodynamic changes:
　Myocardial contractility rarely
　　impaired; ventricular function
　　normal
　Changes that do occur include
　　elevation of afterload, decreased
　　cardiac output, increased vascular
　　resistance, reduced ventricular
　　preload, and reduced total blood
　　volume.
Hematologic changes:
　The primary hematologic change is
　　hemoconcentration; the plasma
　　volume contracts during decreased
　　regional perfusion.
　Other changes include
　　thrombocytopenia; decreased
　　clotting factors; and red blood cell
　　destruction characterized by
　　hemolysis.
Endocrine and metabolic changes:
　During pregnancy, plasma levels of
　　renin, angiotensin II, and
　　aldosterone increase. In
　　preeclampsia, these levels often
　　return toward prepregnancy range.
　Increase in levels of antidiuretic
　　hormone and atrial natriuretic
　　factor
Fluid and electrolyte changes:
　Extracellular volume increases as a
　　result of increased capillary
　　permeability.
　In eclampsia, bicarbonate levels
　　decrease owing to lactic acidosis
　　and compensatory respiratory
　　alkalosis.
Renal changes:
　During pregnancy, renal blood flow
　　and glomerular filtration rate (GFR)
　　increase. In preeclampsia, these
　　factors are reduced toward
　　nonpregnant levels.
　Other changes include sodium
　　retention, increased plasma
　　creatinine, increased uric acid,
　　decreased urinary excretion of

calcium, increased permeability to large–molecular-weight proteins leading to proteinuria, and endothelial damage to renal vasculature.

Hepatic changes:
HELLP (see p. 141) occurs in 10% of women with severe preeclampsia.
Serum transaminase levels increase.
Hepatic rupture is possible but rare, requires surgical intervention, and is associated with a high (70%) mortality rate.

Uteroplacental perfusion: Vasospasm causes compromised placental perfusion and can result in poor fetal growth or even death.

Central nervous system (CNS):
Headaches and visual disturbances (blurred vision and scotomata) occur because of retinal artery spasm. Retinal detachment occurs rarely.
Reflexes can become hyperactive.
CNS signs and symptoms may indicate a high risk of seizure.

**What are the signs and symptoms of preeclampsia?**

Elevation of blood pressure
Proteinuria, which may follow hypertension
Excessive weight gain from extravascular fluid accumulation and edema
Dyspnea: May result from pulmonary edema secondary to cardiac failure (rare) or volume overload (more common)
Abdominal pain/tenderness: RUQ or epigastric pain may indicate hepatic subcapsular swelling from edema (common) or hematoma (rare); hepatic rupture is rare but can occur.

**On what is the diagnosis of preeclampsia based?**

Demonstration of hypertension, proteinuria, and edema

**What laboratory evaluations are appropriate after a diagnosis of preeclampsia?**

Hematocrit
Platelets
Blood urea nitrogen
Creatinine

Carbon dioxide
Uric acid level
Transaminase levels to test for liver
  damage
Total protein
Albumin
24-Hour urine protein
Protime and bilirubin to test for liver
  function
Nonstress test (NST)
Ultrasonography to evaluate growth and
  amniotic fluid level

**What is important to
remember about the
alkaline phosphatase level?**

It is increased in pregnancy owing to
placental production.

**What are the sequelae of
preeclampsia?**

Pulmonary edema
Hepatic hemorrhage, infarction, or
  necrosis
Intracerebral hemorrhage
Abruptio placentae
HELLP syndrome (see p. 141)
Acute renal failure
Shock
Ventricular arrhythmias
IUGR/Intrauterine fetal demise (IUFD)

**How is preeclampsia
managed?**

The only definitive treatment is delivery.
Other objectives of therapy include
seizure prevention with anticonvulsant
agents, delivery of an infant that
subsequently thrives, and restoration of
maternal health.

**How is mild preeclampsia
managed?**

Hospitalization, including bed rest,
  frequent monitoring of vital signs and
  fetal monitoring by NST, as indicated
At less than 37 weeks, continued
  maternal and fetal observation with
  seizure prophylaxis
Past 37 weeks, begin seizure prophylaxis
  and induction of labor

**How is severe
preeclampsia managed?**

Consideration of prompt delivery is
warranted, regardless of fetal age. Some
forms of severe illness may not indicate
delivery when the fetus is very immature.

When immediate delivery is not
performed, monitoring for organ
system impairment, as previously
outlined, must be continued.

Vaginal delivery is preferable. Labor
induction using IV oxytocin can be
attempted and cesarean section can be
reserved for those patients in which it
fails.

Seizure prophylaxis should be instituted
immediately using anticonvulsant
medication. Antihypertensive
medications should be used if DBP
rises above 110 mmHg. Intake and
output should be closely monitored.

**What is the appropriate
pharmacologic
management of
preeclampsia?**

Anticonvulsant medication:
Seizure prophylaxis should be
instituted in all preeclamptics
during labor and delivery and
should be continued for 48 hours
after delivery.

Magnesium sulfate is the agent of
choice. It can be initiated at 8 g/
hour for the first hour, reduced to
4 g/hour for the second hour, and
then maintained at 2 g/hour with a
controlled infusion device. In
patients with normal urine output,
the level of magnesium in this
protocol is predictable and does not
require checking.

Monitoring of deep tendon reflexes
(DTR), which should be present,
can be followed to prevent toxic
levels of this medication.

Therapeutic levels = 8 mg/dl. The
following occur at the indicated
blood magnesium levels:
Loss of DTR: 10 mg/dl
Respiratory suppression: 15 mg/dl
Cardiac arrest: < 25 mg/dl

For overdose, treat with 1 g calcium
gluconate IV push.

Antihypertensive medication:
Indicated for systolic blood pressure >
170 mm Hg or diastolic blood

pressure > 110 mm Hg to decrease
risk of intracranial or hepatic
hemorrhage and abruptio placentae

Acute control of high blood pressure
may be achieved with IV labetalol
5–15 mg slow push every 10
minutes, not to exceed a dose of
300 mg/day.

Alternative medications include
hydralazine 5–10 mg every 20–30
minutes as needed, and nifedipine
10 mg sublingually repeated after
30 minutes.

For refractory hypertension, sodium
nitroprusside 0.5–3 U/kg/minute in
a controlled infusion may be given,
but not to exceed 800 U/kg/minute.

## HELLP SYNDROME

**What is HELLP syndrome?**

A syndrome of **H**emolysis, **E**levated
**L**iver enzymes, and **L**ow **P**latelet
count

A distinct subset of preeclampsia that
occurs in 2%–12% of preeclampsia
patients

Can occur without associated
hypertension or proteinuria

Can occur antepartum or postpartum,
usually within 48 hours; 30% of cases
occur after delivery

**What are its signs and
symptoms?**

Nausea
Vomiting
Malaise
Headache
Epigastric or RUQ pain

**What are its differential
diagnoses?**

Gastritis
Hepatitis
Reflux
Cholecystitis
Pyelonephritis
Appendicitis
Thrombotic thrombocytopenic purpura
Immune thrombocytopenic purpura
Acute fatty liver of pregnancy

**What are the etiologic factors of HELLP syndrome?**

Unclear; clinical and pathologic manifestations result from an insult that leads to intravascular platelet activation and microvascular endothelial injury.

**What laboratory findings are associated with HELLP syndrome?**

Hemolysis:
    Abnormal peripheral smear
    Increased bilirubin > 1.2 mg/dl
    Increased lactate dehydrogenase (LDH) > 600 IU/ml
Elevated liver enzymes:
    Increased LDH
Low platelet count: < 150 ($10^3/\mu$l)

**What are the complications of HELLP syndrome?**

Perinatal and maternal mortality rates are significant.
Maternal morbidity includes complications from coagulopathy and liver disease

**What is the treatment of HELLP syndrome?**

Delivery
    If immediate delivery is not feasible because of fetal immaturity and the aberrations are mild, steroids can be given to promote better neonatal performance. Steroids may temporarily reverse some of the laboratory findings.
    Patients must be followed closely while being managed before delivery.
    Rapid delivery is mandated by fetal instability; vaginal delivery is preferred, but C/S is not contraindicated.
Maternal condition should be assessed and stabilized, particularly coagulation abnormalities. Although seldom necessary, frozen plasma may be required to correct coagulation abnormalities.
Seizure prophylaxis with magnesium sulfate should be given.

## ECLAMPSIA

**What is eclampsia?**

The occurrence of convulsions or coma, unrelated to other cerebral conditions, with signs and symptoms of preeclampsia

**What is its incidence?**

About 1 in every 1000 deliveries

**What are the signs and symptoms of eclampsia?**

Wide spectrum of signs and symptoms

Gradual onset with weight gain of approximately 2 pounds or greater per week in the last trimester

Hypertension: Hallmark; usually associated with significant proteinuria (> +2).

Seizures: Headache with visual disturbances may herald seizures.

**What form of seizure occurs in eclampsia?**

Tonic–clonic type (grand mal)

**What is the onset of eclamptic seizures?**

Can occur antepartum, intrapartum, or postpartum

Nearly all postpartum cases develop within 24 to 48 hours of delivery. Other diagnoses should be considered with onset of seizures after 48 hours postpartum.

Almost without exception, preeclampsia precedes onset of eclamptic seizures.

**What is the epidemiology of eclampsia?**

Primarily affects young primigravidas, but incidence is also increased in women older than 35 years of age.

Highest incidence occurs in low-income, nonwhite primigravidas.

**What are the morbid sequelae of eclampsia?**

Maternal:

Continued seizure activity despite appropriate magnesium sulfate therapy

Aspiration pneumonitis

Azotemia requiring dialysis

Sublethal intracranial hemorrhage resulting in hemiplegias

Massive intercerebral hemorrhage causing sudden death

Lactic acidosis

Blindness secondary to retinal detachment

Perinatal:

Abruptio placentae

Prematurity
IUGR
Hypoxic episodes during convulsions
Fetal death

**What factors increase the risk for maternal death?**

Early onset of preeclampsia in gestation
(< 28 weeks)
Increased maternal age
Multiple gestations

**What is the treatment of eclampsia?**

Continuous intensive monitoring of
mother and fetus
Large-bore IV access
Magnesium sulfate administration to
control convulsions as previously
outlined
Labetalol or hydralazine to control
severe hypertension as previously
outlined
Prevention of maternal injury during
seizures
Maintenance of adequate airway and
oxygenation; measures to minimize
risk of aspiration
Correction of maternal acidemia
Delivery by induction of labor or C/S
Delivery should be attempted after
seizures are controlled.
Some authorities recommend
reevaluation of the patient after
adequate anticonvulsant therapy is
established to decide the necessity of
delivery.

## CHRONIC HYPERTENSION

**What is chronic hypertension?**

Hypertension present before pregnancy
or diagnosed before 20 weeks'
gestation
Hypertension that persists beyond 42
days after delivery

**What is the etiology of chronic hypertension?**

Primary hypertension:
Also called essential or idiopathic
hypertension
Cause unknown
Accounts for 90% of all cases of
hypertension

Secondary hypertension:
  Renal hypertension (5%)
  Renal parenchymal disease (3%)
    Chronic pyelonephritis
    Acute/chronic glomerulonephritis
    Polycystic kidney disease
    Diabetic nephropathy
    Renin-producing tumors
    Renovascular disease
    Renal vascular stenosis
    Renal vascular infarction
Endocrine hypertension (4%–5%)
  Oral contraceptive usage (4%)
  Primary aldosteronism (0.5%)
  Aldosterone-secreting tumor
  Pheochromocytoma (0.2%)
  Cushing syndrome (0.2%)
  Acromegaly
  Hypercalcemia
  Thyrotoxicosis
Miscellaneous
  Acute spinal cord accident
  Coarctation of the aorta
  Acute intermittent porphyria
  Drugs (alcohol)
Heredity: African-American race, male sex, and strong family history increase risk for development of hypertension.
Environmental factors such as obesity, high-stress occupations, smoking, and so forth play a role in etiology.

**What are the target organs of chronic hypertension?**

The major feature in hypertension is increased total vascular resistance, which in turn affects many organ systems:
Cardiac:
  Increased vascular resistance causes need for increased stroke volume, which in turn may cause left ventricular hypertrophy leading to CHF.
  Hypertension may lead to increased risk of myocardial infarction or CHF.
Retinal: Arterial hemorrhage, appearance of exudates, or papilledema may lead to blurred

vision, scotomata, retinal
detachment, and blindness.
CNS:
The most serious neurologic
complication is vascular occlusion
leading to infarct and stroke.
Other CNS complications include
increased risk for arterial
intracerebral hemorrhage and
encephalopathy.
Renal: Arteriosclerotic lesions resulting
from the damaging effects of
hypertensive disease affect the
afferent and efferent arterioles within
the kidney, leading to decreased GFR
and tubular dysfunction; renal failure
is the ultimate result.
(Note: Because hypertension is a
heterogenous disease, multiple factors
affect its course. Eventually all
hypertension results in end organ
damage. Cardiomegaly, CHF,
retinopathy, pulmonary edema, renal
insufficiency are all possible. If left
untreated, this disease is lethal.)

**What are the
complications of chronic
hypertension in
pregnancy?**

Abruptio placentae
IUGR
IUFD
Increased risk of superimposed
preeclampsia

**What is the management
of chronic hypertension in
pregnancy?**

Early prenatal care
Evaluation of the degree of hypertension
Adequate estimation of the severity of
the individual's disease at initial visit
Education and appropriate counseling
about potential risks that pregnancy
imposes on the mother's medical
condition, risks her disease imposes
on her pregnancy, and the risks versus
benefits of hypertensive medications
during pregnancy
Close monitoring of prenatal course:
Frequent follow-up should occur
throughout prenatal course.
In third trimester, fetus should be
monitored with NST.

At term, induction of delivery should be considered, if feasible; complications may dictate earlier intervention.

## What are the important principles of pharmacologic management for chronic hypertension in pregnancy?

Patients with chronic hypertension who conceive while taking antihypertensive therapy may continue their medication if maintaining adequate control.

In general, studies have shown that mild to moderate hypertension does not require pharmacologic treatment in pregnancy. In patients with severe disease, however, pharmacologic therapy may reduce disease progression during pregnancy.

## What is the pharmacologic management of chronic hypertension in pregnancy?

$\alpha$-Methyldopa:
Remains a first-line agent in the United States, primarily because of its extensive use and well-documented fetal safety.
Initial dose is 1 g followed by a maintenance dose of 1–2 g/day.
Most common regimen is 250 mg three times a day or 500 mg four times a day.
Maximum dosage is 4 g/day.
Labetalol and atenolol (and other $\beta$-blockers):
$\beta$-Adrenergic blockers; labetalol hydrochloride has additional $\alpha_1$ blocking capability.
Initial dose of labetalol is 100 mg by mouth twice daily, increased to a maximum dose of 300 mg twice daily or four times a day.
Initial dose of atenolol is 50 mg daily, increased to a maximum dose of 50 mg twice daily or 100 mg daily.
$\beta$-Blockers are contraindicated in asthmatic patients and should be used with caution in insulin-dependent diabetics because of their ability to mask symptoms of hypoglycemia.
Angiotensin-converting enzyme (ACE) inhibitors: CONTRAINDICATED IN PREGNANCY

ACE inhibitors have been associated with fetal hypocalvaria, fetal renal failure, oligohydramnios, IUGR, and fetal and neonatal death. These drugs induce vasodilatation by inhibiting the enzyme that converts angiotensin I to angiotensin II, and have been found to decrease uteroplacental blood flow in experiments with animals, leading to fetal death.

Thiazide diuretics:

Although often first-line medications in nonpregnant chronic hypertensives, they should probably not be initiated during pregnancy.

Commonly cause hypokalemia, hyponatremia, hyperglycemia, hypercalcemia, and elevated uric acid in the mother; a few cases of thrombocytopenia in fetuses have been reported.

Diuretics work by reducing both plasma and extracellular fluid volume, with a concomitant decrease in cardiac output, which theoretically could have adverse fetal effects.

## PREGNANCY-AGGRAVATED HYPERTENSION

**What is pregnancy-aggravated hypertension?**

Superimposition of preeclampsia on chronic hypertensive disease during pregnancy; has a high perinatal morbidity and mortality rate

**What are its signs and symptoms?**

Typically manifests as a sudden rise in blood pressure that is almost always complicated by proteinuria

**What is its progression?**

Rapid progression of maternal hypertensive disease may occur.

**What is its treatment?**

It should be treated as preeclampsia.

# 16

# Pulmonary Diseases in Pregnancy

## ASTHMA

| | |
|---|---|
| **What is the incidence of asthma in pregnancy?** | Asthma occurs in 3% to 5% of adults. It complicates 1% of pregnancies. |
| **What is the pathophysiology of asthma?** | Airway hyperreactivity and bronchoconstriction |
| **What are the symptoms of asthma?** | Wheezing<br>Chest tightness<br>Shortness of breath<br>May be episodic with various degrees of severity or chronic with persistent dyspnea |
| **What are the criteria for a diagnosis of asthma?** | Physical examination: Tachypnea, use of accessory muscles of respiration<br>Pulmonary examination: Hyperinflation of the chest, diffuse pulmonary wheezing, and rhonchi<br>Response to β-agonist, theophylline, or corticosteroid therapy |
| **What are the etiologic factors of asthma?** | The onset of asthma during pregnancy is rare; most cases of asthma during pregnancy are due to exacerbations of disease.<br>The etiologic factors of exacerbations in pregnancy are the same as those in the nonpregnant state (i.e., noncompliance with medications, respiratory tract infections, allergens, gastrointestinal reflux, and exercise). |
| **What is the effect of pregnancy on asthma?** | Asthma improves in 69% of patients during pregnancy, worsens in 9%, and undergoes no change in 22%.<br>Worsening of asthma occurs in the sixth |

or seventh month of pregnancy; improvement in asthma occurs in the first trimester of pregnancy.

The course of a patient's asthma in one pregnancy is not a predictor of the course of asthma in subsequent pregnancies.

The severity of a patient's asthma before pregnancy correlates with the severity of asthma in pregnancy; asthma usually worsens during pregnancy in women with severe asthma.

Certain obstetric medications (i.e., prostaglandins and ergot derivatives) may exacerbate asthma and should be avoided.

Certain physiologic conditions associated with pregnancy (e.g., gastroesophageal reflux) may increase the frequency of asthma attacks.

**What is the effect of asthma on the mother and developing fetus?**

Mild or moderate asthma: No increase in the rate of fetal malformations or adverse effects

Severe asthma: Increased incidence of low birth weight, neurologic abnormalities, and pregnancy-induced hypertension

**What is the management of asthma?**

Avoidance of asthma triggers (e.g., allergens, exercise)

Yearly influenza vaccinations

Compliance with antiasthmatic medications

**What are the treatments for asthma?**

Differ little from therapy for nonpregnant patients

Aerosolized β-mimetic agents and aerosolized glucocorticoids

**Dosage of β-agonists in pregnancy?**

Metaproterenol, terbutaline, and albuterol are commonly given in two deep inhalations every 4–6 hours.

**Teratogenicity or adverse effects on fetus?**

None

**When is methylxanthine used in pregnancy?**

When intermittent inhalation therapy does not suffice

**Dosage of methylxanthine in pregnancy?**

Theophylline 200–400 mg twice a day; for optimal effect, the dosage should be adjusted to maintain therapeutic serum levels.

**Teratogenicity or adverse effects on fetus?**

Methylxanthines inhibit the force of uterine contractions, and their use is associated with a theorized risk of prolonged gestation or abnormally long labor.

Although they cross the placenta, they have no known harmful effects on the fetus.

Maternal toxicity may be difficult to detect because the symptoms include common symptoms of pregnancy such as nausea, vomiting, and tachycardia.

**When are β-adrenergic oral agents used in pregnancy?**

For patients who continue to have respiratory symptoms despite methylxanthine therapy; or primarily

**Dosage of β-adrenergic oral agents in pregnancy?**

Oral terbutaline 2.5–5.0 mg two to three times per day

**Teratogenicity or adverse effects on fetus?**

Theorized risk of prolonged gestation and inhibition of labor

**Dosage of oral corticosteroids in pregnancy?**

Prednisone 60–100 mg; clinical improvement is usually seen within 6 hours of treatment.

**Teratogenicity or adverse effects on fetus?**

None

**Why is prednisone the oral corticosteroid of choice in pregnancy?**

Most of the drug is inactivated by placental 11-B-OL-dehydrogenase; only a small percentage of the ingested dose reaches the fetus.

**When are intravenous (IV) steroids used in pregnancy?**

Increased doses of IV steroids are used peripartum for the increased stress of labor in patients who are chronic users of oral agents.

What effects does
steroid therapy have on
neonatal adrenal
function?

No evidence of neonatal adrenal
suppression due to chronic maternal
steroid use

## PULMONARY EMBOLUS

What is the incidence of
pulmonary embolus (PE)?

Occurs in 0.09–0.7/1000 pregnancies

Why is PE more common
in pregnancy?

Increased incidence is related to the
sixfold increase in development of a
deep venous thrombosis (DVT) in
pregnancy.

Incidence of
thrombophlebitis (deep
and superficial)?

Occurs in 1/70 pregnancies

When does
thrombophlebitis most
commonly occur during
pregnancy?

In the immediate postpartum period;
may occur antepartum

What are the risk factors
for development of a PE?

Maternal age > 35 years
Obesity
Immobility
Cardiopulmonary disease
Diabetes
Prior history of DVT and/or PE (5%–
12% risk of recurrence)
Prior cesarean section (threefold
increase)

What is a patient's course
after the development of a
PE?

Immediate result: Complete or partial
obstruction of the pulmonary arterial
blood flow to the distal lung
Partial obstruction: Decreased
ventilation, pulmonary infarction
Complete obstruction: Circulatory
collapse

What are the symptoms of
PE?

Dyspnea (most common symptom)
Cough
Hemoptysis
Chest pain
Palpitations
Lightheadedness
Anxiety

**What are the findings on physical examination?**

Tachypnea, low-grade fever, pleural friction rub, rales, or decreased breath sounds

Findings may be deceptively normal because a pleural friction rub or evidence of pleural effusion is not present unless an infarction has occurred.

Patients may exhibit acute right ventricular strain with a right ventricular heave.

**What are the laboratory findings?**

Hypoxia

Arterial blood gas: Decrease in $po_2$ (usually < 80)

Chest x-ray: May show an infiltrate or pleural effusion

EKG:

May show right axis shift or right bundle branch block

Often, only a sinus tachycardia with nonspecific ST-T changes is seen.

Confirming tests: Ventilation–perfusion scan; if equivocal, pulmonary angiogram with abdominal shielding

**What finding in the ventilation–perfusion scan is diagnostic of PE?**

A V-Q mismatch showing normal ventilation but decreased perfusion

**What conditions decrease the specificity of this test?**

Congestive heart failure or chronic obstructive pulmonary disease

**What is the maximum dose of radiation to the fetus in a ventilation–perfusion scan?**

Fifty milliroentgen equivalents man (mrem), which is well below the level that raises concerns

**What is the source of most of the radiation exposure, and how can this exposure be prevented?**

The source of 85% of the radiation exposure is the maternal bladder.

A Foley catheter should be placed to empty the bladder.

**What is the maximum dose of radiation to the fetus in a pulmonary angiogram?**

With abdominal shielding, the radiation exposure may be kept under 0.05 cGy

Level that increases risk to fetus is > 5 cGy

**What is the effect of
pregnancy on PE?**

Pregnancy increases the risk for DVT/
PE.
Risk factors for a DVT/PE include stasis,
hypercoagulability, and vascular injury.
Pregnancy increases stasis secondary
to compression by the uterus on the
inferior vena cava.
Pregnancy produces a hypercoagulable
state; risk for DVT/PE is further
increased in patients who are obese,
who have had pelvic surgery, or
who are on bed rest.
Pregnancy also causes an increase in
coagulation factors and a
suppression of the fibrinolytic
system.

**What are the most
common sites for a DVT?**

Venous sinuses within the soleus
Left iliofemoral venous segment

**What is the effect of PE on
mother and fetus?**

If mother is hemodynamically stable: No
adverse effect
If untreated: Maternal mortality rate
may approach 50% and is related to
the size of the lesion.

**What is the treatment for
PE?**

Heparin is the main therapeutic agent
used during pregnancy.
Risks to fetus: It does not cross the
placenta, does not increase the risk of
fetal malformations, and does not lead
to fetal anticoagulation.
Side effects: Hemorrhage (most
common side effect), bone
demineralization when used for more
than 20 weeks, anaphylaxis, alopecia,
and thrombocytopenia (usually mild
and dose/duration dependent)
Dosage:
10,000 U bolus IV followed by 1000–
2000 U/hour until the partial
thromboplastin time is 2.5–3 times
normal
Dose is then maintained at 1000 U/hr
for 10 days.
After 10 days, dose is changed to
approximately 10,000 U twice daily
by subcutaneous administration.

**What is the most common side effect of heparin therapy?**

Hemorrhage

**What is the incidence of thrombocytopenia that results from heparin therapy?**

Twenty percent

**Why is Coumadin (warfarin) contraindicated in pregnancy?**

It is teratogenic.
It has been associated with hemorrhage in the fetus and placenta.
It has been shown to produce nasal hypoplasia, stippling of bones, ophthalmologic abnormalities, intrauterine growth retardation, variable central nervous system (CNS) defects, anatomic defects, and mental delays.

**What is the risk of perinatal hemorrhage as a result of Coumadin therapy?**

Five percent to ten percent

**What is the risk of congenital disease as a result of Coumadin therapy?**

Fetuses exposed to the drug before 14 weeks' gestation have an estimated 10%–25% risk of congenital disease.

**When do CNS defects occur as a result of Coumadin therapy?**

At any time in the second or third trimester; may be related to bleeding

**When are embolectomy, fibrolytic agents, and vena caval interruption indicated during pregnancy?**

These therapies have not been adequately studied in the pregnant woman.
Fibrinolytic therapy:
  Agents such as streptokinase and urokinase are contraindicated peripartum because of the significant risk of hemorrhage.
  Another risk is allergic reaction.
  The exception is a person at risk for death from a PE who does not respond to heparin therapy.
Embolectomy: May be used in patients who do not respond to heparin

therapy yet demonstrate persistent
hypotension, hypoxemia, or both.
Vena caval interruption: Performed
when anticoagulation is
contraindicated; risk of recurrence is
10%.

## PNEUMONIA

**What are the symptoms of
pneumonia?**

Fever
Chills
Cough
Purulent sputum
Tachypnea

**What are the etiologic
factors of pneumonia?**

Most common cause of pneumonia is
  *Streptococcus pneumoniae* infection.
Another common organism is
  *Mycoplasma pneumoniae*, which
  causes a "community-acquired
  pneumonia."
Other bacteria, such as *Haemophilus
  influenzae*, *Staphylococcus aureus*, and
  *Escherichia coli*, and viruses may
  produce pneumonia.

**What are the criteria for
diagnosis of pneumonia?**

History:
  *S. pneumoniae* has a sudden onset,
    productive cough, and purulent
    sputum.
  *M. pneumoniae* has a gradual onset of
    symptoms with a nonproductive
    cough, headache, myalgias, and
    leukocytosis.
Physical examination: Rales and other
  signs suggestive of consolidation, such
  as decreased breath sounds, rhonchi,
  "e" to "a" changes, and percussive
  dullness
Chest x-ray:
  Lobar consolidation and air
    bronchograms are seen in *S.
    pneumoniae* infection.
  Unilateral or bilateral diffuse patchy
    infiltrates are seen in *M.
    pneumoniae*.
Gram stain of sputum and bacterial
  culture: In a healthy young woman,

the trachea should be free of
leukocytes and bacteria. Leukocytes
and bacteria are consistent with
infection.
Cold agglutin titers: Can help determine
*M. pneumoniae* infection

**What is the effect of
pregnancy on pneumonia?**

No effect

**What is the effect of
pneumonia on the mother
and fetus?**

Increased incidence of preterm labor in
patients who have pneumonia near
term
Perinatal mortality rate is < 10% in
infants delivered during the acute
phase of the disease and depends on
the gestational age at birth.

**What is the treatment for
pneumonia?**

IV or oral antibiotics, depending on the
severity of the disease.
*S. pneumoniae:* Penicillin G for 10 to 14
days
*M. pneumoniae:*
Does not respond to either PCN or
cephalosporins
Erythromycin for 10 to 14 days

**What are the
complications of
pneumonia?**

Poor outcome is related to involvement
of more than two lobes, respiratory
rate > 30, severe hypoxemia,
hypoalbuminemia, and septicemia.
Pneumonia that progresses to adult
respiratory distress syndrome has a
70% mortality rate.
Bacteremia may develop in up to 25%
of patients.
Empyema and respiratory failure are
other complications.

## TUBERCULOSIS

**What is the epidemiology
of tuberculosis (TB)?**

Incidence is increasing; it is the most
common communicable disease
among human immunodeficiency
virus-infected individuals.
The risk of acquiring the infection is
highest in large urban settings.
Overall, advanced disease develops in
5%–15% of infected individuals.

| | |
|---|---|
| **What are the stages of TB?** | Primary TB: |
| |     Defined as first infection with tuberculosis agent |
| |     May cavitate and heal spontaneously or progress (called progressive primary TB) |
| | Secondary TB: |
| |     Most common presentation in adults |
| |     Represents a delayed reactivation of infection or exogenous reinfection |
| **What are the symptoms of primary nonprogressive TB?** | Most patients are asymptomatic, have no cough, and produce little sputum; only sign is a positive tuberculin skin test. |
| | Patients in cavitary stage have a chronic cough and produce mucopurulent sputum. |
| **What are the manifestations of progressive primary TB?** | Miliary tuberculosis, sometimes with meningitis; pulmonary disease of the apical and posterior segments of the upper lobes; or lower lobe disease |
| **What are the symptoms of reactivation?** | Night sweats |
| | Chills |
| | Fatigue |
| | Fever from 39°C to 40°C occurring in the late afternoon and evening |
| | Malaise |
| | Weight loss |
| | Hemoptysis |
| **What is the etiologic factor of TB?** | Infection with *Mycobacterium tuberculosis* |
| **How is TB transmitted?** | Inhalation of aerosolized droplets of liquid containing the bacteria from an infected patient with cavitary pulmonary tuberculosis |
| **What is the pathophysiology of TB?** | The bacteria travel to the lung alveoli. |
| | Once local invasion has occurred, the infection can be disseminated hematogenously, thereby seeding multiple organs and establishing latent foci. |
| | These latent foci are the sites of delayed reactivation. |

**What are the criteria for a diagnosis of TB?**

Positive PPD test:
  Defined as a wheal of induration of at least 10 mm
  Suggests a history of exposure to TB but not necessarily active TB
  False-negative reactions may occur in pregnant patients.
Chest x-ray:
  In primary TB, shows patchy or lobular infiltrates in the anterior segment of the upper lobes or in the middle lobes, often with associated hilar adenopathy
  In secondary TB, may show cavitary lesions with infiltrates
Acid-fast stain of the sputum: Definitive test
Culture: May also be performed but results take 6 weeks
Physical examination: Unremarkable or reveals dullness and rales in the upper lung fields

**What is the effect of TB on mother and fetus?**

TB has no adverse effect on pregnancy if adequate treatment is implemented.
Transplacental passage of TB is extremely rare.
Congenital infection of liver or regional lymph nodes may occur in the presence of maternal bacillemia.

**What is the effect of pregnancy on TB?**

No effect

**What is the treatment for TB?**

Two or three sputum samples for culture before starting antituberculous drug treatment
Baseline evaluation of liver function before the administration of potentially hepatotoxic drugs (isoniazid, rifampin, pyrazinamide)
Administration of multiple antimicrobials to prevent the growth of resistant organisms

**What antibiotics are used to treat TB?**

Isoniazid and rifampin for initial treatment in patients with susceptible organisms

A third agent, such as streptomycin, ethambutol, and pyrazinamide, for patients with resistant organisms

**How long should antibiotic therapy last?**

The current minimal acceptable duration of treatment for adults with culture-positive tuberculosis is 6 months.

**What are the risks of TB medications to the fetus?**

The risk of untreated tuberculosis is far greater to a mother and fetus than toxicities of medications.

Isoniazid: No increase in risk of congenital abnormalities

Ethambutol: No increase in risk of congenital abnormalities; the mother risks retrobulbar neuritis.

Rifampin: No associated fetal malformations are known; it readily crosses the placenta and may theoretically inhibit DNA-dependent RNA polymerase and injure the fetus.

Streptomycin: This drug should be avoided if possible in pregnancy because it may interfere with development of the ear, causing congenital deafness; it may be both ototoxic and nephrotoxic to the mother.

**Is breast-feeding contraindicated during TB antibiotic therapy?**

No

**When is prophylactic therapy indicated in pregnancy?**

If patient has a positive PPD and recent conversion

**What agent is used for prophylaxis?**

Isoniazid

# 17

# Renal Diseases in Pregnancy

**What normal renal changes occur in pregnancy?**

Dilatation of the collecting system and ureters:
  Occurs as early as 10 weeks' gestation
  Is due to both mechanical compression of the ureters by the enlarging uterus and the relaxing effect of progesterone on smooth muscle.
Increased renal plasma flow:
  Exceeds prepregnant levels by 50%–75% at the end of the first trimester
  The mean value of renal plasma flow is 840 ml/minute at 16 weeks and 750 ml/minute at term.
Fifty percent increase in glomerular filtration rate (GFR)
Decreased renal threshold for glucose:
  Sometimes causes glycosuria in patients with a normal blood glucose
Decreased serum levels of creatinine and blood urea nitrogen (BUN):
  Nonpregnant levels are 0.8 mg/100 ml and 13 mg/100 ml.
  Pregnant levels are 0.6 mg/100 ml and 9 mg/100 ml (mean values).

## ASYMPTOMATIC BACTERIURIA

**What is the incidence of asymptomatic bacteriuria in pregnancy?**

Occurs in 2%–7% of all pregnancies

**What are the criteria for diagnosis of asymptomatic bacteriuria?**

Greater than 100,000 colonies/ml of a single organism in a clean-catch sample of urine
Unlike typical urinary tract infections in nonpregnant women, pregnant

patients commonly do not experience dysuria.

Polyuria, urgency, and nocturia are symptoms common to both pregnancy and urinary infection and therefore are not diagnostic of infection.

**What are the common organisms that cause asymptomatic bacteriuria?**

*Escherichia coli*:
The most common organism found in urine specimens
Responsible for 75%–90% of bacteriuria cases during pregnancy
Other bacteria: *Klebsiella, Proteus*, and *Enterobacter* sp

**What are the complications of asymptomatic bacteriuria?**

If untreated, asymptomatic bacteriuria may lead to pyelonephritis or acute symptomatic cystitis in 25%–40% of patients.

Approximately 15% of patients treated for asymptomatic bacteriuria have a recurrence.

**What is the treatment of asymptomatic bacteriuria?**

Antibiotic therapy specific to the organisms involved

**What antibiotics are commonly used in pregnancy?**

Sulfa drugs: Avoid using near term because they can cause kernicterus by competitively inhibiting the binding of bilirubin to albumin.

Nitrofurantoin:
Empiric therapy for 7 days is effective in most cases.
Contraindicated in patients with glucose-6-phosphate dehydrogenase deficiency

Ampicillin

Cephalosporins

## PYELONEPHRITIS

**What is the incidence of pyelonephritis?**

Most common serious medical complication of pregnancy
Occurs in 1%–2% of all pregnancies
Right-sided in more than one-half of cases and bilateral in one-fourth

**What are the symptoms of pyelonephritis?**

Fever
Chills
Nausea
Vomiting
Anorexia
Dysuria
Flank pain
Frequency, urgency, and dysuria may not be present.

**What are the criteria for the diagnosis of pyelonephritis?**

Physical examination: Costovertebral angle tenderness and fever
Urinalysis: An increased number of white blood cells and numerous bacteria
Urine culture: Grows the infecting organism.
Urine leukocyte esterase and nitrite: Positive
GFR: Temporarily decreased in ~25% of patients
Blood creatinine: Temporarily increased in ~25% of patients

**What are the etiologic factors of pyelonephritis?**

The same organisms that cause asymptomatic bacteriuria cause pyelonephritis; pyelonephritis is an ascending infection.

**What is the effect of pregnancy on pyelonephritis?**

Increased incidence of pyelonephritis in pregnant women is related to the increased incidence of asymptomatic bacteriuria during pregnancy.
Increased urinary stasis caused by dilatation and compression of the urinary system during pregnancy contributes to increased risk of infection.

**What is the effect of pyelonephritis on the mother and fetus?**

Possible increased risk of preterm labor
Possible increased risk of fetal death and intrauterine growth retardation (IUGR) as a result of recurrent pyelonephritis

**What are complications of pyelonephritis?**

Approximately 15% of patients with pyelonephritis have bacteremia.
Pregnant women are more vulnerable to

endotoxins than are nonpregnant
women.

Up to 2% of bacteremic patients
develop endotoxin-mediated
alveolar injury with resulting
pulmonary edema or adult
respiratory distress syndrome.

Some patients with pyelonephritis
develop acute anemia as a result of
endotoxin-induced hemolysis.

Some women have a considerable
reduction in GFR that is reversed by
effective treatment.

**What is the treatment for
pyelonephritis?**

Intravenous (IV) hydration and IV
antibiotic therapy for at least 24–48
hours; oral therapy may follow.

Lack of improvement by 72 hours
suggests inadequate use or an
underlying anatomic problem; empiric
treatment should begin with an
extended-spectrum antibiotic such as
cefuroxime, pending culture results.

## UROLITHIASIS

**What is the incidence of
urolithiasis?**

Occurs in 0.03% of pregnancies (same as
that for the general population).

**What are the symptoms of
urolithiasis?**

Colicky abdominal pain, hematuria;
these symptoms are far less common in
the pregnant patient.

**What is the
pathophysiology of
urolithiasis?**

Calcium salts make up about 75% of
renal stones; in half these cases,
idiopathic hypercalciuria is the most
common predisposing cause.

Struvite stones are associated with
infection, and *Proteus* is often
cultured from the urine.

Uric acid stones are less common.

**How is a diagnosis of
urolithiasis made?**

History and physical examination

Ultrasound can also be used to detect
stones and hydronephrosis or urinary
tract dilatation proximal to the stone.

The patient's urine can be strained for
stones.

Patients with persistent pyelonephritis despite antibiotic therapy should be evaluated for a possible obstructing renal stone.

**What is the effect of pregnancy on urolithiasis?**

No effect

**What is the effect of urolithiasis on mother and fetus?**

No known adverse effects
Increased frequency of urinary infections

**What is the management/ treatment of urolithiasis?**

Expectant management
Acute event:
    Hydration and narcotic analgesia
    Because of the hydroureter that occurs in pregnancy, over one-half of patients spontaneously pass the stone.
    Approximately one-third of patients with symptomatic stones need cystoscopy, ureteral catheterization, percutaneous nephrostomy, basket extraction, or surgical exploration for ureteral obstruction.
Lithotripsy: Contraindicated in pregnancy
Aggressive treatment for coexisting infection

## GLOMERULONEPHRITIS

**What is the incidence of glomerulonephritis in pregnancy?**

Occurs in 1/40,000 pregnant women

**What are the signs and symptoms of glomerulonephritis?**

Hypertension
Edema (including periorbital edema)
Proteinuria
Hematuria (usually microscopic)
These signs and symptoms may be difficult to distinguish from those of preeclampsia.

**How is glomerulonephritis diagnosed?**

History, physical examination, and laboratory evaluation
Definitive test: Renal biopsy

**How is glomerulonephritis distinguished from preeclampsia?**

Patients with glomerulonephritis have red blood cell (RBC) casts in urine sediment and depressed serum complement levels.

**What are the etiologic factors?**

Acute glomerulonephritis:
  Usually but not always streptococcal in origin
  Other causes include other bacterial, viral, and parasitic infections; multisystem disease such as systemic lupus erythematosus; Henoch-Schönlein purpura; or primary glomerular disease.
Chronic glomerulonephritis: Secondary to a known episode of acute glomerulonephritis, IgA nephropathy, membranoproliferative glomerulonephritis, focal glomerulosclerosis, or systemic lupus erythematosus.

**What is the effect of pregnancy on glomerulonephritis?**

No effect; urinary protein excretion may transiently increase because of the increased renal plasma flow in pregnancy.

**What is the effect of glomerulonephritis on the mother and fetus?**

Increased incidence of fetal demise, IUGR, and preterm delivery
Fifty-two percent of patients have hypertension.
Fifteen percent have impaired renal function.
Patients with hypertension or impaired renal function (creatinine > 1.5) have a higher incidence of complications.

**What are the complications of acute glomerulonephritis?**

Chronic glomerulonephritis with resulting end-stage renal failure
Chronic proteinuria
Hypertension

**What is the management/ treatment of glomerulonephritis?**

Blood pressure control
Restriction of salt intake
Appropriate seizure prophylaxis if preeclampsia is suspected

## CHRONIC RENAL DISEASE

| | |
|---|---|
| **What is chronic renal disease?** | A syndrome that results from progressive and irreversible destruction of nephrons, regardless of cause |
| **What is the criterion for a diagnosis of chronic renal failure?** | Reduced GFR for at least 3 to 6 months |
| **What are the criteria for a diagnosis of chronic renal disease?** | Renal function may be normal. Signs and symptoms include hypertension, proteinuria, or abnormal renal sediment. Diagnosis is supported by the finding of bilateral reduction of kidney size. Casts in the urinary sediment are consistent with chronic renal failure. Proteinuria and hematuria are frequent but nonspecific findings. Other symptoms and laboratory values differ depending on the cause of the renal dysfunction: Moderate proteinuria ($<$ 2 g/day) is seen in glomerular disease (most commonly lipoid nephrosis), systemic lupus erythematosus, and in glomerulonephritis. RBC casts and microscopic hematuria (RBCs > 1–2/hpf) are seen in glomerular disease or collagen vascular disease. Cellular casts are seen in renal tubular disease. |
| **What is the effect of chronic renal disease on mother and fetus?** | In women with preexisting renal disease, the prognosis for a favorable pregnancy outcome is closely related to renal function at the time of conception. Effects include increased incidence of hypertension, superimposed preeclampsia, IUGR, and preterm birth. Obstetric outcome is usually successful provided renal function is only moderately compromised and hypertension is absent or minimal. |

**What is the effect of pregnancy on renal function?**

Patients with baseline creatinine < 1.5: Pregnancy has little effect on long-term prognosis.

Patients with creatinine > 1.5:

Deterioration of renal function is more frequent, especially in patients with diffuse glomerulonephritis.

If renal function deteriorates significantly during pregnancy, pregnancy termination may not reverse the initial process.

Hypertension:

Fifty percent of patients with chronic renal disease have worsening hypertension.

A diastolic blood pressure > 110 occurs in 20% of patients.

Patients with diffuse proliferative glomerulonephritis and nephrosclerosis are at greatest risk for development of severe hypertension.

Increased incidence of pyelonephritis

**What are the causes of sudden deterioration of renal function?**

Infection
Dehydration
Obstruction

**What is the management/ treatment of chronic renal disease?**

Frequent urine monitoring for creatine clearance and protein excretion

Frequent visits

Serial ultrasonography to evaluate possible IUGR

Antepartum fetal heart rate testing

Anemia secondary to chronic renal disease: Erythropoietin

Hypertension: Methyldopa, β-blockers

**When is dialysis indicated?**

Severe abnormalities in fluid and electrolyte balance such as fluid overload, acidosis, and hyperkalemia

Symptoms of uremia

Renal function 5% or less of normal, regardless of symptoms

**What precautions should be taken during dialysis of the pregnant patient?**

Avoidance of sudden volume shifts

Continuous fetal heart rate monitoring in late pregnancy

|  | Avoidance of prolonged periods in the supine position due to compression of the vena cava |
|---|---|
| **What are the complications of dialysis during pregnancy?** | Polyhydramnios<br>Preterm birth<br>Other common problems: Clotting and infection of the vascular access |

## PREGNANCY IN THE INDIVIDUAL WITH A RENAL TRANSPLANT

| **Which individuals with a renal transplant should attempt pregnancy?** | Individuals in whom surgery was performed 2 or more years previously (risk of graft rejection is greatest during first 2 years)<br>Individuals with no evidence of rejection, hypertension, or proteinuria<br>Creatinine < 2 |
|---|---|
| **What is the effect of a renal transplant on pregnancy?** | Ninety percent of pregnancies that continue beyond the first trimester have a successful outcome.<br>Increased incidence of:<br>  Preeclampsia (1/3 of patients)<br>  Preterm labor (1/2 of patients)<br>  IUGR<br>  Premature rupture of membranes<br>  Urinary and viral infections<br>  Cephalopelvic disproportion due to pelvic osteodystrophy<br>Fifteen percent of patients experience a significant decrease in renal function in late pregnancy that usually reverses after pregnancy. |
| **What is the effect of pregnancy on a renal transplant?** | The incidence of rejection is 9%, which is the same as that in the nonpregnant population. |
| **What two conditions can the symptoms of rejection mimic?** | Acute pyelonephritis or severe preeclampsia |
| **What test can distinguish rejection from acute pyelonephritis or severe preeclampsia?** | Renal biopsy |

**What is the management/ treatment of the renal transplant patient?**

Continuation of immunosuppressive therapy (glucocorticoids, azathioprine, and cyclosporin)

Frequent assessment of renal function

Monitoring for worsening of underlying hypertension and superimposed preeclampsia

Urinalysis at each prenatal visit

Urine culture each trimester

Bacteriuria: Requires aggressive treatment; the transplanted kidney is denervated and therefore the patient may have pyelonephritis or urosepsis without pain

**What is the cesarean section rate in this population?**

Fifty percent

**Why does obstruction of labor occasionally occur in this population?**

The transplanted kidney is located in the pelvis and can obstruct labor.

**What are the risks to the fetus associated with immunosuppressive therapy?**

Glucocorticoids are metabolized in the placenta and are not known to cause any adverse fetal effects.

Azathioprine has reported fetal complications of IUGR and a decrease in IgG and IgM in the fetus.

Cyclosporin may cause hypertension and is associated with IUGR.

Concerns persist about the possibility of late effects in offspring subjected to immunosuppressive therapy in utero, including malignancy, germ cell dysfunction, and malformations in the offspring's children.

## ACUTE RENAL FAILURE IN PREGNANCY

**What is acute renal failure?**

The production of < 400 ml of urine in a 24-hour period

**What is the incidence of acute renal failure?**

Occurs in 1/10,000 pregnancies

**When do most acute renal failure cases occur during pregnancy?**

Postpartum

**What are the etiologic factors of acute renal failure in pregnancy?**

Sudden, severe volume depletion due to blood loss occurring in placenta previa, placental abruption, and postpartum uterine atony

Marked volume contraction due to preeclampsia and acute fatty liver of pregnancy

Sepsis

Complicated preexisting renal problems

**What are the most common obstetric causes of acute renal failure?**

Placental abruption and preeclampsia

**What are the signs and symptoms of acute renal failure?**

Oliguria followed by a period of polyuria

Increased BUN and creatinine

Acidosis

Uremia

**What are the complications of acute renal failure?**

The immediate maternal mortality rate with acute renal failure is 20%.

Acute renal failure with mild ischemia: Quickly reversible prerenal failure

With prolonged ischemia: Reversible acute tubular necrosis

With severe ischemia: Irreversible acute cortical necrosis

**Incidence of acute cortical necrosis?**

Occurs in 15%–30% of all cases of acute renal failure in pregnancy

**Mortality rate of acute cortical necrosis?**

One hundred percent if untreated

**Treatment of acute cortical necrosis?**

Dialysis

**How is acute cortical necrosis differentiated from early acute tubular necrosis?**

Differentiation is not possible.

**What is the management/
treatment of acute renal
failure?**

Correction of underlying cause of acute
    volume loss
Balance of volume and electrolytes
Prompt treatment of acidosis, if present
Dialysis if the patient has hypernatremia,
    hyperkalemia, severe acidosis, volume
    overload, or worsening uremia

**Why should diuretics be
avoided?**

They increase urine flow without
correcting the cause, and may contribute
to volume depletion.

# 18

# Teratogenicity

**What is teratogenicity?**

Strict definition: Production of physical defects in the developing embryo. The definition over time has expanded to include functional and behavioral deficits.

**What is the incidence of major congenital malformations in a newborn?**

Three percent

**What are the causes of developmental defects in humans?**

Genetic transmission: 20%
Chromosomal aberrations: 5%
Environmental
    Ionizing radiation: 1%–2%
    Infections: 1%–2%
    Maternal metabolic imbalances: 1%–2%
    Drugs and environmental chemicals: 4%–6%
Unknown: 65%–70%

**What is the incidence of drug use during pregnancy?**

Eighty-six percent of women take medications during pregnancy.
They take an average of five medications.

**What are the most commonly used drugs in pregnancy?**

Analgesics
Antibiotics
Antacids
Diuretics
Laxatives

**What two stages described fetal exposure to medications?**

Preimplantation and implantation

**What is the usual effect of a drug on the embryo preimplantation?**

Any chemical present in the tubal or uterine fluids potent enough to cause irreparable injury usually kills the affected embryo.

**What determines the effect of drugs on the fetus after implantation?**

Placental transfer: Because most drugs have a molecular weight of 250–500 daltons, placental transfer is readily accomplished.
Fetal dosage
Duration of exposure of fetus to drug
Gestational age at time of exposure
During embryogenesis (2–8 weeks' gestational age), teratogens can cause structural defects; an example is neural tube defect.
After embryogenesis, drugs mainly cause adverse effects in the fetus.

**How can teratogenic effects be identified antenatally?**

Amniocentesis is normally **not** helpful because most drugs do not damage the fetal chromosomes.
α-Fetoprotein testing of maternal serum can detect 85% of all open neural tube defects.
Ultrasound may be able to detect malformations or intrauterine growth retardation (IUGR).

**What steps can be taken to decrease congenital anomalies from medications?**

Minimize drug exposures
Avoid polydrug regimens
Use lowest drug dose for shortest duration possible

**For what purpose are the Food and Drug Administration (FDA) Use-in-Pregnancy Ratings intended?**

To provide guidelines on the use of drugs during pregnancy and discourage medication use

**What are the different FDA Use-in-Pregnancy ratings?**

A: Controlled studies show no risk
B: No evidence of risk in humans
C: Risk cannot be ruled out
D: Positive evidence of risk
X: Contraindicated in pregnancy

**For each medication below, list its teratogenicity and/or adverse effect.**
**Phenytoin**

Teratogenicity: Ten percent of newborns may have cleft lip and palate, heart disease, and microcephaly.

Children born to mothers with seizures receiving no medications also have an increased incidence of congenital anomalies.

Considerable controversy exists about the true incidence of teratogenicity from phenytoin, if any.

**Carbamazepine**

Teratogenicity: Growth and developmental delay, minor craniofacial anomalies, neural tube defects in the first trimester ($< 1\%$ incidence)

**Valproic acid**

Teratogenicity: Neural tube defects ($1\%$–$3\%$ incidence), developmental delays, and craniofacial anomalies

**Metronidazole**

Teratogenicity: Mutagenic in bacteria, but no problems have been reported in humans

Because of this **theoretical** risk, it should be given only for clear-cut indications.

**Ciprofloxacin**

Teratogenicity: Not recommended in pregnant women and children

Human studies have **not** shown an association between quinolone use in the first trimester and an increased risk of malformations or musculoskeletal problems.

However, immature dogs and guinea pigs treated with quinolones have developed arthropathy.

**Sulfamethoxazole/ trimethoprim**

Adverse effect: When given in the third trimester, may compete with bilirubin for albumin-binding sites and contribute to increased risk of hyperbilirubinemia

**Tetracycline (doxycycline, minocycline, tetracycline)**

Teratogenicity: Staining of fetal teeth when used after 20th week; enamel hypoplasia and inhibition of fibula growth in premature infants

**Aminoglycosides**

Adverse effect: Hearing loss appears to be dose related; if used, maternal serum levels should be monitored and the course of therapy kept short.

**Other antibiotics (penicillins, cephalosporins, erythromycin, nitrofurantoin and clindamycin)**

Teratogenicity: Apparently none

**Warfarin**

Teratogenicity: When used in the first trimester can cause fetal warfarin syndrome (nasal hypoplasia, bone stippling, and ophthalmologic abnormalities); when used beyond first trimester, blindness and mental retardation can occur.

**Heparin**

Because it is a large molecule and does not cross the placenta, it is the drug of choice or anticoagulation in pregnancy.
Teratogenicity: Apparently none
Adverse effects: Bleeding (2% incidence), bone demineralization with doses > 20,000 U/day

**Enoxaparin**

Because it is a large molecule, it does not cross the placenta.
Teratogenicity: Appears safe, but not as much information exists about this drug as exists for heparin.

**Alcohol**

Teratogenicity: Fetal alcohol syndrome (IUGR, mental retardation, as well as ocular, facial, and skeletal anomalies) occurs when large amounts of alcohol are ingested.
A threshold for safety has not been established, and it is best to avoid any exposure.

**Antihistamines**

Teratogenicity: Apparently none

| | |
|---|---|
| **Decongestants** | Teratogenicity: Apparently none<br>Ventral wall defects have been reported with pseudoephedrine use in the first trimester.<br>If a decongestant is necessary, a topical nasal spray subjects the fetus to lower doses than a systemic medication.<br>Because antihistamines and decongestants provide only symptomatic therapy for the common cold, other remedies such as a humidifier, rest, and fluids should be recommended.<br>If drugs are necessary, only one should be used. |
| **Meclizine** | Teratogenicity: Apparently none |
| **Dimenhydrinate** | Teratogenicity: Apparently none |
| **Metoclopramide** | Teratogenicity: Apparently none |
| **Trimethobenzamide** | Teratogenicity: Apparently none |
| **Promethazine** | Teratogenicity: Apparently none |
| **Acetaminophen** | Teratogenicity: Apparently none when used as an antipyretic and analgesic |
| **Aspirin** | Teratogenicity: Apparently none<br>Adverse effects: Inhibits prostaglandin synthesis and can decrease uterine contractility and cause delayed onset and longer duration of labor<br>May also decrease platelet aggregation in newborn |
| **Nonsteroidal anti-inflammatory drugs** | Teratogenicity: Apparently none, but when used in third trimester may prolong labor and cause premature closure of the fetal ductus arteriosus |
| **Codeine** | Teratogenicity: Apparently none<br>Adverse effect: Fetal/newborn addiction with prolonged use |

**Narcotic analgesics (morphine, hydrocodone, oxycodone, meperidine, hydromorphone)**

Teratogenicity: Apparently none
Adverse effect: Fetal/newborn addiction with prolonged use; at term may cause neonatal respiratory depression

**Methyldopa**

Teratogenicity: Apparently none

**Hydralazine**

Teratogenicity: Apparently none

**Digoxin**

Teratogenicity: Apparently none

**Nifedipine**

Teratogenicity: Apparently none
Experience in human pregnancy is limited.

**β-Blockers**

Teratogenicity: Apparently none

**Angiotensin-converting enzyme inhibitors**

Teratogenicity: **Contraindicated** in pregnancy
Use of these drugs in the second and third trimesters has been associated with fetal injury and death.
Risks to the fetus include potential fatal hypotension, anuria, and renal failure.
Decreased renal function can lead to oligohydramnios, which can result in fetal limb contractures, craniofacial deformities, and hypoplastic lung development.

**Caffeine**

Teratogenicity: Apparently none
Conservative consumption is recommended.

**Hydrochlorothiazide**

Teratogenicity: Apparently none

**Furosemide**

Teratogenicity: Apparently none

**Diuretics**

Adverse effects: Fetal electrolyte disturbances have been observed in some cases when used in the third trimester.
Diuretics are normally not recommended during pregnancy.

**Progesterone (natural)**

Teratogenicity: Apparently none

**Medroxyprogesterone**   Teratogenicity: Apparently none

**Estrogens**   Teratogenicity: Apparently none
Controversy exists.

**Diethylstilbestrol (DES)**   Teratogenicity: **Contraindicated** in
pregnancy
Female fetuses exposed to DES have an
increased risk of adenocarcinoma of
the vagina and cervix.
May also cause uterine anomalies
affecting reproductive capacity.
DES may also affect the reproductive
tract of exposed male fetuses.

**Oral contraceptives**   Teratogenicity: Apparently none
Controversy exists.
Patient should be informed that a
possible risk to the fetus exists if the
drug is continued during pregnancy.

**Vaccines (general)**   Most vaccines contain toxoids or killed
organisms and present a low risk to
the fetus.
Vaccines containing live attenuated
viruses present a slightly higher
**theoretical** risk.
If a vaccine or a toxoid is indicated
during pregnancy, it should be given
during the second or third trimester.
In general, the advantages of
immunization usually outweigh the
potential risks.
**The best time to receive
immunizations is before
pregnancy.**

**Measles, mumps, and
rubella (MMR) vaccine**   Teratogenicity: Although the
recommendation is not to give during
pregnancy, evidence does not support
vaccine-associated malformations.
Give immediately postpartum.

**Influenza vaccine**   Teratogenicity: Apparently none
It is not routinely given to people who
are otherwise healthy.
It is indicated for women in high-risk
groups (the immunocompromised).

**Hepatitis B vaccine**　　Teratogenicity: Pregnancy should **not** be considered a contraindication.

**Tetanus and diphtheria vaccine**　　Teratogenicity: Apparently none

**Docusate**　　Teratogenicity: Apparently none

**Docusate/casanthranol**　　Teratogenicity: Apparently none

**Serotonin reuptake inhibitors (general)**　　Experience is limited.
Unanswered questions include effects on infant behavior and intellect or problems with newborn adaptation.

**Fluoxetine**　　Teratogenicity: Apparently none

**Sertraline**　　Teratogenicity: Apparently none

**Paroxetine**　　Teratogenicity: Apparently none

**Smoking**　　Teratogenicity: Associated with IUGR and preterm labor, but not malformations.
Children may also be at increased risk for sudden infant death syndrome, although the data do not make it clear if smoking before pregnancy, after pregnancy, or both, is the cause.

**Corticosteroids (general)**　　Teratogenicity: Apparently none
All steroids cross the placenta to some degree.

**Prednisone / Prednisolone**　　Teratogenicity: Apparently none
Both drugs are inactivated by the placenta, and less than 10% of the drug reaches the fetus.
Drug of choice for diseases such as asthma

**Betamethasone/ dexamethasone**　　Teratogenicity: Apparently none
These drugs cross the placenta and are preferred for stimulating fetal lung maturity.

# 19

# Diabetes in Pregnancy

| | |
|---|---|
| **What is the most common medical complication of pregnancy?** | Diabetes mellitus |
| **What is the incidence?** | Three percent |
| **What is the perinatal mortality rate in diabetic pregnancy?** | Approximately the same as that of nondiabetic pregnancy |
| **How is nongestational (preexisting) diabetes classified?** | As Type I (insulin-dependent diabetes mellitus) or Type II (non–insulin-dependent diabetes mellitus) |
| **What is gestational diabetes mellitus?** | Carbohydrate intolerance first recognized during pregnancy and not persisting after delivery |
| **How is diabetes that predates pregnancy classified?** | According to the degree of maternal metabolic control and the presence or absence of vasculopathy |

## PREEXISTING DIABETES IN PREGNANCY

| | |
|---|---|
| **What are the benefits of normalization of maternal blood glucose levels during diabetes in pregnancy?** | Decreased congenital anomaly rate (otherwise increased fourfold) if the diabetes is established before conception<br>Decreased risk of neonatal macrosomia<br>Decreased mortality and morbidity rates |
| **Why do infants of diabetic women have high anomaly rates?** | Glucose is a teratogen |
| **What specific anomalies are associated with diabetes in pregnancy?** | Cardiac anomalies<br>Transposition of great vessels<br>Ventricular septal defect<br>Atrial septal defect<br>Caudal regression<br>Neural tube defect<br>Renal anomalies |

**What are the risks associated with preexisting Type 1 diabetes mellitus during pregnancy?**

Higher risk of preeclampsia
Higher risk of pyelonephritis
Hypoglycemia (with tight glucose control) ·
Progression of proliferative retinopathy (but not progression of renal disease)

**What are the goals of maternal metabolic control?**

Glucose levels that do not exceed 90 milligrams per deciliter (mg/dL) at fasting or 105 mg/dL prior to meals
Hemoglobin A or $A_{lc}$ within the normal range

**How can these goals be achieved?**

Patient glucose monitoring
Carefully regulated dietary intake
Carefully regulated insulin administration usually requiring multiple injections of variously acting insulins; insulin pumps can be used

**Why are oral hypoglycemic agents avoided during pregnancy?**

They may produce fetal hyperinsulinemia.

**What is a carefully regulated dietary intake for a woman with diabetes in pregnancy?**

Intake of 2200 kcalories/day
20% protein
50% carbohydrate
30% fat
Consumption: 25% of calories at breakfast, 30% at lunch, 30% at dinner, and 15% as a bedtime snack
Day-to-day consistency in dietary behavior and activity

**What should the prenatal workup of a woman with preexisting diabetes consist of?**

History and physical examination
Standard prenatal laboratory tests
Twenty-four-hour urinalysis for creatinine clearance and protein excretion (usually requires a repeat test)
Ophthalmologic examination
Thyroid function tests

**What does the fetal work-up consist of?**

Early ultrasound to clearly establish gestational age
Ultrasound at approximately 20 weeks' gestation to screen for anomaly
Triple screen or α-fetoprotein (maternal serum) to screen for neural tube defect

Fetal echocardiography (controversial)
Surveillance for fetal well-being (in the
  third trimester)
  Nonstress test (NST)
  BPP
  Ultrasound
  Kick count
  CST
  Determination of lung maturity when
    delivery is considered

**Why is fetal surveillance necessary?**

Intrauterine death from placental insufficiency is common in women with poor glucose control. Surveillance prevents unnecessary early delivery of a healthy fetus.

**When should the fetus be delivered?**

When fetal maturity is determined
Prematurely, when risk in utero exceeds neonatal risk, i.e., when the fetus appears ill by surveillance techniques

**How is maturity determined?**

By amniotic fluid assay

**How is amniotic fluid assessed?**

Lecithin/sphingomyelin ratio is the standard assessment.
The presence of phosphatidylglycerol is helpful.
Both are assayed by thin-layer chromatography.

**What is the preferred method of delivery?**

Vaginal, although rates of cesarean section are high

**How is labor managed?**

Cervical ripening techniques (prostaglandin) are probably acceptable but are used infrequently.
Oxytocin induction is often used.
Maternal euglycemia can be maintained with insulin/glucose infusion (usually 1–2 units per hour with 125 milliliters of 5% dextrose in Ringer's lactate solution or normal saline).
Frequent blood glucose assays should be performed, with a goal of approximately 100 mg/dL.

**What complications of delivery are associated with diabetes in pregnancy?**

Cephalopelvic disproportion
Shoulder dystocia (while not predictable, anticipation allows preparation)
Trauma

**How should the woman be managed postpartum?**

The patient should return to her preconception insulin dose and hypoglycemia should be avoided.

**What newborn complications can occur?**

Hyperbilirubinemia
Hypoglycemia
Hypocalcemia

**What contraception methods are appropriate for women with diabetes?**

Oral contraceptive pills can be used but with caution and probably not in women with vasculopathy.
The intrauterine device (IUD) is acceptable according to the usual guidelines.
Barrier methods are probably optimal.
Bilateral tubal ligation is acceptable for permanent contraception.

## GESTATIONAL DIABETES MELLITUS

**Because it is asymptomatic, how is gestational diabetes mellitus detected?**

With a modified glucose tolerance test

**How is the modified glucose tolerance test performed?**

A 50-gram (g) oral glucose load is given. Blood is then sampled for glucose measurement 1 hour after the glucose load.

**When is this test usually performed?**

At approximately 28 weeks' gestation

**What is an abnormal blood glucose level result of the modified glucose tolerance test?**

> 135 mg/dL

**Is this result diagnostic of gestational diabetes?**

No

**What test is used to diagnose gestational diabetes?**

Standard glucose tolerance test

**How is this test performed?**

A 100-g glucose load is given after morning fasting. To ensure accurate test results, the patient must be healthy and eating an appropriate diet. Blood samples are taken immediately following the glucose load (fasting value) and at 1, 2, and 3 hours after the glucose load.

**What are the normal values of a glucose tolerance test?**

Fasting: < 105 mg/dL
1 hour: < 190 mg/dL
2 hour < 165 mg/dL
3 hour < 145 mg/dL

**What results are diagnostic of gestational diabetes?**

Abnormal fasting value or two abnormal values in either the 1-, 2-, or 3-hour samples

**What are the risk factors for gestational diabetes?**

Obesity
Age > 30
History of large infant(s)
History of unexplained stillbirth
Ethnicity (American Indians)

**Who should be screened for gestational diabetes?**

Women with risk factors
Some experts advocate universal screening.

**How is gestational diabetes managed?**

Dietary and/or insulin management to achieve euglycemia
Fetal surveillance:
  At term if diet controlled
  At 32 weeks if insulin is required

**What percentage of women with gestational diabetes "become" Type II diabetics?**

Fifty percent if obese and stay that way

**How is diabetes after pregnancy diagnosed?**

With a modified or standard glucose tolerance test at 8 weeks postpartum

# 20

# Obstetrics Infections

## INTRODUCTION

**What are the "TORCH" infections?**

"TORCH" is an acronym for the common nonbacterial congenital infections that can lead to a variety of fetal and neonatal problems.

T = Toxoplasmosis
O = Other [e.g., varicella-zoster virus (VZV), parvovirus, and other organisms]
R = Rubella
C = Cytomegalovirus (CMV)
H = Herpes simplex virus (HSV)

**What is the incidence of TORCH infections?**

Cause disease in about 1% of all births and lead to serious disease in about 10% of infected infants

**What are the characteristic neonatal signs and symptoms of TORCH syndrome?**

Prematurity
Intrauterine growth retardation (IUGR)
Microcephaly
Hepatosplenomegaly with jaundice
Thrombocytopenia
Hemolytic anemia
Chorioretinitis
Adenopathy
Rash

**How are perinatal infections diagnosed?**

By isolating or detecting the organism in question or documenting seroconversion (the presence of antibodies to the organism in question) with one or more of the following tests:
Elevated titers of IgM antibodies to the organism in question (in maternal or fetal blood samples) via enzyme-linked immunosorbent assay (ELISA) or other techniques
Amniocentesis with culture
Chorionic villus sampling with

Southern blotting or polymerase chain reaction (PCR)

Ultrasound in combination with the clinical picture

**What are possible consequences of infection to the fetus and mother?**

Interference with organogenesis with consequent structural anomalies with infection in the first trimester

Neurologic impairment secondary to interference with nervous system development (generally occurs throughout the pregnancy and thus impairment can occur late in pregnancy)

Depression and acidosis at birth

Poor sucking reflex, vomiting, or abdominal distension at birth

Respiratory insufficiency at birth

Lethargy or jitteriness at birth

Hypothermia at birth

Depressed total leukocyte or neutrophil counts at birth

**Via which immunoglobulin does the fetus respond to infection?**

The fetus synthesizes IgM as the primary response to infection.

Development of fetal cell-mediated and humoral immunity begins at 9 to 15 weeks' gestation.

**How does the mother contribute to fetal immunocompetence?**

Maternal IgG passes transplacentally and provides passive immunity.

Transfer of IgG begins at 16 weeks' gestation.

By 26 weeks, $[IgG]_{fetal} = [IgG]_{maternal}$.

**By what routes can the fetus/neonate become infected?**

Some agents (e.g., VZV, rubella, and CMV) move transplacentally to cause intrauterine infection.

Other routes of access include ascending chorioamnionitis (intrauterine), maternal exposure (intrapartum), external contamination (intrapartum), and neonatal human or nosocomial exposure.

## TOXOPLASMOSIS

**What is toxoplasmosis?**

A protozoal infection that can be transmitted from mother to fetus by the organism *Toxoplasma gondii*.

**Where is *Toxoplasma gondii* found?**

In undercooked meat as infective tissue cysts and in cat feces as oocysts, which can become aerosolized

**How is *Toxoplasma gondii* transmitted?**

By ingestion of infected meat or exposure to infected cat feces

**How common is infection in adults and in pregnancy?**

Approximately 15% to 40% of adult women in the United States have toxoplasmosis antibodies (IgG) and, hence, immunity.

About 1 in 1000 pregnancies are affected by acute toxoplasmosis infection.

**How does congenital infection and outcome differ in the first and third trimesters?**

In general, congenital infection in the third trimester is more common, whereas infection in the first trimester is more severe.

Third-trimester infection is associated with a 65% congenital infection rate, with most infections subclinical or mild.

First-trimester infection is associated with a 15% congenital infection rate, but two-thirds of these fetuses have severe symptoms. Five percent of first-trimester infections result in perinatal death or stillbirth.

Second-trimester infection is associated with a 25% risk of transmission.

**What are the maternal signs and symptoms of toxoplasmosis?**

Usually asymptomatic, but careful documentation can reveal a mononucleosis-like syndrome with symptoms such as fever, chills, headache, fatigue, muscle pains, and lymphadenopathy in 60% to 90% of patients.

**What are the fetal and neonatal signs and symptoms of toxoplasmosis?**

The classic triad of hydrocephalus, intracranial calcifications, and chorioretinitis is rarely seen.

Seventy-five percent of infected newborns are asymptomatic at birth.

Twenty-five percent of infected newborns have low birth weight, hepatosplenomegaly, icterus, anemia, convulsions, intracranial calcifications, hydrocephaly or microcephaly, microphthalmia, and chorioretinitis.

**How is toxoplasmosis diagnosed in the mother?**

Toxoplasma antibodies indicate acute disease or prior infection.

Antibodies can be detected using hemagglutination, immunofluorescence, or ELISA techniques.

Anti-toxoplasma IgG antibody titers can be obtained, but cannot differentiate between a prior toxoplasmosis infection (which confers immunity) and an infection acquired during pregnancy (which can pose a threat to the fetus).

High IgG titers suggest recent or current infection, whereas lower titers should be followed to determine if a rise in titer occurs, which suggests active infection (a fourfold increase in IgG titer over 2–3 weeks).

Toxoplasma-specific IgM testing can differentiate acute illness from prior exposure.

**How is toxoplasmosis diagnosed in the fetus?**

Culture and serologic testing of fetal blood and amnionic fluid (cord blood IgM is indicative of fetal infection)

Serial fetal brain ultrasound

PCR assays, which may soon be commonly employed to study amnionic fluid when infection is suspected

Placental culture (positive in 90% of infections)

**How is toxoplasmosis prevented?**

Avoidance of undercooked meat, unpasteurized goat's milk, and cat litter or feces

**How is toxoplasmosis treated?**

Proper antimicrobial therapy: either spiramycin alone or pyrimethamine plus sulfadiazine

**What are the recommendations for prenatal screening of toxoplasmosis?**

Routine prenatal screening of toxoplasmosis is not recommended.

## RUBELLA

**What is rubella and what is another name for the virus?**

Also known as German measles, rubella is caused by a single-stranded RNA togavirus capable of causing severe fetal and neonatal problems.
Infection is not threatening in the nonpregnant state.

**Why is rubella infection so rare today?**

The incidence of rubella in the United States has decreased as a result of a massive vaccination program.

**Is the incidence of congenital rubella syndrome (CRS) increasing or decreasing?**

Data suggest a recent resurgence of cases of CRS from an all-time low of 225 cases in 1988 to annual totals of 1093 cases from 1988 to 1990.

**What may account for this change in incidence?**

Six percent to eleven percent of postpubertal women remain seronegative despite attempts at uniform vaccination, according to premarital screening programs.
Greater than 50% of CRS cases may be caused by missed testing or vaccination opportunities.

**What are the signs and symptoms of maternal rubella infection?**

Rash can be the sole presenting symptom.
The remainder of cases are asymptomatic (25%–50% of infections are subclinical despite viremia and embryo or fetal infection).
Outcomes of maternal infection include normal infant, spontaneous abortion, or CRS.

**What are the signs and symptoms of fetal rubella infection (CRS)?**

Cataracts and other eye problems (chorioretinitis, microphthalmia)
Cardiac malformations (patent ductus arteriosus, septal defects, and pulmonary artery hypoplasia)
Sensorineural deafness (detected after 1 year of age)
Central nervous system (meningoencephalitis, microcephaly, psychomotor retardation, brain calcifications)

Symmetric IUGR
Hematologic problems
(thrombocytopenia, hemolytic anemia)
Hepatic problems (hepatitis,
hepatosplenomegaly, jaundice)
Chronic interstitial pneumonitis
Bony changes
Chromosome abnormalities

**What are the signs and symptoms of childhood rubella infection?**

Panencephalitis and type I diabetes
(extended rubella syndrome) in up to
one-third of infants asymptomatic at
birth
May not develop until second or third
decade of life

**When is maternal rubella infection most likely to result in congenital infection?**

The congenital infection rate with
maternal rash/infection in the first
trimester is 80% to 90%.
The risk of congenital infection at 13 to
14 weeks' gestation is 54%.
The risk of congenital infection by the
end of the second trimester is 25%.

**When is maternal rubella infection most likely to result in congenital defects?**

Infected fetuses are most prone to
develop serious defects from infection
prior to 11 weeks' estimated
gestational age.
Fetuses infected after 13 weeks'
gestation have almost no risk of in
utero defect formation.
No studies have demonstrated
congenital defects when maternal
infection occurred after 20 weeks'
gestation.

**How is rubella diagnosed?**

Diagnosis in the pregnant state is usually
made after the appearance of a rash
with conversion from absent rubella
antibodies to positive titers.
Viremia precedes clinically evident
disease by 1 week.

**What is the temporal relationship between infection and antibody detection?**

Peak antibody titers occur 1 to 2 weeks
after rash or 2 to 3 weeks after viremia.
IgM and IgG antibody titers increase with
rash onset; IgM disappears by 1 to 2
months, whereas IgG is present for life.

**What specific serologic findings are diagnostic of maternal rubella infection?**

Either a fourfold increase in acute and convalescent sera of total of IgG rubella antibody titers over 2 weeks, or the presence of rubella IgM antibody

**What specific serologic findings are diagnostic of maternal rubella infections?**

High IgG antibody titers are present in 15% of the normal population.
Acute IgG titers should be saved and tested later in parallel with convalescent specimen of IgG titers to determine a rise in IgG titer.

**Why is rubella-specific IgM useful in diagnosis of rubella?**

Rubella-specific IgM may distinguish acute rubella from prior immunization or infection (peaks at 7 to 10 days after onset of illness and persists for 4 weeks).

**How are IgG and IgM antibodies quantitated?**

Hemagglutination inhibition
ELISA
Indirect immunofluorescent assays

**How is rubella diagnosed in the fetus?**

Fetal IgM can be detected in cord blood (sensitivity, 98%; specificity, 100% after 22 weeks' gestation)
Amniotic fluid isolation of the virus has been used.
RNA identification via in situ hybridization or PCR is a promising technique to detect rubella.

**When should prenatal diagnosis be undertaken?**

Between weeks 8 and 18 gestation, if infection is suspected
Establishment of a diagnosis is not necessary if infection occurs after midgestation, as fetal complications are rare.

**Does the absence of rubella-specific IgM antibody rule out active infection?**

Absence of IgM does not definitively rule out acute rubella infection.
In the presence of acute infection, it is possible to have a false-negative IgM titer because the antibody may decrease to undetectable before the typical 4-week persistence of antibody.
In women with previously documented rubella-specific antibody presence, a rise in rubella IgG antibody titer in the absence of detectable IgM should

be interpreted as potential symptomatic reinfection and consultation with a clinical virologist or other expert in diagnosis of rubella is warranted.

**Does the presence of rubella-specific IgM antibody rule in active infection?**

False-positive IgM assays, although rare, are possible with indirect assays such as ELISA or indirect fluorescent immunoassay.

Diagnosis of acute rubella infection should be based on the appropriate clinical scenario in conjunction with IgG and IgM testing.

**How is rubella infection screened for and prevented?**

All pregnant women should be screened for rubella immunization at their first prenatal visit and non-immune women should be given the vaccine postpartum.

Non-immune women should be given the live attenuated rubella vaccine at routine medical, gynecologic, and family planning clinic visits and after childbirth and abortion.

Children 12 to 15 months of age should be vaccinated and all school children without record of previous rubella vaccination should be vaccinated.

Infants born with congenital rubella syndrome should be isolated from other infants to prevent spread of rubella.

Because the vaccine contains live, attenuated virus, it cannot be administered shortly before (pregnancy should be delayed for three months after receiving vaccine) or during pregnancy.

**What are the risks of administering rubella vaccine to pregnant women?**

All women with positive rubella-specific antibody documentation prior to pregnancy can be presumed to be immune.

Although there is no proven risk of vaccine administration to pregnant women, this recommendation that pregnant women should not be

vaccinated remains on theoretic
grounds.

**Can women vaccinated
postpartum breast-feed?**

Postpartum vaccination should not
prevent breast-feeding, although vaccine
virus may be excreted in milk and cause
infant seroconversion.

**How is rubella infection
treated?**

There is no known treatment for active
rubella infection.
Abortion can be offered with early
infection.

**What is cytomegalovirus
(CMV)?**

CMV is a member of the DNA
herpesvirus family.
It is a commonly acquired infection in
daycare centers.

**How is CMV transmitted?**

Horizontally by droplets, saliva, and urine
Vertically from mother to fetus (via
transplacental infection, delivery, and
breast-feeding)
Via sexual contact and through blood
transfusions

**How common is CMV?**

It is the most common cause of
perinatal infection (0.5% to 2% of all
neonates).
The risk of seroconversion in susceptible
women during pregnancy is 1% to 4%.
One percent to two percent of all infants
excrete CMV in their urine.
Thirty percent to sixty percent of school-
age children and sixty percent of all
pregnant women are seropositive.

**What important factor
predisposes adults to CMV
infection?**

Risk is increased in
immunocompromised individuals.

**What are the maternal
signs and symptoms of
CMV infection?**

A mononucleosis-like syndrome (fever,
pharyngitis, lymphadenopathy, and
polyarthritis) is present in 15% of
cases.
The remainder of cases are
asymptomatic.
Presentation is not affected by
pregnancy.

**What are the fetal and neonatal signs and symptoms of CMV infection?**

Fetal (cytomegalic inclusion disease): symmetric IUGR, nonimmune hydrops, low birth weight, microcephaly, hydrocephaly, microphthalmia, intracranial calcifications, chorioretinitis, psychomotor retardation, deafness, hepatosplenomegaly, jaundice, hemolytic anemia, and thrombocytopenic purpura

Neonatal: 90% of infected newborns are asymptomatic at birth, but may have later onset of hearing loss, mental retardation, visual impairment, or delayed psychomotor development.

**How often do infected infants manifest evidence of congenital CMV syndrome?**

Congenital cytomegalovirus infection (cytomegalic inclusion disease) leads to syndrome in 10% of 40,000 infected neonates born annually and later onset of hearing loss and intellectual impairment in 10% to 15%.

**How does CMV infection vary with socioeconomic status?**

Approximately 55% of high-income pregnant women are immune to CMV.

Approximately 85% of low-income pregnant women are immune to CMV.

**Why is it important to determine if the infection is primary or recurrent?**

Most congenital infections are acquired from maternal reactivation.

Recurrent infection is associated with a low (.15%–2%) risk of transmission and a small number (.1%) of infants with clinically apparent disease or sequelae.

Primary infection is associated with an approximately 40% to 50% transplacental transmission rate; 10% to 20% of these infants are symptomatic at birth.

High-income women have a high risk of developing primary infection and thus are more susceptible to having infants with clinically apparent disease.

**How is CMV screened for and diagnosed in the mother?**

Primary infection is suggested by fourfold increased IgG titers in paired acute and convalescent sera measured simultaneously.

IgM detection in maternal serum is also generally predictive of primary infection, as IgM is usually not produced in recurrent infection (peaks 3–6 months after infection and disappears in 1 to 2 years).

**How is CMV screened for and diagnosed in the fetus?**

Ultrasound: intracranial calcifications, symmetric IUGR, nonimmune hydrops or ascites and CNS anomalies (nonspecific findings)

Amniotic fluid culture

Total IgM (CMV-specific) and elevated γ-glutamyl transferase by cordocentesis

CMV-specific DNA in chorionic villi (PCR)

CMV-specific IgM may not be a reliable test; amniotic fluid cultures are probably the best test (80%–100% sensitivity) while DNA results show good correlation with cultures and clinical outcome.

**How is CMV infection treated?**

There is no effective treatment for maternal infection, although intrauterine treatment with ganciclovir or other antiviral agents may prove safe and effective.

Abortion is an option.

**How can CMV infection be prevented?**

Serologic screening for CMV during pregnancy is not recommended.

Good hygiene and hand-washing practices, avoidance of kissing and nuzzling infants, and use of latex gloves may prevent transmission among health care workers.

**Can personnel in dialysis and neonatal units work while pregnant?**

There is no evidence that transfer to another unit or to a different patient population decreases the risk of CMV infection.

Compliance with universal precautions should be emphasized.

Routine screening of hospital employees for serologic testing of CMV is not recommended.

## HERPES SIMPLEX VIRUS

**What is herpes simplex virus (HSV)?**

HSV is a herpesvirus and can be either type 1 (HSV-1) or type 2 (HSV-2).

**Approximately what percentage of HSV infections are caused by type 1 and type 2?**

Approximately 85% of primary genital herpes infections in adults are caused by HSV-2 and the remainder by HSV-1. HSV-1 causes most nongenital herpetic infections.

Neonatal infection is more commonly caused by HSV-2 (75%); approximately 25% of isolates from infected neonates are HSV-1.

**What is the incidence of HSV in the general population?**

A national study of serology revealed that 20% of all women have HSV-2 antibodies.

**What are the risk factors for presence of HSV antibodies?**

African-American race
Previous marriage

**How is HSV transmitted?**

Via intimate mucocutaneous contact

**How common is HSV infection in pregnancy?**

HSV infection is thought to have the same frequency in pregnancy as in the nonpregnant state.

Estimates vary from shedding in 0.1% to 0.4% of all deliveries to positive cultures in 0.2% to 7.4% of asymptomatic women.

**Does pregnancy alter the course of HSV infection?**

No

**What is the typical duration of primary versus recurrent HSV outbreaks?**

Primary SHV infections last approximately 2 to 3 weeks.

Recurrent HSV infections have a shorter 5 to 10 day course.

Asymptomatic infections also occur and their course is unknown.

**How does the neonate acquire HSV?**

Proposed mechanisms include the following:
During delivery (passage through infected birth canal)
Prior to delivery [ascending infection (90% of cases), especially with rupture of membranes or via transplacental passage of virus]
After delivery (close contact with an infected mother, relative, or health care worker)

**Does neonatal risk of HSV infection vary in primary versus recurrent HSV?**

Primary infection is associated with 50% transmission to the neonate in vaginal delivery.
Recurrent infection is associated with only a 4% transmission rate.
This difference may be related to virus shedding for 1 to 2 weeks during primary infection compared with 3 to 6 days during recurrent infection, or to the protective effect of maternal antibodies in recurrent infection.
Overall, neonatal herpes occurs in 0.01% to 0.04% of deliveries (two-thirds of which are preterm infants).

**What is the mortality rate of neonatal HSV?**

Approximately 60% in infants infected with HSV delivered vaginally by a mother with a primary outbreak

**What is the incubation period for HSV?**

Prodromal symptoms after primary infection with HSV occur within 3 to 6 days of infection.

**What are the varied maternal signs and symptoms of HSV infection?**

Asymptomatic
Prodrome: tingling, burning, or pruritus in vulvar area
Inguinal adenopathy and flu-like symptoms
Painful vesicular lesions on an erythematous base that eventually ulcerate primarily on the labia minora, but can be found anywhere on the vulva, vagina, or cervix
Urinary retention if pain is significant
Disseminated disease: rare and has a high mortality rate; may result in

hepatitis, thrombocytopenia, coagulopathy, meningitis, and encephalitis

**What complications of pregnancy are associated with HSV infection?**

Spontaneous abortion and preterm labor

**What are the fetal signs and symptoms of HSV infection?**

Death (60% of those infected at vaginal delivery from a mother with primary HSV infection)

Disseminated infection involving major viscera

Sequelae include microcephaly, mental retardation, seizures, microphthalmia, retinal dysplasia, chorioretinitis, meningitis, encephalitis, hypertonicity, apnea, and coma

**How is HSV diagnosed?**

Clinical diagnosis is made by identification of the typical lesion.

Viral isolation by tissue culture is highly accurate, with a sensitivity of 95% and few false-positive results.

Occasionally, the Pap smear report will cite cytopathic effects consistent with HSV, but these effects are not as accurate as direct isolation of the virus.

Likewise, the Tzanck preparation (scrapings from the lesion base) can be used for rapid diagnosis (findings include large multinucleated cells and eosinophilic viral inclusion bodies), but it is not as accurate as viral culture.

Antibodies appear within 7 days of the primary outbreak, peak in 2 to 3 weeks, and remain for life.

ELISA assays are available, but have low sensitivity, and PCR techniques are on the horizon.

**What special tests should be done during prenatal care for women with a history of HSV?**

Weekly surveillance cultures from 36 weeks' gestational age to term and amniocentesis to detect intrauterine infection are currently not recommended because they do not decrease the incidence of neonatal HSV and are not cost-effective.

Current recommendations are to obtain viral cultures of an active lesion on any pregnant woman with a reported history of HSV infection not proven by cultures or with new onset of a characteristic herpetic genital lesion for the first time in pregnancy.

**How are women with a history of HSV managed in labor and delivery?**

Careful internal and external genital examination to rule out the presence of any vulvo-vaginal lesions is extremely important.

Any woman with a lesion in labor or with ruptured membranes should undergo cesarean delivery to decrease the risk of neonatal HSV.

If no lesions are present, culture is not necessary and vaginal delivery is acceptable.

**Should women with ruptured membranes undergo cesarean section?**

This topic is controversial.

The "four hour rule" suggests that if the membranes have been ruptured for more than 4 hours in a woman in whom herpes infection is strongly suspected, cesarean section should not be performed because the fetus has already been exposed to the virus through an ascending route from the vagina into the uterus.

However, practitioners now perform cesarean sections in cases of suspected infection regardless of the duration of membrane rupture because a clear cause–effect relationship between the duration of membrane rupture and neonatal infection has not been established.

**How is HSV infection treated?**

Because herpes virus resides in nerve ganglia, it is currently impossible to be completely "cured" of the virus.

Acyclovir has been used to treat primary HSV infections, recurrent HSV infections, and as prophylaxis against developing recurrent infections.

Because of uncertainty regarding teratogenicity in pregnancy, acyclovir is currently recommended in pregnancy only for life-threatening infections.

Disseminated HSV should be treated with parenteral acyclovir.

Symptoms such as urinary retention or pain may be treated with a Foley catheter or lidocaine gel if needed and may require hospitalization.

## OTHER VIRAL INFECTIONS

### VARICELLA-ZOSTER VIRUS

**What is varicella-zoster virus (VZV)?**

Varicella-zoster virus (VZV) is 1 of 6 human herpesviruses.

It is comprised of double-stranded DNA surrounded by a lipid and protein envelope.

**How is VZV infection transmitted?**

It is highly contagious and is transmitted via household contacts and other routes of exposure (respiratory secretions and droplets, direct contact, indirect contact with secretions).

The attack rate of VZV is 90%.

Enters the host via the conjunctivae and mucosa. Moves into the bloodstream and replaces the skin via capillaries, and finally enters the dorsal root ganglia of sensory nerves where it remains latent.

**What diseases does VZV cause?**

Varicella (chickenpox) and herpes zoster (shingles, a reactivation of the virus)

**How common is chickenpox in general and in pregnancy?**

Chickenpox is the second most commonly reported communicable disease in the United States.

It is uncommon in pregnancy (it occurs approximately 1 in 7500 pregnant women).

Prenatal serology shows that 95% of women in the United States are immune.

**What is the mortality rate of infection in nonpregnant adults?**

Approximately 50/100,000

**What is the incubation period of VZV?**

Ten to twenty-one days

**What are the maternal signs and symptoms of VZV infection in pregnancy?**

Prodrome (2–3 days): fever, malaise, myalgia, arthralgia, and headache

Lesions: initially vesicular and intensely pruritic maculopapular lesions that break open and crust over, causing pustules and scabs on the face, scalp, and trunk

Pneumonia: may develop 1 to 6 days after rash with cough, dyspnea, fever, pleuritic chest pain, hemoptysis; chest x-ray reveals diffuse bilateral infiltrates

Encephalitis: potential complication in infected adults

VZV has been implicated in preterm labor.

**What are the fetal signs and symptoms of VZV infection?**

Can result in asymptomatic seroconversion, congenital varicella syndrome, or neonatal varicella

Congenital varicella syndrome (varicella embryopathy) affects the following systems:

Extremities: hypoplasia or contractures

Skin: cutaneous scars

Eye: chorioretinitis, microphthalmia, cataracts

Central nervous system: cervical or lumbosacral cord involvement, cerebral cortical atrophy, microcephaly

Gastrointestinal system

Genitourinary system: hydronephrosis

Can also cause mental retardation and death

**What are the neonatal signs and symptoms of VZV infection?**

Disseminated visceral and central nervous system disease, which can be fatal if untreated

| | |
|---|---|
| **What is the infection rate of neonates if delivered to a VZV-infected mother?** | Twenty-five percent to fifty percent of neonates are infected.<br>Neonatal infection is possible if the mother develops a rash in the 5 days preceding or 2 days following parturition. |
| **What are typical incubation periods in maternal and neonatal infection?** | Maternal incubation period: 11 to 21 days (mean 15 days)<br>Average incubation period in the neonate: 11 days |
| **When is the fetus most susceptible to maternal VZV infection?** | Twenty-five percent to fifty percent of fetuses are infected during maternal infection with a 2% to 5% risk of congenital varicella syndrome (the risk is 10% if VZV is acquired in the first trimester).<br>Most cases of congenital varicella syndrome result from maternal infection occurring at less than 20 weeks' gestation. |
| **When is the infectious period of VZV infection?** | From 2 days prior to the appearance of the rash until all lesions are crusted |
| **How common is varicella pneumonia in pregnancy and why is it so important?** | It occurs in 10% to 30% of all cases of VZV infection in pregnancy.<br>Mortality rates for varicella pneumonia in pregnancy have been quoted as high as 20% to 40%. |
| **How is VZV diagnosed in the mother?** | Clinical assessment<br>Tzanck prep (multinucleated giant cells with intranuclear inclusions for varicella, zoster, and HSV)<br>Culture: vesicular fluid within 3 to 4 days of appearance of rash (virus grows easily in culture)<br>Fluorescent antibody to membrane antigen of ELISA techniques to determine varicella serology and confirm a prior infection |
| **What are the typical changes in antibody titers in VZV infection?** | IgM rises within 2 weeks of infection.<br>IgG rise in paired sera taken 2 weeks apart indicates infection. |

**How is VZV diagnosed in the fetus?**

Ultrasound (microcephaly, limb deformities, polyhydramnios, liver hyperechogenicities, fetal hydrops)
VZV-specific IgM in fetal cord blood (cordocentesis)
Amniotic fluid culture
CVS with PCR

**How is VZV diagnosed in the neonate?**

Characteristic findings include limb hypoplasia, cutaneous scars, chorioretinitis, cataracts, cortical atrophy, microcephaly, and symmetric IUGR.

**How is VZV infection treated?**

All pregnant women with acute VZV infection require chest x-ray to rule out pneumonia.

Treatment is recommended for maternal infection with visceral involvement (pneumonia or encephalitis) or high fever using acyclovir (12.4 mg/kg or 500 mg/m$^2$ every 8 hours) within 72 hours of rash onset or onset of respiratory symptoms.

Some advocate abortion if desired by the mother in the presence of limb abnormalities on a 20-week ultrasound.

All women without a history of chickenpox should be passively immunized with varicella-zoster immune globulin (VZIG) within 96 hours of an exposure to chickenpox.

Neonates exposed peripartum should receive VZIG and/or acyclovir within 72 hours of birth if born to mothers with infection onset from 5 days before until 2 days after delivery.

Exposed infants should be isolated.

**How can VZV infection be prevented?**

Avoidance of persons known to have chickenpox
Isolation of the affected patient from other pregnant women if hospitalized
Isolation of the neonate from an infected mother
Passive immunization (VZIG) in susceptible patients within 96 hours of a significant exposure

| | |
|---|---|
| **How effective is VZIG in preventing VZV infection?** | Eighty percent of susceptible patients given VZIG remain symptom-free. Eighty-nine percent of susceptible patients not given VZIG have symptoms. Varicella vaccine is a live attenuated virus and should not be given in pregnancy. |

## HUMAN IMMUNODEFICIENCY VIRUS

| | |
|---|---|
| **What is human immunodeficiency virus (HIV)?** | HIV is an RNA retrovirus that uses reverse transcriptase to transcribe DNA from its native RNA. HIV DNA is incorporated into the infected cell's genome. It enters cells via the CD4 antigen. The primary target cells of HIV are the T-helper lymphocytes, but macrophages, CNS neurons, and even placental cells can be infected. |
| **What are risk factors for HIV infection in women?** | Illicit drug abuse (especially IV drug use) Current or previous multiple sexual partners or prostitution Transfusion of blood products prior to 1985 Sexual intercourse with bisexual men or IV drug users Origin in endemic countries (e.g., West Africa) History of or current sexually transmitted diseases (STDs) |
| **What is the significance of the CD4 count?** | The CD4 count is inversely related to the immunocompetence of the HIV-infected individual. The lower the CD4 count, the less cell-mediated immunity and the more likely the risk of acquiring opportunistic infections that attack the immunosuppressed susceptible individual. The Centers for Disease Control (CDC) has designated a CD4 count lower than 200 as one definition of "AIDS." |

**What constitutes the diagnosis of AIDS?**

Serologic evidence of HIV infection and a history of characteristic, ARDS-related opportunistic infections, or Pathognomonic-associated illnesses without serologic evidence of HIV, or A CD4 count of less than 200

**What are some opportunistic infections associated with AIDS?**

Extrapulmonary cryptococcus (i.e., cryptococcal meningitis)
Cryptosporidiosis-associated diarrhea
Disseminated *Mycobacterium avium* complex (MAI)
Tuberculosis
*Pneumocystis carinii* pneumonia (PCP)
Cerebral toxoplasmosis
Disseminated coccidioidomycosis
CMV retinitis
Disseminated histoplasmosis

**What are some neoplasms commonly associated with AIDS?**

Kaposi's sarcoma
Brain lymphoma
Small noncleaved cell lymphoma
Some non-Hodgkin's lymphomas

**What noninfectious, nonmalignant conditions are associated with HIV?**

Progressive multifocal leukoencephalopathy
HIV encephalopathy ("HIV dementia"; "AIDS dementia")
HIV wasting syndrome ("slim disease")

**What serologic tests are used to diagnose HIV infection?**

ELISA testing for HIV antibody (sensitivity > 99%)
Western blot assay for HIV antibody (sensitivity = 99% and specificity = 99.8%); used to confirm a positive ELISA test
"HIV-positive" status requires either two positive ELISA tests followed by a positive Western blot or a positive HIV antigen test or a positive HIV culture.

**What is the "window phase"?**

The time between initial HIV infection and demonstration of antibodies in the blood of the infected individual
The appearance of HIV antibodies typically occurs 6 to 12 weeks after infection, but may take up to 6 months or longer.

**What are the initial signs and symptoms of HIV infection?**

Can be asymptomatic or associated with an acute mononucleosis-like syndrome that may be associated with an aseptic meningitis

**How is HIV virus acquired?**

Through parenteral exposure to blood, sexual activity, and vertical transmission from mother to fetus

**What is the prevalence of HIV in pregnant women?**

A 1990 study suggested 1.5/1000 pregnant women were HIV positive, but this number may be much greater today.

**Is prenatal HIV testing compulsory?**

Prenatal compulsory screening for HIV has not yet been accepted by society.
Some states have laws that require offering HIV testing to all pregnant women and explaining the possible benefits to the patient and her fetus with treatment.
Screening should be offered to all pregnant women.

**How does pregnancy affect HIV-infected patients?**

Pregnancy does not affect disease progression, immune status, or morbidity or mortality rates.
Rates of preterm birth, low-birth–weight neonates, and complications in pregnancy likewise have not been proven to be markedly different in asymptomatic HIV-infected individuals compared with individuals not infected with HIV.

**How is HIV passed from mother to fetus?**

Unknown, but may be transmitted by both transplacental and intrapartum pathways

**What is the perinatal transmission rate of HIV from mother to fetus?**

Maternal–fetal transmission of HIV infection occurs in 25% to 35% of pregnancies.
The transmission rate may be increased in women with low CD4 counts and advanced disease.

**How does zidovudine (ZDV) affect the perinatal transmission rate of HIV?**

A monumental study in 1994 found a 67.5% decrease in risk of HIV transmission from mother to infant with antepartum and intrapartum use of zidovudine.

The 25.5% transmission rate in the placebo group was reduced to 8.3% in the treated group.

Women included in the study had CD4 counts greater than 200 and had not received previous antiretroviral therapy.

ZDV was administered orally from the end of the first trimester until delivery and intravenously during labor and delivery.

Neonates were given ZDV for 6 weeks from 12 hours of life.

**Should cesarean section be performed in HIV-positive women?**

Current evidence does not suggest a benefit in reducing maternal–fetal transmission of HIV by routine cesarean section.

Indications for cesarean should be obstetrical.

**Are scalp monitors, episiotomies, and forcep deliveries appropriate for HIV-positive women?**

Currently, no consensus exits about whether or not scalp monitor placement, episiotomy, or delivery via forceps affects maternal–fetal transmission.

On theoretic grounds, use of these invasive procedures should be limited as much as possible in HIV-infected parturients.

## HEPATITIS VIRUSES

**What are the hepatitis viruses?**

A group of viruses, both DNA and RNA, that cause perturbation of liver function by preferentially invading hepatocytes and causing acute and chronic problems and sometimes death

Responsible for the most common serious liver disease in pregnancy

**How is hepatitis infection diagnosed clinically?**

Symptoms of acute hepatitis include malaise, fatigue, anorexia, nausea and vomiting, headache, and right upper quadrant or epigastric pain.
Physical examination may reveal jaundice, upper abdominal tenderness, and liver enlargement.
Encephalopathy and coagulopathy may be present in severe cases.

**What are common laboratory findings in viral hepatitis?**

Elevated liver aminotransferase (AST and ALT) levels (400–4000 U/L) and elevated serum bilirubin levels (5–20 mg/dl) in acute hepatitis
Coagulation abnormalities and hyperammonemia in severe cases

**What illness associated with pregnancy must be ruled out with liver-associated symptoms?**

Acute fatty liver of pregnancy, a rare condition characterized by nausea, vomiting, malaise, anorexia, epigastric pain, and jaundice and commonly associated with hypertension, proteinuria, edema, and coagulopathy in late pregnancy should always be differentiated from viral hepatitis.
The maternal mortality rate of 25% and fetal mortality rate of 50% in acute fatty liver of pregnancy emphasize the need for proper diagnosis.
Differentiation can be made by serologic studies and liver biopsy (viral hepatitis is characterized by a pattern of extensive hepatocellular injury and inflammatory infiltrate, whereas acute fatty liver of pregnancy causes microvesicular fat deposition) if needed.

## Hepatitis A virus (infectious hepatitis)

**What is hepatitis A virus, how is it transmitted, what is the incubation period, and what is the incidence in pregnancy?**

Hepatitis A virus is an RNA picornavirus and causes approximately one-third of all cases of acute hepatitis in the United States
Transmission: usually via fecal–oral contamination and is increased with poor hygiene, poor sanitation, and intimate contact

Incidence in pregnancy: affects about 1/1000 pregnancies.

**How is hepatitis A diagnosed serologically?**

Hepatitis A virus IgM antibodies
Demonstration of IgG hepatitis A antibodies suggest prior infection.

**How is hepatitis A infection prevented and treated?**

An inactivated hepatitis A vaccine is effective in 97% of cases.
The vaccine appears to be safe for use in pregnancy and should be administered to women with risk factors for infection.
Immunotherapy with hepatitis A virus immune globulin is also used in both nonpregnant and pregnant women, especially those traveling to endemic areas and for postexposure prophylaxis.

**What is the perinatal transmission rate of hepatitis A infection?**

Associated with perinatal transmission

## Hepatitis B virus (serum hepatitis)

**What is hepatitis B virus, how is it transmitted, and what is the incidence in pregnancy?**

Hepatitis B virus is a DNA hepadnavirus that causes approximately 40% of hepatitis cases in the United States.
Transmission: The virus is carried in vaginal secretions, semen, blood, saliva, and breast milk and is transmitted via contact with body secretions; risk factors include IV drug use, sexual promiscuity, and exposure to blood (health care workers, hemodialysis technicians, transfusion recipients), especially in endemic areas (Asia and Africa).
Incidence in pregnancy: occurs in 1 to 2/1000 pregnancies acutely, and 5 to 15/1000 pregnant women are hepatitis B virus carriers in the United States.

**What is the composition of the hepatitis B virus and the associated antigens?**

The hepatitis B virus, also known as the Dane particle, is composed of an outer shell, a middle portion, and the viral genome.

Hepatitis B surface antigen (HBsAg) is found on the outer viral shell, but can also circulate free in the serum and is the first marker of infection.

Hepatitis B core antigen (HBcAg) lies in the middle portion of the Dane particle and is found only in hepatocytes (it does not circulate freely like HBsAg).

Hepatitis B e antigen (HBeAg) has its messenger RNA transcribed on the same part of the genome as the core antigen, and it is found when a significant amount of Dane particle is present in the serum; thus, HBeAg correlates with infectivity.

**How is hepatitis B infection diagnosed serologically?**

Acute infection is diagnosed by an immunoglobin M response to the core antigen (anti-HBc) and the presence of the surface antigen.

Detection of HBeAg in acute infection implies severe infection.

Chronic infection is suggested by detecting HBsAg without an IgM antibody response to the core antigen.

**What is the perinatal transmission rate of hepatitis B virus?**

Women who test positive for the hepatitis B surface antigen have a 10% to 20% risk of transmitting the virus to the fetus in pregnancy.

Ninety percent of women with HBeAg transmit the virus to the fetus.

Ten percent of women infected in the third trimester transmit the virus to the fetus.

**What is the mechanism for fetal and neonatal infection?**

The majority of cases of perinatal transmission are the result of exposure of the fetus during labor to blood and vaginal secretions.

Other mechanisms for infection that occur less frequently include transplacental infection, breast-feeding, and close contact between the neonate and mother.

**What are the maternal effects of hepatitis B infection?**

Death in approximately 1% of cases
Resolution of symptoms and complete recovery in 85% of cases
Chronic infection in 14% of cases
Hepatitis and cirrhosis in about 10% to 30% of persons with chronic infection with persistently high HBeAg levels
Chronic infection is a significant risk factor for hepatocellular carcinoma.

**What are the fetal effects of hepatitis B infection?**

Fulminant hepatitis (rare)
Prematurity, low birth weight, and death
Eighty-five percent to ninety percent become chronic carriers.
Twenty-five percent develop hepatocellular carcinoma and cirrhosis.

**How is hepatitis B infection prevented and treated?**

Hepatitis B virus vaccine is the most effective method to prevent infection and is recommended for high-risk women, especially health care workers.
Vaccine administration is believed to be safe during pregnancy.
Hepatitis B immune globulin (HBIG) should be administered after high-risk contact in the pregnant or nonpregnant state.
All infants should receive hepatitis B vaccine after birth, with the second and third vaccine doses given to the infant at 1 and 6 months of age.
Administration of active (hepatitis B vaccine) and passive (HBIG) immunization within 12 hours of birth to neonates of carrier mothers decreases the perinatal transmission rate by 80% to 90%.
Interferon may also be used to treat acute hepatitis.

**What are current prenatal screening recommendations?**

Both the American College of Obstetrics and Gynecology (ACOG) and the CDC recommend universal hepatitis B screening of pregnant women at an early prenatal visit or at the first opportunity in a woman who presents later in pregnancy or in labor with no prenatal care.

High-risk women should be rescreened in the third trimester if the initial screen is negative.

Liver enzyme (AST and ALT) levels and a hepatitis panel should be tested in women who test positive.

Hepatitis B vaccine should be encouraged in women who test negative and have risk factors for future infection.

## Hepatitis C virus

**What is hepatitis C virus, how is it transmitted, and what is the incubation period?**

Hepatitis C virus is a single-stranded RNA virus of the flaviviridae family; it causes a parenterally transmitted non-A, non-B hepatitis.

It is responsible for 10% to 20% of cases of hepatitis in the United States.

Transmission: transmitted parenterally; risk factors for infection include a history of blood transfusions, use of IV drugs, and sex with an infected partner (transmission is the same as that of hepatitis B)

Incubation period: approximately 15 weeks

**How is hepatitis C diagnosed serologically?**

Demonstration of hepatitis C virus antibody

It is possible for the antibody production to be delayed for 2 to 4 months after the initial hepatitis flare.

**What is the risk of perinatal transmission of hepatitis C?**

Can be transmitted vertically, but the exact incidence is not known.

**How is hepatitis C infection treated?**

With interferon-α

Improvement occurs in 30% to 40% of patients, but relapse occurs in half of these patients.

Newborns can be given immune serum globulin in cases of seropositive mothers, although good data are not available regarding its effectiveness.

## Hepatitis D virus

**What is hepatitis D virus, how is it transmitted, and what is the incidence in pregnancy?**

Hepatitis D (delta) virus is an RNA virus that requires hepatitis B virus infection to exert its effects on the host.

It is composed of a hepatitis B surface antigen and a delta core.

It coinfects about 1 in 4 patients infected with hepatitis B simultaneously.

It can cause superinfection (acute hepatitis D infection in a chronic hepatitis B carrier) with sequelae of chronic hepatitis, cirrhosis, and portal hypertension with a 25% mortality rate.

Transmission: same as that of hepatitis B virus

Incidence: rarely affects pregnancy

**How is hepatitis D infection diagnosed serologically?**

Presence of D antigen in liver tissue or blood and anti-hepatitis D IgM antibody

Chronic infection with hepatitis D is diagnosed with continued D antigen presence in the presence of IgM anti-D antibody.

**How is hepatitis D infection prevented and treated?**

Prevented with vaccination and immune prophylaxis against hepatitis B infection

**Is hepatitis D infection transmitted vertically?**

Can be transmitted vertically in pregnancy

Prevention tactics are the same as those used for hepatitis B (hepatitis B vaccination and immune globulin administration).

## PARVOVIRUS B19

**What is parvovirus B19?**

A single-stranded DNA virus

The only known host of this virus is human beings.

**What disease does parvovirus B19 cause, what are its symptoms, and what is its incubation period?**

Causes erythema infectiosum, or "fifth disease"

Symptoms include a red macular facial rash, trunk rash, flu-like symptoms, and symmetric polyarthralgias (especially the hands)

Twenty percent of infections are asymptomatic.

The incubation period for parvovirus infection is about 1 week.

**How is parvovirus transmitted?**

Can be found in respiratory secretions and is thought to be transmitted via these secretions and hand-to-mouth contact, as well as possibly by infected blood products or transplacentally.

**How is parvovirus infection diagnosed?**

The presence of parvovirus IgM antibodies suggests current infection (IgM antibodies persist for several months) and they appear 2 weeks after infection.

The presence of IgG antibodies suggests a history of parvovirus exposure and immunity in the absence of IgM; they appear 3 weeks after infection.

**How common is parvovirus infection and how often is it transmitted to the fetus?**

Approximately 50% of pregnant women show parvovirus immunity.

About 1% of pregnant women seroconvert to show parvovirus IgG antibodies during pregnancy.

The transmission rate of parvovirus infection during pregnancy is estimated to be 20%.

Parvovirus is most commonly transmitted between 10 to 20 weeks' gestation.

**What are fetal effects of parvovirus infection in pregnancy?**

Associated with spontaneous abortion in the second trimester following maternal first-trimester infection

Also linked to the rare development of nonimmune hydrops fetalis, which can resolve spontaneously or lead to fetal death

Typically, the fetus is not affected by maternal parvovirus infection.

| | |
|---|---|
| **How is parvovirus-associated hydrops treated?** | Intravascular transfusion may have a beneficial effect on parvovirus-associated nonimmune hydrops fetalis. |

## BACTERIAL INFECTIONS

## GROUP B STREPTOCOCCUS

| | |
|---|---|
| **What is group B streptococcus (GBS) and what is its importance in perinatology?** | Group B streptococcus (*Streptococcus agalactiae*) is a bacterium commonly found in the vagina and rectum of pregnant women.<br>It is responsible for more life-threatening neonatal infections than any other organism.<br>It is also a common pathogen in chorioamnionitis and postpartum endomyometritis. |
| **What is the incidence of GBS colonization in pregnancy?** | Estimates for vaginal GBS colonization range from 3% to 30%, depending on the population studied.<br>Most experts agree that approximately 1 in 4 women has vaginal GBS colonization in pregnancy. |
| **Where does colonization occur?** | Primarily occurs in the rectum, with secondary genitourinary (bladder, vagina, and cervix) colonization; colonization of the throat and skin also occurs in healthy women |
| **What are the signs and symptoms of maternal GBS colonization?** | Usually asymptomatic |
| **What are the maternal–fetal transmission rates of GBS?** | Range from 35% to 70%<br>Heavily colonized women are at greater risk of transmission.<br>It is important to differentiate fetal colonization (the presence of GBS without ill effects) from fetal infection (outlined as follows) |
| **What are the fetal effects of GBS infection?** | GBS infection in the neonate can lead to respiratory distress, neonatal sepsis, pneumonia, meningitis, shock, and death. |

The mortality rate of early-onset (within 7 days of birth) infections is approximately 15%.

Thirty percent of infants with early-onset GBS sepsis and eighty percent of infants with late-onset GBS sepsis develop meningitis.

One-third of survivors of neonatal meningitis have long-term neurodevelopmental sequelae.

The majority of early-onset neonatal infections are diagnosed within 6 hours of birth.

**What are the fetal effects of fetal GBS colonization?**

Preterm infants colonized with GBS have a 10% risk of developing sepsis; sepsis causes 90% of deaths reported from this disease.

Term infants colonized with GBS have only a 1% to 2% risk of sepsis.

**What are the attack rates and modes of transmission of early-onset versus late-onset neonatal GBS infection?**

Early-onset neonatal sepsis:
  Attack rate: 1.8/1000 live births
  Transmission: primarily via colonization at birth
Late-onset neonatal sepsis:
  Attack rate: 0.5–1/1000 live births
  Transmission: via intrapartum exposure (50%) and nosocomial or community exposure

**What are the maternal effects of GBS colonization?**

Can lead to GBS infection with chorioamnionitis, endomyometritis (20% of all cases, with onset within 48 hours of delivery and typical fulminant course), wound infection, and early postpartum febrile morbidity

Heavy colonization of the genitourinary tract increases the risk of infection for both the mother and fetus.

Presence of GBS in the urine implies heavy vaginal colonization, which increases the rate of neonatal infection to 10/1000 live births.

**How is GBS colonization diagnosed?**

Culture and latex agglutination or ELISA identification of the characteristic polysaccharide antigen

Cultures are accurate, but time-
consuming and thus are not suitable for
immediate decision making in labor
and delivery

Rapid immunoassays appear inadequate
for intrapartum detection of GBS as
they are limited by low sensitivities.

**How are cultures
performed for GBS?**

It is not necessary to culture samples
from the cervix.

The lower vagina and rectum should
both be swabbed and the swab placed
in a selective culture medium.

**What are the risk factors
for neonatal GBS
infection?**

GBS colonization with each of the
following:

Preterm labor (< 37 weeks)

Preterm premature rupture of the
membranes (< 37 weeks)

Prolonged rupture of the membranes
(> 18 hours)

Sibling affected by symptomatic GBS
infection

Maternal fever during labor

**What is the rationale for
intrapartum antibiotic
prophylaxis against GBS?**

Neonatal GBS infection can have grave
consequences (15% mortality rate;
33% risk to long-term
neurodevelopmental problems after
meningitis).

The attack rate is increased tenfold in
neonates born to mothers with
perinatal vaginal colonization.

Group B streptococcus is the most
prevalent cause of serious neonatal
infection.

Intrapartum antibiotic use decreases the
risk of early-onset GBS disease by
thirtyfold.

Antibiotics are inexpensive and have few
side effects.

**What are current
recommendations
regarding GBS prevention
in neonates from ACOG,
the CDC, and by the
American Academy of
Pediatrics (AAP)?**

Clinical risk-factor strategy: intrapartum
antibiotic use for women with risk
factors including preterm labor,
preterm premature rupture of the
membranes, prolonged rupture of the
membranes, previous child with GBS
disease, GBS bacteriuria in the

current pregnancy or maternal fever
(T ≥ 38° C), with the stipulation that
patients may request cultures at 35 to
37 weeks' gestation

Culture-based strategy: intrapartum
antibiotic use based on late prenatal
culture (35–37 weeks' gestation) as
the primary risk determinant;
antibiotics given with positive cultures
or if the mother has had a previous
infant with invasive GBS disease, GBS
bacteriuria in the current pregnancy,
or preterm delivery

One of the above strategies (culture-
based or clinical risk-factor strategy)
should be chosen and consistently
used.

**What is the drug of choice
for chemoprophylaxis of
GBS?**

Intravenous penicillin G, 5 million units
initially followed by 2.5 million units
every 4 hours

Ampicillin is an acceptable alternative
and is given as an initial 2-g dose
followed by 1 g every 4 hours.

## LISTERIA MONOCYTOGENES

**What is *Listeria
monocytogenes*?**

A gram-positive aerobic rod found in
soil, water, sewage, unpasteurized milk
or milk products, and carrier animal (pig
and chicken) feces

**How is *Listeria* transmitted
and what is the incidence
of infection?**

Listeria can be transmitted via food
products including cabbage,
pasteurized milk, and fresh Mexican-
style cheese.

Vertical transmission from mother to
fetus occurs via transplacental passage,
intrapartum, and via ascending
infection.

Listeriosis affects 2 to 3 million people
annually.

**What are the maternal
signs and symptoms of
*Listeria* infection?**

Asymptomatic

A general febrile illness that can be
confused with the flu or
pyelonephritis, usually mild and self-
limited

|  | Can be associated wtih preterm labor, chorioamnionitis (murky brown amniotic fluid), and spontaneous abortion |
|---|---|

**What are the signs and symptoms of *Listeria* infection?**

Stillbirth
Respiratory infection and pneumonitis
Sepsis and disseminated infection
Granulomatous lesions with microabscesses
Meningitis, conjunctivitis, and skin rash

**What is the mortality rate of neonatal listeriosis and how is late-onset disease manifest?**

The neonatal mortality rate for listeriosis has been estimated at 50%.
Late-onset disease is characterized by meningitis about 1 month after delivery.

**How is *Listeria* screened for and diagnosed?**

Listeria is relatively rare in pregnancy and does not have a characteristic clinical presentation; thus, it is often difficult to diagnose.
It is often diagnosed via blood or other cultures (with selective media) sent with a high index of suspicion in a pregnant patient.
It should be suspected in the presence of an unusual illness in a pregnant woman.
Women who ingest contaminated food should have vaginal, rectal, stool, cerebrospinal fluid (CSF), urine, and blood cultures.

**How is *Listeria* infection treated?**

Either ampicillin and gentamicin or Bactrim in penicillin-allergic patients

## SEXUALLY TRANSMITTED DISEASES

### SYPHILIS

**What is *Treponema pallidum*?**

*Treponema pallidum* is the spirochete responsible for causing the chronic infection known as syphilis.
Venereal Disease Research Laboratory (VDRL) and rapid plasma reagin (RPR) tests nonspecific antibodies and have good sensitivity 4 to 6 weeks after infection but lack specificity.

The fluorescent treponemal antibody absorption test (FTA-ABS) and the microhemagglutination assay for antibodies to *Treponema pallidum* (MHA-TP) are specific tests that confirm a positive VDRL or RPR test.

**What are recommendations for screening in pregnancy?**

Screening for syphilis in pregnancy is required by law.
CDC recommend an additional screening in the third trimester in women at high risk for syphilis infection.

**What are risk factors for syphilis in pregnancy?**

Include drug abuse (especially crack use) and lack of prenatal care
Syphilis appears to be increasing in incidence in both

**What is the transmission rate for syphilis in pregnancy?**

Fifty percent to eighty percent; occurs transplacentally

**What are the effects of *Treponema pallidum* on pregnancy and on the fetus/neonate?**

Infection in pregnancy has been linked to preterm labor, fetal death, and neonatal infection via transplacental or intrapartum transmission.
Early congenital syphilis is characterized by infection of fetal organs, which leads to marked hepatomegaly, ascites, nonimmune hydrops, anemia and thrombocytopenia, skin lesions, rash, osteitis and periostitis, pneumonia and hepatitis and is associated with a 50% perinatal mortality rate.
Late congenital syphilis (after 2 years of age) causes dental abnormalities, saber shins, nasal septum destruction, interstitial keratitis, cranial nerve VIII deafness, and failure to thrive.
The placenta becomes large and pale with a decrease in the number of blood vessels.

**How is *Treponema pallidum* treated in pregnancy?**

Penicillin is used to treat syphilis; treatment is aimed at maternal cure and prevention of congenital syphilis.

Benzathine penicillin G is the CDC drug of choice and use of alternative nonpenicillin therapy is discouraged with recommendations for penicillin desensitization and subsequent penicillin treatment.

Follow-up VDRL or RPR titers should be obtained.

Infants symptomatic for syphilis, seropositive for syphilis, or with CSF studies suggestive of infection should also be treated with penicillin.

## GONORRHEA

**What is *Neisseria gonorrhoeae* and how is it detected?**

The causative organism of gonorrhea infection

It is detected via an endocervical swab, which can be used for DNA probe analysis or culture on selective media (e.g., Thayer-Martin medium)

**To what drug is the organism resistant?**

Penicillin and tetracycline

**What are the effects of *Neisseria gonorrhoeae* on pregnancy?**

Has been linked to septic spontaneous abortion, stillbirth, preterm delivery, premature rupture of the membranes, chorioamnionitis, postpartum infection, first-trimester pelvic inflammatory disease [(PID); rare], and maternal disseminated gonorrhea

Maternal disseminated disease can lead to gonococcal arthritis, dermatitis, endocarditis, and meningitis.

Fetal infection occurs in 25% to 50% of cases in pregnancy if not treated.

Neonatal gonococcal ophthalmia, sepsis, and arthritis may result.

**How is *Neisseria gonorrhoeae* treated in pregnancy?**

High penicillin resistance in Neisseria strains mandates treatment with ceftriaxone or spectinomycin.

Erythromycin or azithromycin should also be prescribed if chlamydia cultures are not performed due to high coincidence of infection with chlamydia.

Infants should all be given prophylactic ophthalmic erythromycin or silver nitrate to prevent possible blindness from gonococcal ophthalmia neonatorum.

## CHLAMYDIA

**What is *Chlamydia trachomatis* and how is its presence diagnosed?**

An obligatory intracellular bacterium that attaches to columnar or transitional cell epithelium

It is the most common sexually transmitted bacteria in the United States.

Diagnosis is made with culture on selective media (cycloheximide-treated McCoy cells), rapid antigen detection, or DNA probe analysis.

**What are risk factors for chlamydia infection?**

Age less than 20 years
Unmarried status
Inner-city population
Multiple sexual partners
History or presence of other sexually transmitted diseases

**What are the effects of *Chlamydia trachomatis* on pregnancy?**

Most cases are asymptomatic.

Mothers can have chlamydial cervicitis, urethritis, proctitis, salpingitis (rare), or conjunctivitis.

Neonates manifest infection primarily as conjunctivitis, pneumonitis, and otitis media.

Links have been suggested to antepartum chlamydia infection and preterm labor, premature rupture of membranes, increased perinatal mortality, and late postpartum endometritis.

**How is *Chlamydia trachomatis* treated in pregnancy?**

Pregnant women should be treated with erythromycin or azithromycin to prevent teratogenic consequences of tetracycline-based therapy (fetal teeth and long bone anomalies).

Should receive erythromycin ophthalmic ointment or silver nitrate drops to treat chlamydial conjunctivitis/ophthalmia neonatorum.

# 21

# Neurologic Disorders in Pregnancy

| | |
|---|---|
| **In general, how does pregnancy affect preexisting neurological disease?** | Most neurologic disorders are compatible with normal pregnancy. Pregnancy seldom exacerbates neurologic disease. |

## USE OF NEUROLOGIC IMAGING TECHNIQUES DURING PREGNANCY

| | |
|---|---|
| **Is computed tomography (CT) safe to use during pregnancy?** | Yes, with appropriate abdominal shielding |
| **When is CT is most useful?** | To evaluate acute intracerebral hemorrhage |
| **Is magnetic resonance imaging (MRI) safe to use during pregnancy?** | Because MRI does not employ radiation, it has no known fetal risk. |
| **When is MRI most useful?** | To diagnose atrioventricular malformations, posterior fossa lesions, and spinal cord disease |
| **Is angiography safe to use during pregnancy?** | Can be used if necessary, with shielding of the abdomen |
| **Is positron emission tomography (PET) safe to use during pregnancy?** | No, because PET uses radioisotopes |

## SEIZURE DISORDERS

| | |
|---|---|
| **What is the prevalence of seizure disorders in pregnancy?** | Four in every 1000 pregnancies |

| | |
|---|---|
| **For each type of seizure disorders, give its distribution (in percentages) in pregnancy.** | Complex partial: 60%<br>Generalized tonic–clonic: 30%<br>Petit mal (absence): 5% |
| **What causes seizure disorders?** | Injury<br>Structural lesion<br>Drugs<br>Biochemical<br>Idiopathic |
| **Does pregnancy worsen seizures?** | No |
| **Is pregnancy outcome adversely affected by seizure disorders?** | Some data indicate increases in:<br>   Pregnancy-induced hypertension<br>   Preterm delivery<br>   Low-birth–weight infants<br>   Cerebral palsy<br>   Seizure disorders in children<br>   Mental retardation<br>   Congenital anomalies |
| **How should management of seizures be changed when the patient is pregnant?** | Drug use should be minimized but must be effective. |
| **For each of the following seizure medications, list the possible adverse effects in pregnancy:**<br>   **Phenytoin** | Interferes with vitamin K-dependent clotting factors and contributes to impaired clotting mechanism in the newborn<br>May cause craniofacial anomalies, although it is not clear whether these abnormalities result from the drug or the seizure disorder |
| **Carbamazepine** | Associated with a 1% risk of neural tube defect |
| **Phenobarbital** | Has not been associated with anomaly |
| **Valproic acid** | Associated with a 2% risk of neural tube defect |

## CEREBROVASCULAR DISEASE

| | |
|---|---|
| **What percentage of maternal deaths are caused by cerebrovascular accident?** | Ten percent |
| **Are ischemic or hemorrhagic strokes more commonly associated with pregnancy?** | Hemorrhagic |
| **What condition is associated with thrombotic stroke during pregnancy?** | The presence of lupus anticoagulant |
| **What two conditions are associated with hemorrhagic strokes during pregnancy?** | Hypertension or atrioventricular malformation |

## MIGRAINE HEADACHES

| | |
|---|---|
| **What is the definition of migraine headache?** | Periodic, hemicranial, throbbing headaches usually accompanied by nausea, paresthesia, and scotomata |
| **Does pregnancy influence incidence or severity?** | Yes; both commonly improve |
| **Can ergot derivatives be used during pregnancy?** | No |
| **Can beta-blockers and calcium channel–blockers be used during pregnancy?** | Yes |
| **Can sumatriptan be used in pregnancy?** | The safety of sumatriptan during pregnancy has not been evaluated. |

## MULTIPLE SCLEROSIS

| | |
|---|---|
| **Does multiple sclerosis worsen during pregnancy?** | Yes, in 10% of affected women |
| **Does multiple sclerosis impair pregnancy outcome?** | No |

**Can epidural anesthesia be used in women with multiple sclerosis?**   Yes

## MYASTHENIA GRAVIS

**Does pregnancy affect the course of myasthenia gravis?**   Yes. Myasthenia gravis worsens in one-third of affected women and improves in two-thirds of women.

**Is magnesium sulfate contraindicated?**   Yes, except under extreme circumstances

**What neonatal problems may occur as a result of myasthenia gravis during pregnancy?**   Fifteen percent have neonatal muscle function impairment.

## NEUROPATHIES

**Does the incidence of Bell's palsy increase during pregnancy?**   Yes

**What is the incidence of carpal tunnel syndrome during pregnancy?**   Twenty-five percent of women have some symptoms of median nerve compression.

**What serious complication of cord injury is especially important in pregnancy?**   Autonomic dysreflexia

**What circumstances trigger this complication?**   Labor and bladder or bowel distention

**What consequence of this complication is extremely dangerous to the mother and fetus?**   Hypertension

# Section II

## Gynecology

# 22

## Gynecologic Glossary

**Abdominal Incisions**

The abdominal incision may be either vertical or transverse.

Cherny: the rectus bellies are dissected off pubic symphysis

Mayllard-transverse: divides the rectus bellies horizontally to increase the diameter of the incision

Midline-vertical: used most commonly in gynecologic oncology to allow access to the upper abdomen

Pfannenstiel (low transverse): most common for cesarean section; performed approximately two fingerbreadths above the pubic symphysis

**Adenomyosis**

Endometrial tissue within the myometrium

**Adnexa**

The fallopian tubes, ovaries, and other structures attached to the uterus

**Adrenarche**

Normal development of axillary and pubic hair as a result of increases in 17-ketosteroids, dehydroepiandrosterone (DHEA), and dehydroepiandrosterone sulfate (DHEA-S)

**Barr bodies**

One less than the number of X chromosomes in a cell

**Bartholin gland**

Vulvar-vaginal glands located at both sides of the fourchette; analogous to the bulbourethral glands in the male

**Blighted ovum**

Gestational sac with diameter > 3 cm with absence of fetal pole

| | |
|---|---|
| **Culdocentesis** | Diagnostic maneuver in which the peritoneal cavity is entered through the posterior cul-de-sac; used in the diagnosis of pelvic inflammatory disease and ectopic pregnancy |
| **Curettage** | Scraping of the uterine lining (endometrium); used diagnostically in the event of bleeding to evaluate pathology and therapeutically after abortions to remove products of conception |
| **Danazol** | Derivative of 17-ethinyl testosterone used to create a "pseudomenopause" in endometriosis therapy |
| **D&C** | Dilation and curettage |
| **Dysmenorrhea** | Pain with menstrual periods |
| **Dyspareunia** | Pain with intercourse<br>Multiple etiologic factors, including psychosocial, secondary to endometriosis, scar tissue from obstetric trauma, and sexual dysfunction |
| **Decidua basalis** | Area of endometrium that separates the placenta from the myometrium and maintains the embryo during early pregnancy |
| **Ectopic pregnancy** | Any pregnancy located outside of the uterine cavity |
| **Endometriosis** | Condition in which endometrial glands are located outside the uterine cavity |
| **ERT** | Estrogen replacement therapy; also known as hormone replacement therapy |
| **Fibroid (leiomyoma)** | Common benign muscle cell tumors that occur in approximately 50% of African-American women and 25% of white women; associated symptoms include bleeding, pain, dyspareunia, dysuria, premature labor, and infertility |

| | |
|---|---|
| **Fitz-Hugh–Curtis syndrome** | Perihepatic adhesions most often secondary to chlamydia or gonorrhea infection |
| **FSH** | Follicle-stimulating hormone |
| **GnRH** | Gonadotropin-releasing hormone |
| **HPV** | Human papillomavirus |
| **HSG** | Hysterosalpingogram |
| **Hysteroscopy** | Fiberoptic evaluation of the endometrial cavity |
| **Imperforate hymen** | Occlusion of the outflow tract of the vagina; possible cause of primary infertility, and may be associated with hematocolpos (vaginal cavity filled with blood) |
| **IUD** | Intrauterine device used for contraception |
| **Kallmann syndrome** | Inappropriate GnRH secretion that may be associated with anosmia; a cause of primary amenorrhea |
| **Kleinfelter syndrome** | 47XXY male; associated with tall stature, mental retardation, small testes, decreased testosterone, and increased FSH and LH |
| **Koilocytosis** | Cellular changes associated with HPV infection consisting of perinuclear cavitation |
| **Krukenberg tumor** | Metastatic signet-ring cell ovarian tumor; primary tumor located in gastrointestinal tract; other locations include breast, cervix, and bladder |
| **Laparoscopy** | Fiberoptic evaluation of the peritoneal cavity |
| **Laparotomy** | Surgical entry into the peritoneal cavity |

**LH**                    Luteinizing hormone

**Meigs' syndrome**       Benign ovarian tumor, most likely an
                          ovarian fibroma; also associated with
                          ascites and pleural effusions

**Menarche**              Onset of menses

**Menopause**             Cessation of menses secondary to
                          ovarian failure or removal
                          The perimenopausal period is associated
                          with other complaints, such as
                          insomnia, mood swings, fatigue,
                          forgetfulness, depression, and hot
                          flushes

**Mittelschmerz**         "Middle pain"; abdominal pain
                          associated with ovulation

**Necrotizing fasciitis** Anaerobic infection that affects the
                          underlying layers of fascia; occurs most
                          commonly in diabetic patients with
                          perineal infections

**OCP**                   Oral contraceptive pill

**Pap**                   Papanicolaou smear (cervical cytology)
                          used as a screening test for cervical and
                          uterine malignancy

**PID**                   Pelvic inflammatory disease

**PCO**                   Polycystic ovary

**POF**                   Premature ovarian failure

**Premarin**              PREgnant MARe urINe; a form of
                          estrogen most commonly used for
                          hormone replacement therapy

**Provera**               Medroxyprogesterone acetate

**Puberty**               Physical changes and sexual maturation
                          occurring as a result of the maturation
                          of the hypothalamic–pituitary axis and its
                          effects on the gonads

**RKH**

Rokitansky-Küster-Hauser syndrome; also called Mayer-Rokitansky-Küster-Hauser syndrome; uterovaginal agenesis leading to amenorrhea

**Spinnbarkeit**

Clinical test performed on cervical mucus to evaluate the degree of estrogenization

**Stein-Leventhal syndrome**

Polycystic ovary syndrome

**Tanner staging**

Tanner defined five stages of breast and pubic hair development
Refer to Chapter 34

**Testicular feminization**

Androgen insensitivity (male pseudohermaphrodite) XY karyotype; characterized by blind vaginal canal, absent uterus, primary amenorrhea, and the presence of male gonads

**Thelarche**

Onset of development of breast tissue

**TOA**

Tubo-ovarian abscess

**Vaginitis**

Inflammation of vaginal mucosa due to infection, contact or chemical irritation, or atrophy

**Vaginismus**

Involuntary constriction of the outer muscles of the vagina, which can lead to sexual dysfunction and dyspareunia

# 23

# Gynecologic Infections

## INFECTIONS OF THE LOWER GENITAL TRACT

### ACUTE URETHRAL SYNDROME AND BACTERIAL CYSTITIS

**What are the three classic symptoms?**

Dysuria, frequent urination, and urinary urgency

**Diagnosis?**

Pelvic exam to rule out dysuria secondary to vulvovaginitis
Urinalysis
Urine culture with antibiotic sensitivities

**How is acute urethral syndrome differentiated from bacterial cystitis?**

Acute urethral syndrome: Dysuria, urinary frequency, and $< 10^2$ organisms/ml
Bacterial cystitis: Dysuria and $> 10^2$ organisms/ml

**What is the most common cause of acute urethral syndrome?**

*Chlamydia trachomatis*

**What is the treatment for acute urethral syndrome?**

Seven days of a tetracycline

**What are the most common organisms that cause cystitis?**

*Escherichia coli*, *Klebsiella* sp, *Pseudomonas* sp, and *Proteus* sp

**What is the treatment for bacterial cystitis?**

Single dose or 3-day course of:
    Trimethoprim–sulfamethoxazole
    Nitrofurantoin
    Amoxicillin or ampicillin
    First-generation cephalosporin
    Ciprofloxacin
Phenazopyridine hydrochloride (Pyridium) may be used as a urinary analgesic

## INFECTIONS OF THE BARTHOLIN GLANDS

**Where are the Bartholin glands located?**

At the vaginal introitus at 5 and 7 o'clock
Normally not palpable

**What are the three main causes of clinical enlargement?**

1. Cystic dilatation: Usually due to continued secretion of glandular fluid after duct obstruction
2. Abscess: Also follows duct obstruction and is often polymicrobial
3. Adenocarcinoma (rare)

**What are the differential diagnoses?**

Mesonephric cyst, epithelial inclusion cysts, lipoma, fibroma, hydrocele

**Diagnosis of Bartholin gland cyst?**

Usually asymptomatic and found on exam

**Treatment?**

Excision in older women to rule out cancer

**Diagnosis of Bartholin gland infection?**

Presents with acute vulvar pain and dyspareunia

**Treatment?**

Simple incision and drainage are associated with a high rate of recurrence. If true abscess has not yet developed, treat with antibiotics and soaks. If abscess is present, marsupialization creates a permanent opening and prevents recurrence.

## PARASITES

**Describe two parasitic conditions associated with gynecologic symptoms.**

1. Pediculosis pubis: Infestation by the crab louse, *Phthirus pubis*
2. Scabies: Infestation by the itch mite, *Sarcoptes scabiei*

**What are the symptoms of pediculosis pubis and scabies?**

Constant itching, particularly over the mons pubis
Scabies symptoms are often worse at night

**How are pediculosis pubis and scabies diagnosed?**

Visualization of the eggs (nits), excreta, or parasite itself

| | |
|---|---|
| **What are the treatments for pediculosis pubis and scabies?** | Permethrin (Nix Cream) or lindane (Kwell) |

## MOLLUSCUM CONTAGIOSUM

| | |
|---|---|
| **What is molluscum contagiosum and its cause?** | An asymptomatic, benign skin disease of the vulva caused by the poxvirus |
| **What are the signs of molluscum contagiosum?** | Characteristic lesions are small nodules or papules, 1–5 mm in diameter, with an umbilicated center. |
| **What are the treatments for molluscum contagiosum?** | Excision, cryosurgery, or electrocautery of lesions |

## CONDYLOMA ACUMINATUM

| | |
|---|---|
| **What is condyloma acuminatum?** | Genital warts<br>The most common sexually transmitted disease |
| **What is the cause of condyloma acuminatum?** | The highly contagious human papillomavirus |
| **What areas are affected?** | Vulva, vagina, perineum, anus, and cervix |
| **What lesions are associated with condyloma acuminatum?** | Pedunculated, warty excrescences |
| **What is the characteristic cell on Pap smear?** | The koilocyte, a cell with a perinuclear clearing or halo |
| **Why is colposcopy important after the finding of the characteristic cell on Pap smear?** | Koilocytosis is often associated with atypia and dysplasia. |
| **What are the treatment options for condyloma acuminatum?** | Small, external lesions: Topical podophyllin, trichloroacetic acid, or 5-fluorouracil<br>Cryotherapy, electrocautery, or laser therapy |

## GENITAL HERPES

| | |
|---|---|
| **What is the cause of genital herpes?** | The highly contagious herpes simplex virus (HSV)<br>HSV type II is more common than HSV type I as a cause of genital herpes. |
| **What is the incubation period of HSV?** | Two to seven days |
| **What are the duration and symptoms of primary infection with HSV?** | Duration: About 10 days<br>May be accompanied by systemic symptoms of malaise and fever<br>Lesions:<br>  Multiple vesicles that may coalesce and become superficial ulcers<br>  Associated with severe vulvar pain and exquisite tenderness<br>  Often simultaneously involves the vagina and cervix<br>  Possible urinary retention secondary to vulvar pain<br>  Often associated with inguinal adenopathy<br>Fifty percent of infected people never experience the "typical primary outbreak" and are thus unaware that they harbor this virus. |
| **How is the diagnosis of genital herpes made?** | Physical examination: Typical appearance of vesicles and ulcers<br>History: Typical clinical syndrome<br>Cytologic smear and culture of lesions: High rate of false-negative results, depending on the activity of the lesion |
| **What are the characteristics of recurrences?** | Less severe and shorter in duration than primary infection<br>Vary widely in incidence; the virus lies dormant in S2, S3, and S4 nerve roots between recurrences.<br>Viral shedding may occur for several weeks after lesions appear. |
| **What is the treatment for genital herpes?** | Oral acyclovir can reduce viral shedding and shorten the clinical course.<br>Severe cases may require intravenous (IV) acyclovir, especially if patient is immunocompromised. |

Oral acyclovir for prophylaxis is used if frequent episodes occur. Therapeutic procedures include sitz baths and vulvar rinses with Burow solution.

## GRANULOMA INGUINALE

**What is granuloma inguinale?**

Chronic, ulcerative infection of the vulva
The lesion is a painless nodule that progresses to a beefy-red ulcer.
It is uncommon in the United States and more frequent in the Caribbean.

**What is the cause of granuloma inguinale?**

The bacterium *Calymmatobacterium granulomatis*

**What is the classic diagnostic finding?**

The lesion smear shows Donovan bodies, deep-staining bacteria with a bipolar appearance resembling a safety pin.

**What is the treatment for granuloma inguinale?**

Oral tetracycline

## LYMPHOGRANULOMA VENEREUM (LGV)

**What is LGV?**

Chronic infection of lymphatic tissue in the genital region, including the vulva, urethra, rectum, or cervix
Rarely seen in the United States except in the tropical areas

**What is the cause of LGV?**

*C. trachomatis*

**What are the three phases of infection?**

Primary infection: Shallow, painless ulcer on labia
Secondary:
  Painful adenopathy in inguinal and perirectal areas
  If untreated, buboes (matted nodes that adhere to overlying skin) form.
  Classic sign is the double genitocrural fold or "groove sign."
Tertiary: Rupture of bubo, leading to formation of multiple sinuses/fistulas

| | |
|---|---|
| **How is the diagnosis of LGV made?** | Polymerase chain reaction for *C. trachomatis* DNA obtained by swab from lesion |
| **What is the treatment for LGV?** | Oral tetracycline or erythromycin for 2–3 weeks |

## CHANCROID

| | |
|---|---|
| **What is chancroid?** | Acute, ulcerative disease of the vulva Typically, a painful ulcer with ragged edges Solitary or multiple lesions |
| **What causes chancroid?** | *Haemophilus ducreyi* |
| **How is a diagnosis of chancroid made?** | Gram stain shows classic streptobacillary chains. |
| **What is the treatment for chancroid?** | Oral trimethoprim–sulfamethoxazole or erythromycin |

## SYPHILIS

| | |
|---|---|
| **What is the cause of syphilis?** | *Treponema pallidum* |
| **How is a diagnosis of syphilis made?** | Definitive: Dark-field microscopy reveals spirochetes. |
| **What serologic screening tests are available?** | Nonspecific: Venereal Disease Research Laboratory (VDRL) test and rapid plasma reagin (RPR) test Easy and cheap to perform High rate of false-positive results Must confirm with specific test Specific: FTA-ABS (fluorescent-labeled *Treponema* antibody absorption) MHA TP (microhemagglutination assay for antibodies to *T. pallidum*) HATTS (hemagglutination treponemal test for syphilis) |

**What are the three clinical phases of syphilis?**

Primary: Hard chancre or painless ulcer
Secondary: Hematogenous dissemination
causing systemic disease
Classic rash of red macules and
papules on palms and soles of feet
Condyloma latum, or large, raised,
gray areas on vulva or other mucous
membranes
Latent phase ranges from 2 to 20
years.
Tertiary: Optic atrophy, tabes dorsalis,
paresis, aortic aneurysm, gummas
(necrotic abscesses) of skin and bone

**What is the treatment for syphilis?**

Lumbar puncture for women with
syphilis of > 12 months' duration to
rule out neurosyphilis
Penicillin:
Drug of choice
Different regimens for different stages
of syphilis
Tetracycline: For patients allergic to
penicillin
Pregnant patients:
Penicillin regimen appropriate for
stage
Skin testing and desensitization if
patient has a history of penicillin
allergy

## BACTERIAL VAGINOSIS (NONSPECIFIC VAGINITIS)

**What is bacterial vaginosis?**

A symbiotic infection of anaerobic
bacteria and *Gardnerella vaginalis*

**What are the symptoms of bacterial vaginosis?**

Presenting symptom: Vaginal odor
described as "fishy" or "musty"
Discharge: Thin and grayish white
without associated vulvar irritation,
pH > 5, amine-like odor when mixed
with potassium hydroxide (KOH;
positive whiff test)

**How is bacterial vaginosis diagnosed?**

A saline wet smear reveals clue cells,
vaginal epithelial cells with bacteria
clusters that adhere to the epithelial cell
surface.

| **What is the treatment for bacterial vaginosis?** | Oral metronidazole<br>If pregnant, clindamycin or ampicillin |

## TRICHOMONIASIS

| **What is trichomoniasis?** | A protozoan vaginal infection<br>The most prevalent nonviral sexually transmitted disease |

| **What is the cause of trichomoniasis?** | The anaerobic, flagellated protozoan *Trichomonas vaginalis* |

| **What are the symptoms of trichomoniasis?** | Presenting symptoms and signs: Profuse discharge; erythema and irritation of vulva; vulvar pruritus; dysuria; "strawberry cervix"<br>Discharge: Large amount; often frothy and bubbling; malodorous; pH > 5 |

| **How is the diagnosis of trichomoniasis made?** | Light microscopy of vaginal fluid mixed with saline reveals mobile, flagellated organisms and many white blood cells. |

| **What is the treatment of trichomoniasis?** | Oral metronidazole 2 g orally in a single dose or 500 mg twice daily for 7 days<br>If pregnant, the same treatment is used but deferred until the second trimester<br>Treatment of sexual partners |

## CANDIDIASIS

| **What is candidiasis?** | Yeast infection |

| **What is the cause of vaginal candidiasis?** | Primarily *Candida albicans*<br>Other species: *Candida glabrata* and *Candida tropicalis* |

| **What factors predispose a patient to candidiasis?** | Antibiotic treatment that alters the normal vaginal flora<br>Depressed immunity [corticosteroids, acquired immunodeficiency syndrome (AIDS)]<br>Hormonal changes associated with pregnancy and menstruation<br>Diabetes mellitus |

**What are the symptoms of vaginal candidiasis?**

Presenting symptoms: Pruritus, burning, external dysuria, extreme vulvar erythema

Discharge: White; highly viscous; often with clumps or plaques; pH < 5

**How is vaginal candidiasis diagnosed?**

Light microscopy of vaginal fluid mixed with KOH reveals filamentous forms or pseudohyphae.

**What is the treatment for vaginal candidiasis?**

Topical antifungals such as miconazole, clotrimazole, and terconazole as a 3- or 7-day course of intravaginal suppositories inserted at bedtime; can also be used externally for itching

Oral fluconazole as a single 150-mg dose in nonpregnant women

## INFECTIONS OF THE CERVIX

**What are the two diagnostic criteria for mucopurulent cervicitis?**

1. Direct visualization of yellow mucopurulent material on a swab of the cervix
2. Presence of 10 or more leukocytes on Gram-stained smears from cervix

**What are the symptoms of cervicitis?**

Presenting symptoms: Vaginal discharge, dyspareunia, and postcoital bleeding

**Signs?**

Erythema, edema, or friability

**What are the major causes of cervicitis?**

*C. trachomatis* (most common)
*Neisseria gonorrhoeae*
*Mycoplasma hominis* (rare)
*C. trachomatis* and *N. gonorrhoeae* are often found simultaneously.

**What kind of organism is *C. trachomatis*?**

An obligate intracellular bacterium

**How is a diagnosis of *C. trachomatis* infection made?**

DNA probe for the organism in epithelial cells removed from the endocervical canal

**What is the treatment for *C. trachomatis* infection?**

Oral doxycycline 100 mg bid for 10 days (or erythromycin)
Treatment of sexual partners

**What kind of organism is
N. gonorrhoeae?**

Gram-negative, intracellular diplococci

**How is a diagnosis of N.
gonorrhoeae infection
made?**

DNA probe for the organism in
epithelial cells removed from the
endocervical canal
Cultures of rectum, pharynx, or urethra
may be indicated.
Test for sensitivity to penicillin because
of high rate of resistance

**What is the treatment for
N. gonorrhoeae infection?**

Recommended regimen treats both C.
trachomatis and N. gonorrhoeae
infections:
Norfloxacin 800 mg by mouth once,
or
Ceftriaxone 250 mg intramuscularly
once, or
Doxycycline 100 mg by mouth twice a
day for 7 days (for possible
coexisting C. trachomatis infection)
should be given with either.
Repetition of cultures following therapy
to ensure response after treatment of
either or both

## INFECTIONS OF THE UPPER GENITAL TRACT

### PELVIC INFLAMMATORY DISEASE (PID)

**What is PID?**

An infection that ascends from the
vagina and endocervix along the
mucosal surface
May involve any or all of the following
sites: Endometrium (endometritis),
oviducts (salpingitis), ovary
(oophoritis), uterine wall
(myometritis), broad ligaments
(parametritis), and the pelvic
peritoneum

**What pathogens cause
PID?**

Most common pathogens: N.
gonorrhoeae, C. trachomatis
C. trachomatis often causes a longer
standing infection with a more
indolent course.
C. trachomatis infection may lead to
more sequelae because treatment is

often not initiated quickly.
Other pathogens:
Facultative aerobes such as *E. coli*,
coagulase-negative staphylococcus,
and group B streptococcus
Anaerobes such as *Bacteroides* and
*Peptococcus*
Genital mycoplasmas such as
*Mycoplasma hominis*
Key point: PID is almost always a
polymicrobial infection.

**What are the risk factors
for PID?**

Menstruation: Most episodes occur after
menses because of mucosal
susceptibility during this event.
Multiple sexual partners without barrier
protection
Young age and early onset of sexual
behavior
Previous PID
Invasive procedure that penetrates the
mucosal barrier (i.e., iatrogenic)
History of other sexually transmitted
diseases

**What are the symptoms of
PID?**

Often nonspecific and can vary from
mild to severe
High rate of false-positive and false-
negative results occur when diagnosis
is based on history, physical
examination, and laboratory results.

**How is a diagnosis of PID
made?**

Laparoscopy is the ultimate standard for
making the diagnosis by visualization
of the infection and subsequent
cultures.
Often, the physician must rely on
history, physical examination, and
laboratory results because laparoscopy
may be inappropriately invasive.
The main diagnostic criteria (required
for diagnosis) are
Diffuse lower abdominal pain and
tenderness with or without rebound
Cervical motion tenderness
Adnexal tenderness, can be bilateral
or unilateral

Minor criteria:
Fever
Leukocytosis
Purulent material in cul-de-sac
Purulent cervical discharge (defined
as > 6 white blood cells/hpf)
Pelvic abscess or mass detected by
physical examination or ultrasound
(although this obviously is not a
minor problem, it is not an essential
criterion for diagnosis)
Elevated erythrocyte sedimentation
rate
Positive gonorrhea or chlamydia tests
from endocervix

**What is Fitz-Hugh–Curtis syndrome?**

Perihepatic inflammation with associated
right upper quadrant pain
Occurs in 5%–10% of PID cases

**What other tests should be considered?**

β-Human chorionic gonadotropin assay
to rule out ectopic pregnancy
Complete blood count with differential
Cervical cultures
Ultrasonography to investigate any
masses
Culdocentesis to evaluate fluid in the
peritoneal cavity

**What are the differential diagnoses of PID?**

Ectopic pregnancy
Acute appendicitis
Urinary tract infection
Adnexal torsion
Endometriosis
Bleeding corpus luteum
Diverticulosis

**What are the criteria for hospitalization?**

Suspected pelvic or tubo-ovarian abscess
Pregnancy
Temperature > 38°C
Uncertain diagnosis
Nausea and vomiting precluding oral
medications
Upper peritoneal signs, suggesting
spread of peritonitis
Failure to respond to outpatient
antibiotics within 48 hours

| | |
|---|---|
| **What is the inpatient treatment of PID?** | Inpatient and outpatient treatment both require multiple antimicrobials because no single agent is active against entire spectrum of possible pathogens. |
| | Anaerobic coverage is very important: |
| |    Cefoxitin IV 2 g q6h plus doxycycline 100 mg q12h by mouth or IV (or third-generation cephalosporin) |
| |    Clindamycin IV 900 mg q8h plus gentamicin IV 1.5 mg/kg q8h |
| |    Imipenem/cilastin IV |
| |    Treatment of sexual partners |
| **What is the outpatient treatment of PID?** | Ceftriaxone [250 mg intramuscularly (IM)] or cefoxitin (2 g IM) plus doxycycline by mouth for 10–14 days |
| | Ofloxacin 400 mg orally bid for 14 days plus either clindamycin 450 mg orally four times a day or metronidazole 500 mg orally two times a day for 14 days |
| | Reexamination of the patient within 48 to 72 hours |
| **What are the complications of PID?** | Infertility |
| | Ectopic pregnancy |
| | Chronic pelvic pain |
| | Adhesions |
| | Hydrosalpinx |
| | Dyspareunia |
| **What are preventive measures for PID?** | Barrier methods of contraception: Mechanical and chemical |
| | Oral contraception: Thickens the cervical mucus and decreases the duration of menstrual flow, limiting the interval for bacterial colonization |
| | Treatment of sexual partners |

## TUBO-OVARIAN ABSCESS

| | |
|---|---|
| **With what disease are tubo-ovarian abscesses often associated?** | PID; significantly increases the mortality rate from PID |
| **What are some common findings on physical examination?** | Patients are very ill with severe pelvic and abdominal pain, high fever, nausea and vomiting, and possible septic shock. |

Tachycardia
Abdominal rigidity and guarding
Rebound tenderness
Manual examination of adnexa is usually
  difficult because of extreme adnexal
  tenderness, but it may be possible to
  appreciate an adnexal mass.

**How is a tubo-ovarian abscess diagnosed?**

Ultrasound
Computed tomography scan
Exploratory laparoscopy

**What are the differential diagnoses of tubo-ovarian abscess?**

Septic incomplete abortion
Acute appendicitis
Diverticular abscess
Adnexal torsion

**What are the treatment options for tubo-ovarian abscess?**

Conservative treatment with bed rest in
  the hospital, adequate hydration,
  analgesics, and IV antibiotics
  (clindamycin and an aminoglycoside;
  or imipenem/cilastin)
Surgery if no improvement or rupture
  occurs; often requires total abdominal
  hysterectomy and bilateral salpingo-
  oophorectomy

## ACTINOMYCOSIS

**What is actinomycosis?**

Infection with *Actinomyces* sp

**What species of *Actinomyces* causes infection in the urogenital tract?**

*Actinomyces israelii*

**What birth control method is associated with *Actinomyces* abscesses?**

Intrauterine device

**What are characteristic gross and histologic findings?**

"Sulfur granules"
Fistula formation
Chronic draining sinuses

**What is the treatment for actinomycosis?**

Penicillin

## TUBERCULOSIS (TB)

| | |
|---|---|
| **What is the cause of genital tract TB?** | *Mycobacterium tuberculosis* or *Mycobacterium bovis* that has spread hematogenously from either the lung or gastrointestinal tract |
| **What are the symptoms of TB?** | Infertility, abnormal uterine bleeding, and abdominal pain |
| **How is a diagnosis of TB made?** | Should be suspected when patient does not respond to conventional PID therapy<br>Confirmed by endometrial biopsy and culture |
| **What is the treatment of TB?** | Isoniazid and rifampin. Secondary agents may be necessary when resistance occurs. |

## OTHER INFECTIONS

## TOXIC SHOCK SYNDROME (TSS)

| | |
|---|---|
| **What is TSS?** | An acute, febrile illness leading to multiorgan system failure<br>Fifty percent of cases are associated with menses and tampon use. |
| **What is the cause of TSS?** | A bacterial exotoxin from *Staphylococcus aureus* |
| **What are the signs and symptoms of TSS?** | Presenting signs and symptoms: Abrupt onset of high fever, headache, myalgia, vomiting, diarrhea, generalized skin rash, and often hypotension<br>Characteristic rash begins as an intense "sunburn" that evolves into flaky desquamation and sloughing of the skin. |
| **What is the treatment for TSS?** | Intravenous fluids<br>Antibiotics (β-lactamase–resistant penicillin such as oxacillin or nafcillin) |

## ACQUIRED IMMUNODEFICIENCY SYNDROME

**What is the cause and pathophysiology of AIDS?**

Caused by the human immunodeficiency virus (HIV)
HIV attacks CD4+ T-lymphocytes.
Opportunistic infections occur when the CD4+ count drops below 200.

**What are the clinical presentations of AIDS?**

Community-acquired pneumonias and gastroenteritis
*Pneumocystis carinii* pneumonia
TB
*Cryptococcus* infection
Candidiasis
Toxoplasmosis
Cytomegalovirus infection
HSV infection

**Which presentations are most common in women?**

Candidiasis and HSV infections

**How is a diagnosis of AIDS made?**

Two tests:
1. Enzyme-linked immunosorbent assay test for antibodies against HIV; has a high rate of false-positive results.
2. Western blot identifies antibodies to an HIV-specific protein.

**What is the incidence of AIDS in women?**

Approximately 11% of people with AIDS are women.
Fastest growing population

# 24

# Leiomyomas

**What is a leiomyoma?**

Also known as a fibroid
Smooth muscle tumor of the uterus
Most common neoplasm in the female
pelvis

**What causes leiomyomas?**

Thought to arise through somatic
mutations of smooth muscle cells
Possible mutations include translocations
and deletions most commonly
involving chromosome 12.
Individual leiomyomas in the same
uterus arise through different
mutations.

**What receptors are
present in leiomyomas?**

Estrogen and progesterone receptors

**Where in the leiomyoma
are the receptors located?**

In the cell cytosol

**Which has a greater
concentration of receptors:
a leiomyoma,
endometrium, or
myometrium?**

Leiomyomas have greater concentrations
of receptors than endometrium or
myometrium.

**How do leiomyoma
receptor concentrations
vary?**

With the menstrual cycle
Greater concentrations in the first 18
days of the cycle

**What are the locations of
leiomyomas?**

Intramural: within the myometrial wall
Submucosal: grow from myometrium
toward and into the endometrial cavity
Subserosal: grow from myometrium
toward and into the abdominal cavity
Interligamentary: grow from
myometrium into the broad ligament
Parasitic: grow into abdominal cavity,
achieve secondary blood supply from

mesenteric arteries, and detach from
initial blood supply of myometrial
arteries to become autonomous
tumors on bowel or mesentery

Pedunculated: Connected to
myometrium by a narrow stalk and
"float" in the abdominal cavity,
endometrial cavity, or even through
the cervical os in the vagina

**What is the incidence of
leiomyomas?**

Present in 20% to 25% of women of
reproductive age

More common in African-American
women

**What is the surgical impact
of leiomyomas?**

Account for approximately one-third of
all hysterectomies (most common
indication for hysterectomy)

Account for a significant number of
other surgical procedures, including
dilation and curettage; diagnostic and
operative hysteroscopy; laparoscopy
and myomectomy

Abnormal uterine bleeding: most
common symptom associated with
leiomyomas and usually manifests as
menorrhagia

Pelvic pain

**Why do leiomyomas cause
abnormal uterine
bleeding?**

Theories:

Increased surface area of endometrial
cavity mucosa leading to increased
bleeding

Increased anovulatory bleeding (thus
far no link between leiomyomas and
anovulatory status)

Mechanical interference from
leiomyomas on normal myometrial
contractions during menses
preventing blood loss

Compression of endometrial venules
by intramural leiomyomas, causing
venular dilatation and increased
venous blood loss

**Why do leiomyomas cause
pain?**

Theories:

Carneous (red) degeneration:

1. Hemorrhagic degeneration of leiomyoma causing acute pelvic pain, low-grade fever, mild peritoneal signs, and occasionally leukocytosis
2. Often difficult to distinguish from other causes of acute abdominal pain (including placental abruption in pregnancy)

Pelvic pressure: Pressure from a leiomyoma on bladder or rectum can result in urinary frequency, urgency, incontinence, and the sensation of rectal pressure.

**How do leiomyomas interfere with the ability to achieve a term pregnancy?**

Theories:

Prevention of conception (infertility): Bilateral cornual obstruction secondary to cornual leiomyomas leading to complete bilateral tubal occlusion

Other mechanisms

Prevention of implantation or growth of the developing embryo (recurrent pregnancy loss): Conception occurs but submucosal leiomyomas interfere with implantation, placentation, or continued adherence to myometrial wall.

Prevention of progression to term (preterm labor): Leiomyomas cause myometrial irritation, which stimulates the onset of premature uterine activity and premature contractions.

**How are the above-stated effects on pregnancy remedied?**

Interference with the ability to achieve or maintain pregnancy: correction of the structural abnormality imposed by leiomyoma with myomectomy (using laparotomy, hysteroscopy, or laparoscopy)

Myomectomy during pregnancy: Has been accomplished when the size or location may interfere with the ability to carry the pregnancy to

term or lead to other complications
in pregnancy
Is best performed in the nonpregnant
state

**What other complications
in pregnancy are related
to leiomyomas?**

Dystocia:
Can prevent vaginal delivery
Accounts for the increased cesarean
section rate in women with
leiomyomas
Increased risk of uterine inversion with
submucosal leiomyomas
Red (carneous) degeneration occurs
more frequently in pregnancy.

**How does pregnancy affect
preexisting leiomyomas?**

Recent studies suggest that whereas
some leiomyomas grow during
pregnancy, the majority do not and most
shrink in the third trimester.

**What condition could
rapid growth of
leiomyomas indicate?**

Leiomyosarcoma, a malignant sarcoma
that can mimic benign leiomyomas, is
characterized by rapid uterine
enlargement.

**What is the incidence of
leiomyosarcoma?**

Approximately 0.1% to 1% of all
pathologic specimens submitted as
leiomyomas are actually
leiomyosarcoma.
Leiomyosarcoma is more prevalent in
the fifth and sixth decades of life.

**What is the prognosis of
leiomyosarcoma?**

Poor prognosis if discovered after
menopause
More favorable prognosis in early stages
(I or II) in younger women

**What is the management/
treatment of asymptomatic
leiomyomas?**

Serial examinations to determine rate of
growth and careful history to detect new
symptomatology
Rapid enlargement is of concern.
If leiomyomas are not enlarging
rapidly, annual examinations are
sufficient.
Nonsteroidal anti-inflammatory drugs:
decrease blood loss associated with
menses

**What are gonadotropin-releasing hormone (GnRH) agonists?**

Synthetic derivatives of GnRH created by substitutions of amino acids at the sixth and sometimes tenth amino acid residues

Confer a longer half-life and better binding of GnRH to the GnRH receptor

**How do GnRH agonists affect the size of leiomyomas?**

Inhibit GnRH secretion by downregulation after 2 weeks of use, leading to a decrease in gonadotropin secretion and, thus, a decrease in ovarian estrogen synthesis and a hypoestrogenic state

Decrease leiomyoma size approximately 50%, with maximal effect after 12 weeks of use and no decrease in size after that time

**What are the indications for use of GnRH agonists in the management of leiomyomas?**

American College of Obstetrics and Gynecology (ACOG) recommendations:

For treatment of large submucous leiomyomas prior to hysteroscopic resection to facilitate resection and decrease blood loss

For treatment of leiomyomas while awaiting menopause (a hypo-estrogenic state that leads to shrinkage of leiomyomas) in a perimenopausal woman

For treatment preoperatively while awaiting work-up of medical problems or when other considerations prohibit immediate surgery

**How long should GnRH agonist therapy last?**

Use is generally limited to less than 6 months to limit side effects.

**What are the purported benefits of GnRH agonist therapy?**

Reduction in menstrual blood loss

Improvement in anemia prior to surgery

Allowance of time for autologous blood donation

Reduction of operative blood loss

Decrease in the need for hysterectomy

Improvement in chance that a hysterectomy can be done vaginally instead of abdominally

**What are the side effects of GnRH agonists?**

Similar to menopausal symptoms

**What is the definition of myomectomy?**

Removal of individual leiomyomas from an intact uterus

**What are the indications for myomectomy in the treatment of leiomyomas?**

Usually performed when preservation of fertility is an issue
ACOG recommendation: when the leiomyoma is a probable factor in failure to conceive or in recurrent pregnancy loss

**What are the benefits of myomectomy?**

Approximately 80% of women who have a myomectomy have improvement in hypermenorrhea, pelvic pain, or pressure.

**How is myomectomy performed?**

Laparotomy or via hysteroscopy for submucosal tumors
Laparoscopic myomectomies have been performed

**What are the indications for hysterectomy in the treatment of leiomyomas?**

Controversial
General guidelines:
  For treatment of asymptomatic leiomyomas that are palpable abdominally and of concern to the patient
  For treatment of excessive bleeding with either flooding and/or clots for greater than 8 days, or for acute or chronic blood loss
  For treatment of pelvic discomfort when the pain is either acute or severe, causes chronic lower abdominal or back pain, or causes bladder pressure with urinary frequency

# 25

# Pelvic Relaxation

**What is the pelvic floor?**

Paired levator ani muscles are fused to the bony pelvis anteriorly and posteriorly and attached laterally to the white line (the arcus tendineus fasciae pelvis) which overlies the obturator internus muscles.

The normal tone of the levator ani muscles supports the pelvic organs from below and contributes to urinary and fecal continence.

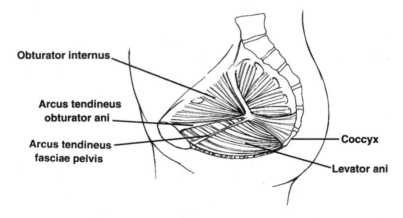

Obturator internus

Arcus tendineus obturator ani

Arcus tendineus fasciae pelvis

Coccyx

Levator ani

**What is the levator hiatus?**    The anterior separation through which
the urethra, vagina, and rectum pass

The vaginal axis of the erect or standing living female is shown. Notice the almost
horizontal upper vagina and rectum lying on and parallel to the levator plate. The latter
is formed by fusion of the pubococcygei muscles (A) posterior to the rectum. The
anterior limit of the point of fusion is the margin of the genital hiatus immediately
posterior to the rectum. (From Nichols DH, Milley PS: Clinical anatomy of the vulva,
vagina, lower pelvis, and perineum. In Sciarra (ed): *Gynecology and Obstetrics,* 1977;
reproduced with permission of Harper & Row.)

**What is endopelvic fascia?**    Visceral fascia investing the pelvic
organs that form bilateral condensations
known as ligaments. For example:
To maintain support of the bladder,
    pubocervical fascia is plicated in the
    midline when repairing a cystocele.
Likewise, to support the rectum,
    perirectal fascia is plicated to repair a
    rectocele.

Stereograph shows the connective tissue septae and paravaginal spaces in relation to
the bladder, uterus, and rectum. The spaces permit these three organs to function
independently of one another (53).

**What are the important ligaments of pelvic support?**

In general, all pelvic ligaments attach organs to the pelvic sidewall and/or bony pelvis.

From caudad to cephalad for the uterus:
Uterosacral
Cardinal
Round

For the bladder and urethra:
pubourethral

Normal anatomy of layers of pelvic supports (vaginal view): Superficial skin and adipose tissue have been removed to expose the *numbered* structural layers. 1, suspensory L. clitoris; 2, clitoris; 3, urethral meatus; 4, hymen; 5, perineal body; 6, anal sphincter; 7, anus; 8, anococcygeal body; 9, ischiocavernosus muscle; 10, bulbocavernosus muscle; 11, vestibular bulb; 12, Bartholin gland; 13, superficial perineal muscle; 14, ischial tuberosity; 15, levator ani muscle; 16, gluteus maximus muscle.

**How does the perineal body help maintain pelvic support?**

It is the central point for attachment of the perineal musculature.
It is inferior to, and serves to support, the urogenital diaphragm. It also supports the distal vagina and rectum.

**What is pelvic relaxation?**

Loss of support for the female urogenital organs
Can include the uterus, vagina, rectum, or small bowel
Primarily occurs in adult women as a result of direct or indirect damage to the vagina, its support systems, or both

**What factors contribute to pelvic relaxation?**

Childbirth: detachments, lacerations, denervations from parturition

Iatrogenic: failed episiotomy repairs, prior surgical repairs

Medical: chronic obstructive pulmonary disease, obesity, strenuous physical activity, ascites, or other situations resulting in chronic increased intra-abdominal pressure

Inherent: hypoestrogenic atrophy of tissues; inherent connective tissue characteristics

**What are the signs and symptoms of pelvic relaxation?**

Generally visceral, sexual, and hernia related

Protrusion of organs; ulceration or bleeding in severe cases (or with procidentia); low back pain; pressure; and heaviness, especially at the end of the day.

Dyspareunia or a complete inability to have intercourse

Bladder: incontinence, inability to void, frequent urinary tract infections

GI: constipation, need to splint the vagina for defecation

**What questions should be asked in taking the patient history?**

In addition to the previously mentioned, ask about:

Prior vaginal/abdominal surgeries

Parity: birth weights, use of forceps, difficult labors, etc.

Interest in future fertility

Hormone replacement

Occupation and activities involving lifting or straining

Cardiac and respiratory problems or obesity in medical history

**What should be included in the physical examination?**

Examination of patient in both lithotomy AND standing positions
Inspection of the genital hiatus:
  Protruding tissues?
  Is the uterus present or absent?
  Does the cervix or vaginal apex descend?
Instruct the patient to bear down (Valsalva) and note any change.
Be as SITE-SPECIFIC as possible.

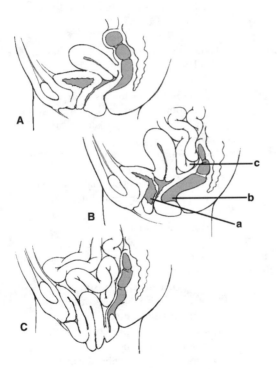

Types of genital prolapse are diagrammatically shown. *A*, Sagittal section of a normally supported pelvis. *B*, Incomplete uterine prolapse is noted along with specific types of herniation, (*a*) cystocele, (*b*) rectocele, and (*c*) enterocele. *C*, Complete uterine prolapse (procidentia) is shown.

**What is a cystocele?**

Relaxation and/or descent of the bladder anteriorly into the vagina

**What is a rectocele?**

Relaxation and/or descent of the rectum posteriorly into the vagina

**What is an enterocele?**

Herniation of the small bowel into the cul-de-sac (or pouch of Douglas)

**How is pelvic organ prolapse graded?**

One common grading system is as follows:
Grade 0: no descent (organs well supported and above the level of the ischial spines)
Grade 1: descent halfway down to the introitus
Grade 2: descent to the introitus
Grade 3: descent halfway out of the introitus

**What is uterine procidentia?**

Grade 4: descent completely outside of the introitus

**What are the nonsurgical treatment options?**

Correction of reversible medical conditions such as obesity, smoking, and asthma
Modification of strenuous activities such as heavy lifting
Estrogen therapy to assist with tissue integrity

**What are Kegel exercises?**

Pelvic muscle exercises (daily repetitions of pubococcygeus muscle contractions) to strengthen the pelvic floor

**What are pessaries?**

Devices placed in the vagina that press against the vaginal sidewalls to support the pelvic organs within the vagina (various shapes and names)

**What is their use in treatment of pelvic relaxation?**

Generally used for the nonsurgical patient; can be used for years

**What problems are associated with pessaries?**

Vaginal irritation and ulceration
Work best in well-estrogenized tissue
Require periodic removal and cleaning

**What are the goals of surgery in the treatment of pelvic organ prolapse?**

Relieve symptoms
Restore normal anatomy
Restore normal visceral function
Allow satisfactory coital function
Obtain a durable result

**What are the considerations in choosing a particular surgical treatment?**

Type of surgery depends on the patient's particular constellation of symptoms and physical findings, along with her interest in future fertility, if any.

**What are some commonly performed vaginal procedures?**

Vaginal hysterectomy, enterocoele plication, anterior and posterior colporrhaphy
Vaginal hysterectomy:
    For patients who have completed childbearing, especially if they have other pelvic defects.
    Will not correct uterovaginal prolapse; proper suspension of the vaginal apex is needed.

**What are the key principles in the repair of an enterocele?**

Same as with repair of any hernia: completely identify the sac, reduce any small bowel found in the sac; perform high ligation and then excision of the distal portion of the sac.

**What is an anterior colporrhaphy (or an anterior repair)?**

Indication: repair of a cystocele
Basic technique: interrupted horizontal
sutures to plicate the endopelvic (or
pubocervical) fascia in order to elevate
and support the urethrovesical
junction and the bladder

A specific supporting suture or two is placed at the level of the urethrovesical junction and anchored to the fibromuscular tissue of the underside of the pubic ramus bilaterally. The bladder neck is elevated when these sutures are tied. The cystocele is then reduced by placement of a series of plicating sutures along the bladder base.

The pubovesical fascia is plicated to the midline, reducing the cystocele.

**What is a posterior colporrhaphy (or a posterior repair)?**

Indication: repair of a rectocele
Basic technique: dissection of the rectovaginal septum up to the vaginal apex, then interrupted horizontal sutures to plicate the perirectal fascia over the rectum

The rectocele repair is initiated by incising the skin of the perineal body along the mucocutaneous junction.

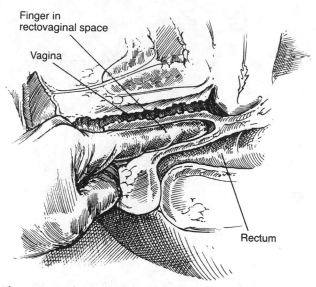

Finger in
rectovaginal space

Vagina

Rectum

The rectovaginal space is bluntly developed once any scar tissue has been incised. The space is developed to a point above the site of the rectocele.

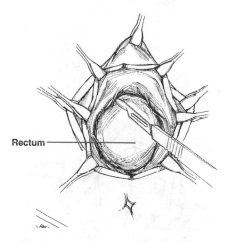

Rectum

The posterior vaginal wall and rectovaginal septum are incised and reflected. The underlying rectum and perirectal fascia are exposed.

The rectocele is reduced by plicating the perirectal fascia to the midline. As the distal vagina is reached, the medial bodies of the levator ani are incorporated into the plicated tissues for additional support.

Excess vaginal mucosa is excised from the posterior vagina, and the vaginal incision is closed.

**What are the choices for correction of prolapse of a post-hysterectomy vaginal vault prolapse?**

Vaginal approaches:
McCall's culdoplasty, which incorporates the strong uterosacral ligaments to the vaginal mucosa
Sacrospinous ligament fixation, which tacks the vaginal apex to the sacrospinous ligament
Abdominal approaches: *sacro-colpopexy,* which uses synthetic mesh to connect the vaginal apex to the sacral promontory

**What other abdominal procedures can be performed to address pelvic organ prolapse?**

Abdominal hysterectomy, if indicated, with particular attention given to reattachment of the cut ends of the cardinal and uterosacral ligaments to the vaginal apex

**What is a Moschcowitz procedure?**

An abdominal procedure used to obliterate the cul-de-sac to prevent an enterocele
Permanent suture is used in a circumferential manner.

**What is a Halban procedure?**

Same as a Moschcowitz procedure, but performed in a vertical fashion

**What is a paravaginal repair?**

Procedure of choice if a cystocele exists as a result of loss of LATERAL support

Can be accomplished from either a vaginal or an abdominal approach

OF ————

———— ATFP

The reparative phase of paravaginal repair. ATFP, arcus tendineus fasciae pelvis; OF, obturator foramen. Defects and suture placement are shown on right and left sides.

The basic technique involves reattaching the lateral fascia of the anterior superior vagina to the "white line," or fascia of arcus tendineus levator ani.

**What are the potential surgical complications from pelvic reconstructive surgery?**

Failure of the procedure, especially if all defects are not addressed or if the patient does not address concomitant medical conditions

Gastrointestinal: small or large bowel injury

Genitourinary: postoperative voiding dysfunction from temporary bladder denervation or edema, urinary retention or incontinence, ureteral injury, unintentional cystotomy

Sexual: vaginal stenosis or shortening of the vagina if too many sutures are placed or if too much vaginal mucosa is excised

Bleeding: pudendal vessel injury with
   sacrospinous ligament fixation,
   presacral vessel injury with abdominal
   sacrocolpopexy
Nerve damage: peroneal damage from
   improper lithotomy positioning (recall
   the nerve that runs lateral to the head
   of the fibula); sciatica from needle
   penetration with sacrospinous
   ligament fixation

**What is the LeFort
procedure?**

A technique of vaginal obliteration,
   mainly used in older, infirm patients
   who are not sexually active
It is important to leave a tunnel between
   the cervix and vagina for exit of
   abnormal discharge or bleeding.

**What are the options for
women who have not
completed childbearing?**

Usually it is better to delay treatment
   until childbearing is complete.
Nonsurgical methods such as Kegel
   exercises or pessaries
Ventral suspensions of the uterine
   fundus are points of historical interest
   only.

# 26

# Pelvic Pain

**What are the differences among nociception, pain, suffering, and pain behavior?**

Nociception refers to the origination and detection of a neurologic signal based on a noxious event.
Pain is the recognition of the signal or event.
Suffering is the affective response to the event.
Pain behavior involves adaptive behavioral changes made as a result of pain.

**What noxious events can lead to pain?**

Thermal stimuli: Heat or cold
Mechanical stimuli: Stretch, distention, muscular contraction
Chemical stimuli: Various biologic pain mediators, neurotransmitters, and ions

**How does the character of pain mediated by slow versus fast pain fibers vary?**

Slow pain fibers characteristically mediate visceral pain, which is usually described as a diffuse burning or aching and is usually the result of inflammation or ischemia (e.g., the referred periumbilical aching in appendicitis).
Fast pain fibers characteristically mediate parietal peritoneal pain, which is usually described as a well-localized, sharp pain (e.g., the sharp pain over the right lower quadrant in appendicitis).

**What are the three main models of pain perception?**

1. Medical Model: Pain perception is the result of anatomic or physiologic abnormalities of tissues that, if corrected, result in the amelioration of pain.
2. Gate Control Model: Pain perception is the result of a complex interaction between peripheral stimuli and cortical variables (mood, anxiety).

Amelioration of pain must target both somatic and psychogenic precipitants.
3. Biopsychosocial Model: Pain perception is the result of nociceptive stimuli, psychological factors, and social determinants. Elimination of nociceptive stimuli leads to symptom shifting, which results in disabling symptoms elsewhere.

**What is pelvic pain?**

A general term that refers to pain of gynecologic or nongynecologic origin perceived by the patient as originating from the female pelvis

**Where is pelvic pain localized?**

Right lower quadrant, left lower quadrant, infraumbilical, deep pelvic, or cervicovaginal

**What percentage of office visits are for pelvic pain?**

The presenting complaint in approximately 10% of gynecologic office visits and comprises a significant percentage of emergency room visits

**What are some common extrauterine gynecologic causes of pelvic pain?**

Adhesions, ectopic pregnancy, pelvis infection, endometriosis, ovarian cysts, ovarian torsion, and residual ovary syndrome

**What are some common uterine causes of pelvic pain?**

Adenomyosis, endometriosis, leiomyomas, intrauterine device, pelvic congestion, pelvic support defects, and polyps

**What are some common urologic causes of pelvic pain?**

Urinary tract infection, interstitial cystitis, chronic urethral syndrome, nephrolithiasis, urethral diverticulitis, detrusor overactivity, and urethritis

**What are some common gastrointestinal causes of pelvic pain?**

Cholelithiasis, appendicitis, constipation, diverticular disease (Crohn's disease or ulcerative colitis), irritable bowel syndrome, and gastrointestinal neoplasm

**What are some common musculoskeletal causes of pelvic pain?**

Gait disorders, postural dysfunction, intervertebral disc disease, degenerative joint disease, fibromyositis, hernias, shingles, pelvic floor spasm (levator ani syndrome), myofascial pain, nerve

entrapment syndromes, strains and
sprains, and coccydynia

**What are some other
causes of pelvic pain?**

History of or current physical or sexual
abuse, heavy metal poisoning, porphyria,
psychiatric disorders (depression, bipolar
disorder, personality disorders),
psychosocial stressors, somatiform
disorders, sickle cell disease, and sleep
disturbances

**What is chronic pelvic
pain?**

Pelvic pain that lasts more than 6
   months, as opposed to subacute (3–6
   months) or acute (less than 3 months)
It presents an often difficult diagnostic
   and management dilemma for the
   gynecologist.

**What is the general
approach in the evaluation
of pelvic pain?**

Initially, a determination of the acuity
   and duration of pain should be made
   to determine if the pain requires
   emergent treatment (i.e., it is
   potentially life-threatening, subacute,
   or long-standing in nature).
History and physical examination are
   particularly important in determining
   the cause of pelvic pain given the
   extensive differential diagnosis.
Once acute causes of pelvic pain have
   been ruled out or appropriately
   treated, diagnosing the cause of
   chronic pelvic pain may require
   numerous office visits and varied
   treatments.
Assessment of pelvic pain requires an
   integrated multidisciplinary approach
   that addresses medical, psychological,
   and social issues.

**What important questions
should be asked when
evaluating the patient with
chronic pelvic pain?**

The character, intensity (often graded
   subjectively on a scale of 1 to 10),
   location, and radiation of the pain
Temporal aspects (typical pattern
   throughout the day/week/month,
   cyclicity, duration) and exacerbating or
   relieving factors
Menstrual symptoms, including
   menorrhagia, colicky dysmenorrhea,

and the relation of the menstrual
complaints to pelvic pain

Sexual history, including contraceptive
history, dyspareunia (if present), and
vaginal symptoms (if present)

Gastrointestinal symptoms, including
changes in bowel habits (constipation
or diarrhea), anorexia, nausea,
vomiting, and bloating

Urologic symptoms, including dysuria,
changes in urinary habits, nocturia,
and incontinence

Musculoskeletal symptoms, including
low back pain

History of prior surgeries and
gynecologic or obstetric problems

Psychological history, including history
of depression, somatization, anxiety
disorders, sexual or physical abuse,
rape or incest, marital or relationship
discord, substance abuse, sleep
disturbances, or other stressors

**What aspects of the physical examination are important in the evaluation of chronic pelvic pain?**

Thorough abdominal examination,
including inspection for deformity,
scars, hernias, distention; auscultation
for bowel sounds; and palpation of the
epigastrium, flanks, back, and inguinal
regions for tenderness and masses

Special attention to pain reproduction
during pelvic and rectovaginal
examination, with an attempt to
determine adnexal or uterine
tenderness and uterosacral ligament or
cul-de-sac nodularity or tenderness

Evaluation for rectal masses or
tenderness, cystocele, pelvic
relaxation, and tenderness or
thickening in the bladder or urethra

Evaluation for spinal and
musculoskeletal anomalies, including
scoliosis, leg asymmetry or motion
restriction, gait dysfunction, and
neurologic examination

Elucidation of trigger points, including
myofascial (especially in the levator
ani and obturator internus),
musculoskeletal, and abdominal

**What laboratory studies are important in the evaluation of chronic pelvic pain?**

Complete blood count to evaluate for infection or hemorrhage

Human chorionic gonadotropin assay to evaluate for intrauterine ectopic or molar pregnancy

Cervical cultures to evaluate for the presence of an infection

Urinalysis and culture to evaluate for kidney stones and cystitis or pyelonephritis

Hepatic transaminases and bilirubin to evaluate hepatobiliary obstruction or hepatitis

Erythrocyte sedimentation rate to evaluate chronic disease states

**How can ultrasound be helpful in the evaluation of pelvic pain?**

Pelvic ultrasound can supplement an inconclusive or limited (usually secondary to obesity) pelvic examination.

Ovarian cysts or masses, uterine fibroids, and tubal pathology (including hydrosalpinx, tubo-ovarian abscess, or ectopic pregnancy) may be seen.

**How is diagnostic laparoscopy helpful in the evaluation of pelvic pain?**

Laparoscopy can be useful in evaluation of acute pelvic pain by identifying hydrosalpinx, tubo-ovarian abscess, pelvic inflammatory disease (PID), ectopic pregnancy, and appendiceal or intestinal pathology.

With chronic pelvic pain, laparoscopy is usually used to rule out the presence of endometriosis, but other infectious or structural lesions may be ruled out as well.

Chronic pelvic pain is the indication for about 25% of all laparoscopies performed in the United States annually.

**What are the two most common gynecologic problems encountered in women undergoing laparoscopic evaluation for pelvic pain?**

Endometriosis is the most common abnormality encountered, and one large study suggested that one in three women undergoing laparoscopy have endometriosis present, although the severity of pain does not seem to correlate with the severity of the lesions present.

Adhesions are the second most common finding. The same study found adhesions in about one in five women undergoing laparoscopic evaluation for chronic pelvic pain, although the role of adhesions in the cause of pelvic pain is controversial.

**What is the role of PID in chronic pelvic pain?**

Chronic pelvic pain is one of the sequelae of PID, along with infertility and ectopic pregnancy.

Some authors have estimated that chronic pelvic pain develops in one in four women with PID.

**What is the most common gastrointestinal diagnosis made in the workup of chronic pelvic pain, and what are the associated symptoms?**

Irritable bowel syndrome (IBS) may be diagnosed in up to half of all patients undergoing workup for chronic pelvic pain.

Pain is often colicky, with a sensation of rectal fullness relieved with bowel movements and intensified with meals.

Pain may be worse during menstruation and associated with dyspareunia.

Associated symptoms include constipation and diarrhea.

**What is the association of physical or sexual abuse and chronic pelvic pain?**

Studies have shown that up to 60% of women with chronic pelvic pain have a history of sexual abuse, and that there is also a significant association between physical abuse and chronic pelvic pain.

**What medications are commonly used to treat chronic pelvic pain?**

Mild pain relievers such as aspirin, nonsteroidal anti-inflammatory drugs, and acetaminophen can be used to treat mild pain.

Stronger agents, including narcotics such as codeine, oxycodone, propoxyphene, pentazocine, and hydromorphone, can be used for relief of more severe pain. Tolerance and physical dependence can develop with opioid use, and thus use of narcotics should be for a defined period of time.

Antidepressants and medications for insomnia can sometimes be helpful.

Standing medications usually are more helpful than prn medications. IBS may respond to bulk-forming agents, anxiolytics, and low doses of antidepressants.

Occasionally, empiric antibiotic treatment is used in the absence of culture-proven infection.

Oral contraceptives can be used to suppress ovulation and regulate the menstrual cycle in cases where dysmenorrhea appears to be a significant component of pain.

Danazol or leuprolide acetate can be used to suppress endometriosis.

**What considerations should be taken into account before surgical treatment of pelvic pain?**

Identifiable causes of pelvic pain should be treated as indicated surgically, but the patient must be informed that removal of the suspected problem does not guarantee relief of the pain.

Patients with a history of unsuccessful attempts to treat pelvic pain surgically have a much higher risk of having persistent pain after another operation.

**What are surgical options for treatment of chronic pelvic pain?**

Laparoscopic uterosacral nerve ablation and presacral neurectomy interrupt the pathways of nerves responsible for pain transmission.

Ablation of endometriotic lesions can be accomplished with laser fulguration, coagulation, or excision.

Lysis of adhesions can be accomplished with laser or sharp dissection.

Hysterectomy is an option provided the patient has had gastrointestinal and urologic sources of pain ruled out and has failed medical management for greater than 6 months.

**How successful is hysterectomy in curing chronic pelvic pain?**

Traditionally, chronic pelvic pain is not thought to respond well to hysterectomy, although recent studies suggest that up to three in four women undergoing hysterectomy for chronic pelvic pain may have complete resolution of pain.

**What are the predictors for persistent pain after hysterectomy?**

Age < 30 years, history of PID, no identified pelvic disease, or having a history of at least two pregnancies

**What conditions are associated with resolution of pain after hysterectomy?**

Resolution occurred in 84%, 77%, and 81%, respectively, with adenomyosis, leiomyomas, or endometriosis.

**What modalities of treatment other than conventional surgical and medical methods are used in the multidisciplinary approach to chronic pelvic pain treatment?**

Addressing and treating the physical, psychological, and social factors involved in chronic pelvic pain has proved to be effective.

Techniques include teaching methods for coping or relaxing, biofeedback, depression therapy, psychotherapy, marital and sexual counseling, nerve blocks, exercise programs, and hypnosis.

# 27

# Endometriosis

**What is endometriosis?**

Ectopic occurrence of hormonally responsive endometrial tissue

**Where is endometriosis most commonly found?**

In or on the ovaries, posterior cul-de-sac, uterosacral ligaments, broad ligament, and anterior cul-de-sac

Can involve the uterine serosa, rectovaginal septum, cervix, vagina, rectosigmoid, ileum, appendix, cecum, bladder, and ureter

Rarely involves the umbilicus, laparotomy or episiotomy scars, lungs, or distant organs

**What problems do endometriosis implants cause?**

Bleeding, inflammation, and adhesions leading to pelvic pain, dyspareunia, and infertility

**How does endometriosis cause infertility?**

Unknown, but proposed mechanisms include:

Adhesion formation:

Leads to distorted anatomy, increased distance from the ovary to the fimbriae, encasement of the ovary by adhesions, and destruction of ovarian and tubal tissue

All can disrupt ovulation and ovum transport.

Altered peritoneal fluid constituents (including hormones, prostaglandins, and immune substances) leading to alterations in ovulation, ovum "pickup" by the tube, tubal function, nidation, and luteal phase adequacy

Interference with ovulation and menstrual cyclicity

Luteinized unruptured follicle syndrome:

A condition in which there is objective evidence of ovulation but the oocyte is not released by the ovary

Increased incidence in women with endometriosis

**What are endometriomas?**

Invasive endometriotic lesions found in the ovary

Also called "chocolate cysts" because of the chocolate-colored blood inside the lesions

Can cause extensive pelvic adhesions, especially periovarian, when repeated leakage results in dense, fibrotic tissue formation

**What are the ultrasound findings suggestive of endometriomas?**

Large cysts with homogenous, low-level internal echoes

**What is the incidence of endometriosis?**

Occurs in 3%–10% of women of reproductive age group and 25%–35% of infertile women

**What three mechanisms have been proposed to cause endometriosis?**

Retrograde menstruation:

Menstrual material flows retrograde through fallopian tubes and implants on pelvic and abdominal structures.

Reinforced by studies that showed that monkeys with cervices surgically altered to empty into peritoneal cavity developed endometriosis.

Coelomic metaplasia:

Peritoneal coelomic epithelium undergoes metaplastic changes to assume characteristics of endometrial tissue.

Reinforced by the finding of endometriosis in prepubertal girls and women who have never menstruated

Hematogenous/lymphatic spread:

Endometrial tissue "metastasizes" by vascular and lymphatic pathways to implant on various pelvic, abdominal, and distant organs.

Explains extrapelvic and pulmonary endometriosis

**Is there a genetic predisposition to development of endometriosis?**

Genetic or immunologic factors may play a role in endometriosis.
Seven percent of first-degree relatives of women with endometriosis have the disease, compared to one percent of control group, in one study.
A polygenic/multifactorial mechanism of heredity has been proposed.

**What are the risk factors for endometriosis?**

Nulliparity
Infertility
Reproductive age (usually, late teens to forties)
A first-degree relative with endometriosis
Regular menstrual cycles less than 27 days
Prolonged menses of 8 or more days

**What is the most common endometriosis symptom?**

Pelvic pain; can manifest as secondary dysmenorrhea, deep dyspareunia (pain on deep penetration), low sacral backache (especially premenstrually), or constant diffuse pelvic pain

**How does endometriosis affect organs adjacent to the uterus?**

Rectosigmoid involvement can lead to perimenstrual tenesmus or diarrhea.
Bladder involvement can result in dysuria or hematuria.

**What physical examination findings are suggestive of endometriosis?**

Tenderness on bimanual examination
Tenderness or nodularity on the posterior vaginal fornix
Uterosacral ligament tenderness or nodularity
Cystic ovarian enlargement
Fixation of adnexal structures
Retroflexed uterus
Episiotomy or cesarean section scar implants

**Is an OCA-125 level helpful in diagnosing endometriosis?**

OCA-125 is elevated (> 35 U/ml) in approximately one-third of women with advanced endometriosis.
Elevated OCA-125 level is neither diagnostic nor an accurate screening test.

| | |
|---|---|
| **Are radiologic studies useful in making the diagnosis?** | Ultrasound or magnetic resonance imaging may reveal endometriomas, but otherwise are not useful in the diagnosis of endometriosis. |
| **Is endometriosis a clinical diagnosis?** | Endometriosis is **not** a clinical diagnosis! Definitive diagnosis of endometriosis can be made **only** by direct visualization of endometriotic lesions at time of laparoscopy or laparotomy **or** tissue diagnosis by pathologist. |
| **What do endometriosis lesions look like?** | "Classic" endometriosis lesions are red, dark brown, dark blue, or black peritoneal implants or "chocolate cysts" of the ovary, but endometriotic lesion appearance varies as follows: "Powder burn" implants from thickened or scarred perilesional peritoneum Clear vesicles White or yellow spots or nodules Normal-appearing peritoneum (microscopic disease) |
| **How is endometriosis classified?** | The American Fertility Society classification system is based on findings at time of laparoscopy or laparotomy to determine severity of disease. Numeric values are assigned to various findings, with higher numbers implying more severe disease. |
| **How is endometriosis staged?** | Stages are determined by the total point assignment for the constellation of findings in a given patient. Stage I: Minimal Stage II: Mild Stage III: Moderate Stage IV: Severe |
| **What are some examples of point assignment for various findings at the time of laparoscopy or laparotomy?** | 1: Filmy adhesions enclosing less than one-third of the ovary *or* filmy adhesions enclosing less than one-third of the tube *or* superficial ovarian endometriotic implants < 1 cm in size 2: Superficial peritoneal endometriosis 1–3 cm in size |

4: Partial cul-de-sac obliteration *or* superficial peritoneal endometriosis ≥ 3 cm in size

6: Deep peritoneal endometriosis ≥ 3 cm in size

8: Dense tubal adhesions with less than one-third enclosure

16: Deep ovarian implants 1–3 cm in size *or* dense tubal adhesions with more than two-thirds enclosure

40: Complete cul-de-sac obliteration

**How useful is classification of endometriosis?**

High intraobserver and interobserver variability limits utility, but classification is helpful in operative report summaries.

**What are the goals of management/treatment of endometriosis?**

Control of symptoms
Treatment of infertility
The disease is progressive and difficult (or impossible) to "cure."

**What are the types of management/treatment of endometriosis?**

Medical (hormonal)
Surgical (conservative or definitive)
Combination of medical and surgical

**How is the choice of management/treatment determined?**

By severity of disease, reproductive considerations, and physician/patient preference

**What medications are used in the treatment of endometriosis?**

Medications suppress estrogenic stimulation of ectopic endometrial tissue:
Combined estrogen–progestin
Progestins
Danazol
Gonadotropin-releasing hormone (GnRH) agonists

**Indications for medical therapy?**

Used only after surgery confirms the presence of endometriosis through viewing classic endometriotic lesions, or a tissue diagnosis is made

**What is danazol, how does it work, and what are its side effects?**

Danazol (Danacrine) is a weak synthetic androgen.
Mechanism of action: Suppresses luteinizing hormone (LH) and follicle-stimulating hormone (FSH) secretion, leading to decreased ovarian steroidogenesis, and directly inhibits

endometrial cells (by androgen receptors), creating a high-androgen/low-estrogen environment

Side effects: Increased liver enzymes, increased low-density lipoproteins, decreased high-density lipoproteins, weight gain, edema, decreased breast size, oily skin, acne, hirsutism, and, rarely, permanent voice deepening

**What are GnRH agonists, how do they work, and what are their side effects?**

GnRH agonists are novel peptides synthesized by substituting the sixth amino acid residue (and sometimes the tenth) of the native GnRH molecule to achieve a longer half-life and better binding to the GnRH receptor.

Mechanism of action:

Initially cause an increase in gonadotropin release from the anterior pituitary (the "flare effect")

After 2 weeks, acts in downregulating the pituitary, leading to a decrease in FSH and LH secretion and thus decreased ovarian estrogen synthesis (hypoestrogenic state), which causes shrinkage of endometrial implants

Side effects:

"Pseudomenopause"

Include hot flashes, sweating, vaginal dryness/vaginitis, headache, decreased libido, depression, emotional lability, and, eventually, bone loss

**What is the effect of oral contraceptive pills (OCPs) and progestins on endometriosis?**

Create a "pseudopregnancy"

OCPs suppress FSH and LH secretion and endogenous estrogen production **and** reduce menstrual volume, which may lead to decreased reflux of menstrual products and decreased formation of new endometriosis lesions.

Progestins (Provera) have similar effects on FSH/LH secretion and estrogen synthesis, but also induce decidual change in endometriosis implants.

**What is the preferred treatment for infertility in a woman with mild endometriosis?**

If endometriosis has just been diagnosed by laparoscopy and the remainder of the infertility workup is negative, no treatment is preferred.

**What is the treatment for infertility in a woman with severe endometriosis?**

Laparoscopic ablation of endometrial implants with or without medical treatment

**What are the goals of conservative surgery (with laparoscopy or laparotomy) for endometriosis?**

Destruction of implants
Drainage and excision of endometriomas
Lysis of adhesions
Relief of pelvic pain through uterosacral ligament ablation or presacral neurectomy

**How do postoperative pregnancy rates after laparoscopy or laparotomy compare in severe endometriosis?**

Fifteen nonrandomized, retrospective studies of 206 patients with severe endometriosis after laparoscopic treatment revealed a mean crude postoperative pregnancy rate of 47.6%.
Fourteen nonrandomized, retrospective studies of 591 patients after treatment with laparotomy revealed a mean crude postoperative pregnancy rate of 38.2%.

**What is the goal of definitive surgery for endometriosis?**

Removal of any potential sites of origin or implantation of endometriosis

**What are the potential sites of origin or implantation of endometriosis?**

Uterus
    Treated with hysterectomy
    Leaving nondiseased ovaries intact is also an option if ovarian function is important.
Ovaries (treated with bilateral oophorectomy)
Cul-de-sac (treated with obliteration)
Bowel (treated with resection of bowel lesions)

**Indications for subtotal hysterectomy?**

Extensive fibrosis and pelvic adhesions, to avoid complications from difficult dissection

**How are medical and surgical therapy used together in endometriosis treatment?**

After surgery, medical therapy can be used to treat severe or extensive endometriosis.

**Options for postoperative medical therapy?**

GnRH agonist
Danazol
Postoperative oral contraceptives

**What is the incidence of recurrence of endometriosis after medical treatment? After surgical treatment?**

Medical therapy: Recurs in 30%–50% of patients treated
Conservative surgical treatment: Recurs in 14%–40% of patients
The more radical the surgery (oophorectomy, hysterectomy), the less likely a recurrence.
In reality, endometriosis is probably never "cured" until the hypoestrogenic postmenopausal state ensues.

# 28

## Contraception

**What are the three general types of reversible contraception?**

Barrier methods (with or without spermicide)
Intrauterine devices (IUDs)
Hormonal agents

**What are the failure rates for the commonly used contraceptives?**

Table 28–1.

| Contraceptive Method | Annual Pregnancy Rate |
|---|---|
| No contraceptive action | 85% |
| Withdrawal | 14.7% |
| Condom | 9.8% |
| Diaphragm | 12.0% |
| Sponge | 16.0% |
| IUD | 2.5% |
| Pill | 3.8% |
| Implants | 0.8% |
| Injectables | 0.4% |
| Tubal sterilization | 0.5% |

## BARRIER METHODS

**What are the most commonly used barrier methods for contraception?**

Condoms, diaphragms, and sponges
All may be used in conjunction with spermicidal compounds.

### CONDOM

**What are the advantages and disadvantages of the condom?**

**Advantages:** No danger to health; rare side effects; instant reversibility; and protection against human immunodeficiency virus (HIV), other sexually transmitted diseases (STDs), and cervical intraepithelial neoplasia
**Disadvantages:** Interference with flow of sexual activity, need for availability, and risk of the condom breaking or slipping off

| | |
|---|---|
| **How effective is the condom in preventing HIV and other STDs?** | One study found a zero HIV transmission rate for couples in which one partner was HIV positive and condoms were consistently used. |

## DIAPHRAGM

| | |
|---|---|
| **What is it?** | A dome-shaped device made of latex rubber; the shape is maintained by a metal spring within the latex rim |
| **How are diaphragms classified?** | By the shape of the spring and rim |
| **What are the different types of diaphragms?** | Arcing spring<br>Coil spring<br>Flat spring<br>Wide seal rim |
| **How does the diaphragm prevent conception?** | Acts as a physical barrier to sperm and serves as a reservoir for spermicide (nonoxynol-9) at the cervix. |
| **How does the diaphragm prevent transmission of STDs?** | The combination of chemical and physical barriers is thought to be involved in the prevention of STDs. |
| **What is the proper placement of a diaphragm?** | A properly placed diaphragm rests posterior to the pubic symphysis and extends backward to the posterior fornix, thereby covering the cervix. |
| **How long before and how long after coitus should the diaphragm be left in place in order to prevent conception effectively?** | The diaphragm containing spermicide on the cervical side should be inserted no more than 6 hours before intercourse, and additional spermicide should be applied if coitus occurs again.<br>The diaphragm should remain in place for 6–8 hours after the last act of coitus. |
| **What are the advantages and disadvantages of the diaphragm?** | **Advantages:** Self-managed method and protection against STDs and cervical neoplasia<br>**Disadvantages:** Increased risk of urinary tract infections secondary to alteration of vaginal flora by spermicide, lack of protection of the entire genital tract against pathogens, |

must be fitted by trained personnel, small risk of toxic shock syndrome

**What are the contraindications for diaphragm use?**

Anatomic abnormalities that impair adequate fit such as vaginal septum, uterine prolapse, vesicovaginal fistulas, severe cystocele or rectocele, and poor vaginal muscle tone

Allergy to rubber, latex, or spermicide

History of toxic shock syndrome

Recurrent cystitis associated with diaphragm use

Inability or unwillingness of the user correctly to use or care for the diaphragm

Lack of trained personnel to fit the diaphragm

## CONTRACEPTIVE SPONGE

**What is it?**

A cup-shaped sponge made of polyurethane foam and impregnated with nonoxynol-9 that is inserted into the vagina

**How long before intercourse can the sponge be inserted?**

Up to 24 hours

**What are the advantages and disadvantages of the contraceptive sponge?**

**Advantages:** Absence of serious side effects, universal size eliminates the need for fitting, available over-the-counter, allows user to engage in multiple acts of coitus without additional preparation, no need to wait after insertion, can be inserted hours in advance of intercourse, and disposability

**Disadvantages:** Availability (currently, the only manufacturer stopped the production of the contraceptive sponge secondary to bacterial contamination problems); toxic shock syndrome

## INTRAUTERINE DEVICES

**What are IUDs?**

The currently available IUDs are T-shaped devices bearing either copper or a slow-release progestin agent.

An IUD is placed by the physician high in the uterine fundus and is thought to interfere with fertilization or implantation.

IUDs have a nylon thread "tail" for the purposes of detection and future removal.

**What is the mechanism of action of copper-containing IUDs?**

Prevent fertilization of the egg within the fallopian tube by reducing the number of sperm in the tube and possibly by an additional effect of copper on fertility of the egg

**What is the mechanism of action of progestin-containing IUDs?**

Act mainly by rendering the endometrium atrophic and thereby interfering with implantation of the fertilized egg

Also, in 50% of women using this type of IUD for at least a year, ovulation is prevented.

**What is the effect on menstruation of progestin-containing IUDs?**

Tend to cause a gradual decrease in menstrual blood loss

May lead to partial or total amenorrhea

**Which patients are good candidates for an IUD?**

Patients should have a monogamous sexual relationship.

Both the patient and her partner should be free of any STDs.

IUDs may be the contraceptive method of choice for women 35 years of age or older involved in a monogamous relationship, who smoke, and who are therefore not candidates for oral contraceptives.

**Do IUDs cause pelvic infections?**

The risk of infection associated with IUDs was overstated in the 1970s and 1980s.

The IUD does not itself cause infection, but contraction of gonococcal and chlamydial infections in an IUD user may lead to a more severe course of infection.

Nonmonogamous women are at greater risk for contracting these illnesses and are therefore not candidates for IUD use.

**What are the contraindications for the use of IUDs?**

Absolute contraindications: Pregnancy, known or suspected pelvic malignancy, and current or chronic pelvic infection

Relative contraindications: History of ectopic pregnancy or pelvic inflammatory disease (PID), debilitating dysmenorrhea, congenital anomalies of the genital tract, and sickle cell anemia (because of increased susceptibility to infection)

Some authorities consider valvular heart disease a contraindication to use of IUDs.

**When during the menstrual cycle should the IUD be inserted?**

During menses so that the spotting and cramping associated with insertion become less noticeable and important to the patient; also, so that the physician can be more confident that the patient is not pregnant.

**What are the possible complications of IUD use?**

Expulsion of the IUD (partial or complete)

Uterine perforation

Dysmenorrhea

Pregnancy (both ectopic and intrauterine)

**What is the significance of the patient not being able to feel the tail of her IUD?**

The IUD may have been expelled from the uterine cavity, especially if the patient cannot feel the tail after a menstrual period.

The patient should see her physician promptly and use a different method of contraception until then.

**What is the significance of elongation or shortening of the IUD tail?**

Elongation of the tail may represent partial expulsion; may indicate that the device has lost its contraceptive effect and pregnancy must be ruled out.

Shortening of the tail may be due to the gradual migration of the IUD out of the uterine cavity; may represent perforation of the uterine wall.

## HORMONAL AGENTS

### ORAL CONTRACEPTIVE PILLS (OCPs)

**What are the two types of OCPs currently available?**

Combination estrogen and progesterone pill (either ethinyl estradiol or mestranol as the estrogenic compound and one of a variety of different progestins as the progestational agent)
Progesterone-only pill

**How do OCPs prevent conception?**

Mainly by suppressing the pituitary–gonadal axis and reducing the secretion of gonadotropins
Also by thickening of the cervical mucus and inhibition of endometrial proliferation, making fertilization and implantation less likely

**What are the contraindications to OCP use?**

Absolute contraindications: Past or present thrombophlebitis or thromboembolism; smoker and 35 years of age or older; cerebrovascular or coronary artery disease; lipodystrophy; current or past breast or endometrial cancer or other estrogen-dependent tumor; impaired liver function; cholestasis of pregnancy, or jaundice before pill use
Relative contraindications: Vascular or migraine headaches, especially with concomitant cigarette use; hypertension (blood pressure ≥ 160/100 mm Hg); gallbladder disease; lactation

**Can women 35 years of age and older who do not smoke use the OCP?**

Yes, provided that they do not have any other significant cardiovascular risk factors (e.g., high-risk lipid profile)

**How is OCP therapy managed in patients undergoing surgery?**

Combination OCPs should not be taken during surgery or any hospitalization involving long periods of immobilization because of the four- to sixfold increased risk of thromboembolic complications.

Patients scheduled for elective surgical procedures that may place them at increased risk for thromboembolic disease should stop using combination OCPs a month before date of surgery and use a different method of birth control during this time.

Progestin-only OCPs pose no increased health risks during surgery and patients can continue taking them.

**What are the beneficial effects of OCPs?**

Decrease the prevalence of menorrhagia, dysmenorrhea, and premenstrual tension

OCP users have lower incidences of benign cystic breast disease (fibroadenoma and chronic cystic disease), ovarian and endometrial cancer, and PID.

**What is the association between OCPs and thromboembolic disease?**

OCPs are associated with an increased incidence of thromboembolism because of estrogen-induced increase in blood levels of clotting factors VII and X and decrease in levels of antithrombin III. Progesterone's fibrinolytic effects oppose, at least in part, the hypercoagulable state produced by estrogen.

The risk of thromboembolism due to OCP use is synergistic with other risk factors such as hyperlipidemia and smoking.

It is believed that the risk of thromboembolic disease outweighs the benefits of OCPs only in predisposed patients (i.e., those with prior history) and in those with multiple risk factors (e.g., women 35 years of age or older who smoke).

**What is the association between OCP use and incidence of myocardial infarction (MI)?**

OCP-associated increases in the risk for MI of zero to fourfold have been reported.

The larger relative risks were reported

in studies of OCPs with higher estrogen content than commonly used today.

As in thromboembolic disease, this risk increases synergistically with other risk factors such as smoking, diabetes, and hypercholesterolemia.

It is believed that smoking represents the major risk factor for MI in OCP users.

**What is the association between OCP use and cerebrovascular disease?**

The major cerebrovascular risk associated with OCP use is that of subarachnoid hemorrhage, which is about six times the risk of nonusers.

Women who smoke and use OCPs have a 22 times greater chance of having a subarachnoid hemorrhage than the control group.

Strokes seem to be limited to older ($\geq$ 35 years of age) women who smoke or have other risk factors.

**What effects do OCPs have on blood pressure?**

About 1%–5% of OCP users have mild to moderate hypertension with elevations of 20–40 and 10–20 mm Hg in the systolic and diastolic pressures, respectively.

Cause of OCP-associated hypertension is thought to involve abnormalities of the renin–angiotensin system, leading to increased aldosterone production and sodium retention.

Incidence increases with age, parity, and obesity.

Hypertension resolves after discontinuation of the pill in the absence of other contributing causes.

**What is the relationship between OCPs and diabetes mellitus?**

Studies have shown that some OCPs can cause a decrease in glucose tolerance that appears to be associated with the progestin component of OCPs.

Incidence of diabetes mellitus is not increased by OCP use.

In predisposed patients, insulin dependence may occur sooner if certain OCPs are used.

In diabetic women with vascular complications of the disease (retinopathy, nephropathy), there may be an increased risk of thrombus formation secondary to OCP use.

In patients at risk, the progestin of choice is low-dose norethindrone or one of the newer progestins (levonorgestrel, gestodene, desogestrel, or norgestimate).

**How is thyroid function affected by OCP use?**

Induces increased production of thyroid-binding globulin, and increases thyroxine levels

Triiodothyronine RU declines, and thyroid index is normal. Patients remain euthyroid.

**What liver disease is associated with OCP use?**

Hepatocellular adenoma, a benign liver neoplasm, is associated with long-term OCP and other exogenous steroid use.

Presents as right upper quadrant pain or a palpable mass

If ruptured, can present as acute abdomen with hemodynamic instability

**What is the management of hepatocellular adenoma?**

Discontinuation of OCP leads to regression of the tumor and is the treatment of choice in most patients.

Pregnancy should be avoided in patients with hepatocellular adenoma because of the associated hyperestrogenic state, which can lead to enlargement and potential rupture of the adenoma.

If pregnancy is desired, patients should first undergo surgery to remove the adenoma.

**What is meant by "breakthrough bleeding" in OCP users?**

Bleeding that occurs at an inappropriate time during the cycle

**What causes it?**

Usually an imbalance between estrogen and progestin levels

| | |
|---|---|
| **How is it managed?** | If it occurs early during OCP use (first 3 months), it usually resolves spontaneously; reassurance and counseling are usually sufficient. Pathologic causes such as spontaneous abortion, neoplasia, ectopic pregnancy, PID, and benign uterine pathology should be considered. If bleeding continues after the first 3–4 months of use, switching to a formulation with a higher estrogen dose or a less potent progestin is advisable. |
| **How is the initial OCP selected?** | General evaluation for risks and contraindications to OCP use is done. Low-dose estrogen pills usually are appropriate. Menstrual characteristics and hormonal sensitivity should be noted. |
| **What signs and symptoms may be present in estrogen-hypersensitive/ progesterone-deficient patients?** | Severe nausea or edema during pregnancy or at mid-cycle<br>Prolonged and heavy menses with severe cramps<br>Severe and prolonged premenstrual symptoms beginning 7–12 days before menses |
| **What signs and symptoms may be present in progesterone-hypersensitive/estrogen-deficient patients?** | Scant menses<br>Mid-cycle spotting |
| **What signs and symptoms are indicative of androgen excess?** | Very oily skin<br>Acne<br>Male-pattern hair loss or hair growth on face and chest<br>Oligomenorrhea<br>Amenorrhea |
| **How do OCP hormones affect acne?** | Progestins increase sebum production (androgenic side effect) and hence cause a worsening of acne; estrogens have the opposite effect. |

**What causes the androgenic side effects associated with OCPs?**

Related to the quantity and quality of the progestin agent in the pill

Include hirsutism and hair loss in addition to acne

Can be treated by using a less androgenic progestin or, if problems persist, increasing the estrogen dosage

**What are the relative androgenic activities of the commonly used progestins?**

The androgenic activities of the common progestins, from highest to lowest, are: Levonorgestrel > norgestrel > desogestrel > norgestimate > norethindrone acetate > norethindrone > ethynodiol diacetate > megestrol acetate = medroxyprogesterone acetate.

**What are examples of the appropriate initial choice of OCP for each of the listed types of patients?**

**Patients with normal menses**

Ethinyl estradiol 35 μg–desogestrel 0.15 mg (e.g., Ortho-Cept, Desogen) or the equivalent (N.B. desogestrel has recently been associated with a higher rate of thrombus)

**Estrogen-hypersensitive/ progesterone-deficient patients**

Require lower estrogenic activity (20–30 μg of ethinyl estradiol)

Examples: Ethinyl estradiol 20 μg– norethindrone acetate 1.0 mg (Lo Estrin), ethinyl estradiol 30 μg– norgestrel 0.3 mg (Lo/Ovral) or the equivalent

**Progesterone- hypersensitive/estrogen- deficient patients**

Require low progesterone dose and progestational activity and slightly higher estrogen dose

Examples: Ethinyl estradiol 35 μg– norgestimate 0.25 mg (Ortho-Cyclen), ethinyl estradiol 35 μg–norethindrone 0.5 mg (Brevicon, Modicon) or the equivalent

**Androgen-hypersensitive patients/patients with polycystic ovary disease**

Pills with high progestational and low androgenic activity are best suited for this group.

Examples: Ethinyl estradiol 30 μg– desogestrel 0.15 mg (Desogen, Ortho-

Cept) or ethinyl estradiol 35 µg–
ethynodiol diacetate 1.0 mg (Demulen
1/35) or the equivalent.

**What should the patient do
if she forgets to take one
or more of her OCPs?**

Use additional contraceptive measures
for the remainder of that cycle.
Missed single pill: Take the missed dose
immediately and the next dose at the
regular time.
Missed two pills: Take two pills
immediately and two the following
day.
Missed three or more pills: Discard the
old packet of pills and start a new
packet on that day.
If menstruation does not occur at the
regular time, a pregnancy test must be
performed.

**What is postpill
amenorrhea?**

Failure to resume menses by 6 months
after termination of OCP use

**What is its incidence?**

One percent of patients
Almost half of these patients have a
history of oligomenorrhea before pill
use.

**What is the management
of postpill amenorrhea?**

Most cases spontaneously resolve within
6 months of the discontinuation of
OCPs.
An endocrinologic workup is not needed
until amenorrhea continues for 6
months unless galactorrhea is also
present; in this case, workup should
occur at 3 months after
discontinuation of the OCP.
Workup should:
Rule out pregnancy because it may
occur before resumption of menses
Rule out other causes of amenorrhea
such as strenuous exercise and
anorexia nervosa
Include progestin challenge test

**What is a progestin
challenge test?**

Helpful in assessing the status of the
hypothalamic–pituitary–ovarian axis.
Medroxyprogesterone acetate 0.5 mg is
given for 5 days.

|  | Presence of bleeding signifies anovulatory dysfunction. Absence of bleeding indicates absence of estrogen or a nonfunctional endometrium. |
|---|---|
| **How is anovulatory dysfunction managed?** | With ovulation-inducing agents such as clomiphene |
| **How is absence of estrogen or nonfunctional endometrium managed?** | Requires further evaluation for pituitary, hypothalamic, and endometrial disorders |
| **What drugs can interfere with OCP action?** | Those that are strong inducers of the liver cytochrome $P_{450}$ system. Include anticonvulsants (e.g., phenobarbital, carbamazepine, phenytoin, primidone) and some antibiotics (e.g., rifampin, isoniazid, neomycin, ampicillin, penicillin V, tetracycline) |
| **What are signs and symptoms of drug interaction with OCP?** | Breakthrough bleeding. Absence of withdrawal menses (due to pregnancy) |
| **How is drug interaction managed?** | Short-term use of interfering drug (e.g., a course of antibiotics): Backup method for contraception. Long-term use (e.g., seizure prophylaxis): Another method of birth control may be advisable. |
| **Do OCPs cause weight gain?** | An equal number of people lose and gain weight on OCPs; however, both estrogens and progestins are capable of causing weight gain. |
| **How can weight gain be minimized?** | By using the lowest effective estrogen–progestin combination with the lowest potency progestin and maintaining a sensible diet |

## INJECTABLE MEDROXYPROGESTERONE ACETATE

| **What is injectable medroxyprogesterone acetate?** | Also known as DMPA and Depo Provera. Similar to naturally occurring progesterone |
|---|---|

Available in the form of microcrystals in an aqueous suspension

**How is medroxyprogesterone acetate absorbed?**

After intramuscular injection, medroxyprogesterone acetate is slowly absorbed over the following 3–4 months.

**What is the dosing schedule for medroxyprogesterone acetate?**

150 mg every 3 months

**What is the mode of action of medroxyprogesterone acetate?**

Inhibits ovulation through the suppression of the pituitary–gonadal axis, decreasing luteinizing hormone and follicle-stimulating hormone, and preventing luteinizing hormone surges

**What are the advantages and disadvantages of medroxyprogesterone acetate?**

**Advantages:** Effective, easy-to-use contraceptive method; decrease in menses and menstrual blood loss (in most patients); decreased incidence of PID, candidal infections, and endometrial cancer; retains efficacy in presence of anticonvulsant medications; and does not affect infant nutrition in women who are breast-feeding

**Disadvantages:** Menstrual changes (number one cause of discontinuation); slight weight gain (1–3 kg); slightly slower return to fertility after discontinuation; minor complaints such as headaches, dizziness, and hair loss in some patients

**What menstrual changes are associated with use of medroxyprogesterone acetate?**

From amenorrhea to heavy bleeding Amenorrhea is more common with continued use.

**What is the incidence of conception after discontinuation of medroxyprogesterone acetate?**

Respectively, 70% and 90% of patients conceive within 1 and 2 years after discontinuation of medroxyprogesterone acetate.

**In what conditions is medroxyprogesterone acetate especially useful?**

Postpartum/lactation

Conditions contraindicating use of estrogen-containing contraceptives (e.g., women 35 years of age or older who smoke)

Conditions that may benefit from a reduction in menstrual blood loss (e.g., menorrhagia, fibroids, hemoglobinopathies)

Concomitant use of drugs that may interact with oral or implantable contraceptives, such as carbamazepine, rifampin, and phenytoin

Conditions associated with poor compliance with other contraceptive methods

Conditions in which pregnancy has catastrophic fetal risks, such as use of teratogenic medications (e.g., isotretinoin, valproate)

## LEVONORGESTREL IMPLANTS (NORPLANT)

**What are levonorgestrel implants?**

Six subdermally placed 34 x 2.4 mm Silastic tubes filled with the progestin levonorgestrel

**How long are the implants effective?**

Recommended period of use is 5 years. As release and plasma levels of levonorgestrel from the implants decrease, the failure rate increases, reaching 2 per 100 users in the sixth year of use.

**What effect does the weight of the user have on implant use?**

Because plasma levels of levonorgestrel vary inversely with the user's weight and the release rate is independent of weight, higher failure rates have been reported for women who weigh more than 70 kg.

**How do levonorgestrel implants prevent pregnancy?**

Inhibition of ovulation

Or, less frequent ovulation

In one-third to one-half of women, cyclic luteal activity and associated menstrual bleeding are observed, indicating lower-than-normal ovulatory progesterone levels.

Luteal insufficiency and disruption of
oocyte maturation have been
hypothesized to prevent fertilization
in this subset of users who ovulate.
Implants may also cause cervical mucus
changes that are hostile to sperm.

**Which medication can
interfere with the
implants' efficacy?**

Anticonvulsants, presumably due to
hepatic enzyme induction by many
members of this class of drugs

**What are the advantages
and disadvantages of
levonorgestrel implants?**

**Advantages:** Low maintenance, high
efficacy
**Disadvantages:** Need for placement
and removal, menstrual irregularities
(main reason for discontinuation),
headache, and weight gain

**What is the effect on
fertility after
discontinuation of
levonorgestrel implants?**

No effect; 86% of women achieve
pregnancy within 1 year of removal.

# 29

# Sexual Differentiation and Development

## NORMAL DEVELOPMENT

**How do the ovaries develop?**

Three weeks' gestation:

Primitive germ cells (oogonia) in the yolk sac of the fetus migrate to the genital ridge, where they are incorporated into sex cords.

Oogonia undergo mitosis to reach a maximum of more than 2 million by week 20; atresia reduces this number to 1 million at birth and 300,000 at puberty.

Four weeks' gestation:

Genital ridge develops medial to the mesonephric ridge.

This genital ridge consists of an inner core of ovarian mesenchyme and an outer layer of proliferating coelomic epithelium.

Five weeks' gestation:

The epithelium sends spoke-like projections into the mesenchyme to form primary sex cords.

Between eight and twelve weeks' gestation:

Oogonia begin meiosis and are arrested in prophase of the first meiotic division; they are then called primary oocytes.

The follicles surrounding primary oocytes are called primordial follicles.

Six months of age:

Formation of primary oocytes is complete.

Primary oocytes remain arrested until puberty when the surge of luteizing hormone (LH) causes ovulation, stimulating some to resume meiosis.

Differentiation of human gonads; A and B: Indifferent stages; C and D: Male development showing the primitive sex cords that develop into the testicular ducts; E and F: Female development showing degeneration of the primitive sex cords, which are replaced by secondary sex cords from the surface epithelium. (From Gilben SF: Developmental Biology, 2nd ed. Sunderland, MA: Sinauer Associates, 1988, with permission of the publisher)

**What changes occur in the ovary at menarche?**

Shortly before ovulation, the primary oocyte completes the first meiotic division to form the secondary oocyte and the first polar body.

First meiotic division is followed by the second meiotic division, which is again arrested (in metaphase) and does not resume meiosis unless fertilization by sperm occurs.

If a sperm cell penetrates the oocyte, meiosis resumes to form the mature oocyte (ovum) and the second polar body.

**How do the fallopian tubes, uterus, and vagina develop?**

All three structures develop from **müllerian ducts** (paramesonephric ducts):

Develop in both sexes during week six of gestation

Appear as grooves in the coelomic epithelium of the paired genital ridges

In males, androgens and müllerian inhibiting factor (MIF) produced by the developing testes induce resorption of the müllerian ducts.

In females, the absence of MIF and androgens stimulates further müllerian development.

Fallopian tube: Each duct opens into the coelomic cavity cranially and becomes a fallopian tube.

Uterus and upper vagina:
Caudally, the two ducts fuse in the midline at the urogenital septum.

Regression of the septum leads to the development of the uterus and upper vagina.

Lower vagina: formed by the vaginal plate and lengthening of the urogenital sinus.

A schematic drawing of the genital ducts in the female at the end of the second month of development. **A.** Note the müllerian tubercle and the formation of the uterovaginal canal. **B.** Genital ducts after descent of the ovary. The only parts remaining of the mesonephric system are the epoöphoron, paroöpharon, and Gartner's cyst. Note the suspensory ligament of the ovary, the ligament of the ovary proper, and the round ligament of the uterus.

## How do the external genitalia develop?

During the seventh week of gestation, the genital tubercle elongates to form the phallus.

Two sets of folds, the lateral genital folds and the medial urogenital folds, differentiate to form the labia majora and labia minora, respectively.

The urogenital folds also form the prepuce of the clitoris.

**What is Tanner staging?**  A classification system for the development of secondary sex characteristics (breast and pubic hair development)

**List the stages.**

### Table 29.1 Tanner staging

| Stage | Breast | Pubic Hair |
|-------|--------|------------|
| 1 | Preadolescent, elevated papillae | None |
| 2 | Breast bud and papillae slightly elevated | Sparse, long, slightly pigmented |
| 3 | Further enlargement of breast mound; increased palpable glandular tissue | Darker, coarser, curly |
| 4 | Areola and papilla project above breast | Adult-type hair; no spread to medial thigh |
| 5 | Papillae projected, mature | Adult-type hair with spread to medial thigh; inverse triangle distribution |

## CONGENITAL ANOMALIES OF THE REPRODUCTIVE TRACT

**What are the main ovarian anomalies?**  The many ovarian anomalies are included under the broad term gonadal dysgenesis.

**What is the definition of gonadal dysgenesis?**  Condition of abnormal gonadal development; denotes the presence of streak gonads regardless of other associated anomalies.
Many chromosomal abnormalities are associated with gonadal dysgenesis.

**What is a streak gonad?**  Nonfunctioning gonadal tissue consisting of dense fibrous stroma and lack of oocytes or spermatocytes

**What are some of the chromosomal abnormalities that cause gonadal dysgenesis?**  Turner syndrome
Abnormal X chromosome

**What is Turner syndrome?**  An abnormality with chromosome count of **45, X**
Chromosome count may also be:
45X/46XX mosaic
45X/46XY mosaic

| | |
|---|---|
| **What is the incidence?** | Occurs in 1 per 2000 live births |
| **What is the cause?** | In the fetus, oogonia migrate normally to the genital ridge but soon undergo rapid degeneration, resulting in **streak ovaries** (no hormones are produced). |
| **What are the associated clinical findings?** | Primary amenorrhea<br>Short stature<br>Lack of secondary sexual characteristics<br>Shield-shaped chest with widely spaced nipples<br>Webbed neck<br>Associated with cardiac anomalies (coarctation of the aorta)<br>Intelligence: usually normal; mental retardation in 10% of patients<br>Urinary **gonadotropins** (follicle-stimulating hormone [FSH] and LH): markedly **elevated** |
| **What is the treatment?** | Secondary sex characteristic development can be promoted with exogenous estrogen treatment. |
| **What is a special consideration of 45X/46XY mosaics?** | **Y** chromosome predisposes to **gonadal malignancy**.<br>Prophylactic surgical removal of the dysgenetic gonads is necessary. |
| **What is abnormal X chromosome?** | Karyotype is **46,XX,** but one of the X chromosomes is **incomplete**.<br>Deletion of long arm (Xq): streak gonads, sexual infantilism, normal stature, sterility; estrogen replacement therapy necessary for breast development<br>Deletion of short arm (Xp): phenotypically similar to Turner syndrome |
| **What are some causes of gonadal dysgenesis that have a normal chromosome complement?** | Pure gonadal dysgenesis<br>Gonadal agenesis (male pseudohermaphroditism) |

**What is pure gonadal dysgenesis?**

Condition in which chromosomal complement is normal (46,XX) but streak gonads are present.

**What are the etiologic factors?**

Occurs when primitive oogonia fail to migrate to genital ridge and ovaries fail to develop

May also be the result of nongenetic factors which affect gonadal tissue such as neoplasm or infarction

**What are the associated clinical findings?**

Primary amenorrhea
Infantile secondary sexual characteristics
Normal stature
No estrogen synthesis (gonads are nonfunctional)

**What is gonadal agenesis (male pseudohermaphroditism)?**

Also called "vanishing testes syndrome"
**Absence of gonads** with normal **male 46,XY** karyotype

**What are the associated clinical findings?**

Ambiguous external genitalia or normal female external genitalia but **NO internal female** reproductive organs
May present at puberty with primary amenorrhea and lack of breast development

**What is the theoretic cause?**

Sometime in embryonic development testicular tissue was present and MIF suppressed müllerian development. Then, for some unknown reason, the testes disappeared after müllerian inhibition.

**What are the etiologic factors of common uterine anomalies?**

Malfusion of the müllerian ducts with varying degrees of septation most commonly due to teratogenesis, genetic inheritance, and multifactorial expression. Often do not have clinical manifestations. Variations are shown in Figure 29-3.

Common clinical manifestation of abnormalities of müllerian duct development. **A.** Normal female. **B.** Septate uterus (failure of dissolution of septum). **C.** Bicornuate uterus (failure of fusion of mid müllerian ducts). **D.** Didelphis anomaly (complete failure of fusion). **E.** Septate uterus with duplication of cervix and vagina (combined failure of fusion and dissolution of septum). **F.** Unicornuate uterus failure of formation of one müllerian duct).

| | |
|---|---|
| **What is Mayer-Rokitansky-Küster-Hauser syndrome?** | Results in a complete lack of müllerian development (müllerian agenesis). Usually incomplete development of the fallopian tubes with absence of the uterus, cervix, and most of the vagina. |
| **What are the common vaginal anomalies?** | Vaginal agenesis **Transverse vaginal septum** **Longitudinal vaginal septum** Imperforate hymen |
| **What is vaginal agenesis?** | Partial or complete absence of vaginal vault Occurs as part of the Mayer-Rokitansky-Küster-Hauser syndrome, or independently |
| **What are the associated clinical findings?** | Since ovaries are present, secondary sex characteristics develop normally. |

**How is the diagnosis made?**

Physical exam confirms absence of vagina

Usually diagnosed in the setting of **delayed menarche**

Pelvic ultrasound to confirm presence or absence of uterus

Intravenous pyelogram is performed to detect urinary tract anomalies (found in 1/3 of patients with müllerian agenesis)

Testosterone level to rule out testicular feminization

Karyotype to confirm patient is 46,XX and to rule out disorders associated with 46,XY (e.g., testicular feminization)

**What is the treatment if the uterus is absent?**

Treatment is aimed at creating a neovagina to allow satisfactory sexual function (assumes *absent* uterus).

**Nonsurgical**: progressive vaginal dilatation if rudimentary vagina present

**Surgical:**

McIndoe procedure—If vaginal atresia is complete, a split-thickness skin graft is used to create a neovagina; graft is placed in the potential space between the bladder and rectum.

Williams vulvovaginoplasty—The labia majora are used to lengthen preexisting rudimentary vagina; does not require skin graft.

**What is the treatment if functioning uterus is present?**

Immediate treatment is crucial to remove obstruction to menstrual flow.

**Surgical** treatment: Neovagina is created using a stent with a central opening to allow flow; stent is left in place for 4 to 6 months.

**What is a transverse vaginal septum?**

A septum composed of vaginal mucosa with or without intervening connective tissue

May be either partial or complete, and can vary in thickness

| | |
|---|---|
| **What are the clinical findings?** | Clinical picture varies depending on extent of septation. |
| | **Partial** septation may present with dysmenorrhea, irregular vaginal spotting, secondary pelvic inflammatory disease (PID) from anaerobic infection, or no clinical symptoms. |
| | **Complete** septation presents with primary amenorrhea and obstruction; surgical treatment is imperative. |
| **What is the treatment?** | Surgery |
| **What is a longitudinal vaginal septum?** | Results from improper fusion of the distal müllerian ducts |
| | May be accompanied by bicornuate uterus with one or two cervices |
| **What are the associated clinical findings?** | May present with obstruction to drainage or dyspareunia |
| **What is the treatment?** | Necessary only if symptomatic or if childbearing is anticipated |
| **What is an imperforate hymen?** | Outlet obstruction which causes build-up of vaginal secretions |
| **What are the associated clinical findings?** | **Newborns:** mucocolpos |
| | **Adolescents:** hematocolpos; usually diagnosed in setting of primary amenorrhea |
| **What is the treatment?** | Surgery at the time of diagnosis |

## ABNORMAL SEXUAL DIFFERENTIATION

| | |
|---|---|
| **What causes abnormal sexual differentiation?** | Many of these disorders are the result of a defect in the steroid hormone biosynthetic pathway. |
| **What is female pseudohermaphroditism?** | Masculinization of the female fetus in utero |
| **What is male pseuohermaphroditism?** | Feminization of the male fetus in utero |

Obstetrics and Gynecology Recall

**What is congenital adrenal hyperplasia?**

Autosomal recessive defect in steroid biosynthesis
Karyotype is **46,XX**
Causes female pseudohermaphroditism
Most frequent cause of ambiguous genitalia in the newborn

**What is the incidence?**

Occurs in 1 in 5000 live births

**What are the etiologic factors?**

**21-hydroxylase deficiency** most common
Also caused by 11-hydroxylase deficiency (associated with hypertension) and 3B-ol-dehydrogenase deficiency (usually fatal due to severe adrenal insufficiency)

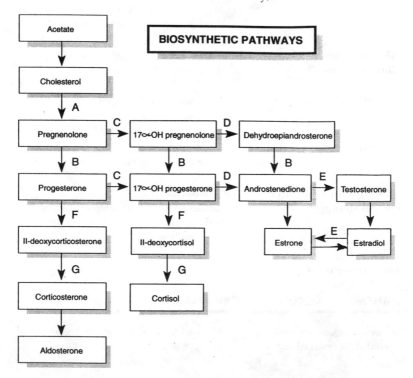

Summary of important adrenal and gonadal biosynthetic pathways. Letters designate enzymes required for the appropriate conversions. **A.** 20α-hydroxylase, 22R-hydroxylase, and 20,22-desmolase. **B.** 3β-ol-dehydrogenase. **C.** 17α-hydroxylase. **D.** 17,20-desmolase. **E.** 17-ketosteroid reductase. **F.** 21-hydroxylase. **G.** 11β-hydroxylase. (Simpson JL: Disorders of Sexual Differentiation. Etiology and Clinical Delineation. New York, Academic Press, 1976)

**Describe the pathophysiology of congenital adrenal hyperplasia.**

Lack of 21-hydroxylase (or others)→**decreased cortisol→increased ACTH**→accumulation of intermediate compounds in the pathway prior to the enzyme defect (17-hydroxyprogesterone and 17-hydroxypregnenolone)

These intermediates are converted to the "adrenal androgens" dehydroepiandrosterone (DHEA) and androstenedione, which are then converted peripherally into testosterone.

**What are the clinical findings?**

Presents as **ambiguous genitalia** in the newborn (clitoromegaly and accentuation of labial folds)

Chromosomes, gonads, and internal genitalia are female.

**How is the diagnosis made?**

Increased plasma levels of 17-hydroxyprogesterone or increased urinary levels of 17-ketosteroids (breakdown product of most androgens)

**What is the treatment?**

Hydrocortisone administered indefinitely

**What is 5α-reductase deficiency?**

Also called incomplete male pseudohermaphroditism

Autosomal recessive genetic defect

**46,XY** karyotype

**Describe the pathophysiology of 5α-reductase deficiency.**

5α-reductase normally converts testosterone to a more active steroid, dihydrotestosterone (DHT), which is necessary for the androgen target tissues of the urogenital sinus (development of external genitalia).

5α-reductase deficiency leads to **decreased DHT** and **normal testosterone** levels.

**What are the associated clinical findings?**

**Ambiguous genitalia** or phenotypic female, with or without palpable labial/inguinal testes

At puberty, testosterone production increases and is converted to DHT, causing virilization with growth of the penis and descent of the testes; pronounced muscle development may also occur.

After puberty, some patients may have penile erection, ejaculation, and fertility.

**What is the treatment?**

Important to establish diagnosis early, as late diagnosis may have profound psychological impact.

In most circumstances, individual should be raised as a female with gonadectomy and reduction clitoroplasty performed as soon as diagnosis is made.

**What is 17α-hydroxylase deficiency?**

Karyotype is **46,XX.**

**Describe the pathophysiology of 17α-hydroxylase deficiency.**

17α-hydroxylase is an enzyme in cortisol and steroid hormone synthesis (androgens and estrogens).

Decreased 17α-hydroxylase results in **increased ACTH** (in effort to produce more cortisol-negative feedback).

Mineralocorticoid pathway (to aldosterone synthesis) does NOT require 17α-hydroxylase, so the increase in ACTH causes **increased aldosterone** production, resulting in sodium retention, hypertension, and low potassium.

**What are the associated clinical findings?**

Similar to pure gonadal dysgenesis with no estrogen production

**What are some disorders of sexual differentiation that are NOT associated with defects of the steroid hormone biosynthetic pathway?**

Androgen insensitivity syndrome (testicular feminization)
True hermaphroditism
**Female pseudohermaphroditism of maternal origin**

**What is androgen insensitivity syndrome (testicular feminization)?**

X-linked recessive disorder resulting in **46,XY** genotype and **female phenotype** (male pseudohermaphroditism)

**Describe the pathophysiology.**

Androgen receptors are absent or defective.

Fetal testosterone and MIF production by the testes are normal.

However, because the **receptors** are defective, **male external genitalia do not develop.**

Normal MIF causes müllerian regression; results in absent fallopian tubes, uterus, and upper vagina (vagina ends as a blind pouch).

**What are the associated clinical findings?**

Secondary sex characteristics:

These patients produce some estrogen; therefore, breast development may be normal. Pubic and axillary hair, however, are sparse or absent (they rely on testosterone).

Presents as primary amenorrhea

The testes are located in the labia or in the inguinal canal (presenting as inguinal hernia) and should be removed after puberty because of increased risk for **gonadal malignancy.**

Patients are often reared as females.

**What is true hermaphroditism?**

Very rare condition

Dual gonadal development (both male and female gonadal tissue)

Genotype is usually **46,XX.**

**What are the associated clinical findings?**

External genitalia may appear male, female, or ambiguous; masculinization of the external genitalia depends on the amount of testicular tissue present.

Uterus is usually present

Cryptorchidism is frequent, usually with some degree of labioscrotal fusion.

At puberty, about 75% of patients develop gynecomastia and more than half menstruate.

**What is the treatment?**

Sex assignment should depend on the dominant appearance of the external genitalia (75% raised as males).

**What is female pseudohermaphroditism of maternal origin?**

Female pseudohermaphroditism due to exogenous or endogenous androgens

# 30

# Menstrual Cycle and Dysfunction

## NORMAL MENSTRUAL CYCLE

**What is the mean duration of the menstrual cycle?**
Mean: 28 days
Range: 24–32 days

**What is the average duration of menses?**
Three to seven days

**What is the normal estimated blood loss?**
Approximately 30 ml
About 80% of total loss occurs in first 2 days.

**When does the menstrual phase occur?**
From day 1 to day 4

**What uterine changes occur during menses?**
Glandular and stromal degradation with sloughing of the functionalis (inner endometrial layer)

**What are the hormonal levels during the menstrual phase?**
Estradiol and progesterone levels are low from the regressing corpus luteum of the previous cycle.
Follicle-stimulating hormone (FSH) level begins to rise in response to declining estradiol and progesterone levels.
Luteinizing hormone (LH) level rises slowly several days after FSH begins to increase.

**What is the follicular phase?**
Ovarian phase that begins with menses on day 1 of the menstrual cycle and ends with ovulation
The cumulus oophorus and fluid-filled antrum form.
A cohort of ovarian follicles begins maturation, but only one reaches maturity.

**When does ovulation occur in the menstrual cycle?**

Usually on day 14 within 30 to 38 hours after the onset of the mid-cycle LH surge

**What is the proliferative phase?**

Endometrial phase occurring at approximately day 4 to 14

**What uterine changes occur during the proliferative phase?**

Proliferation of the endometrial glands
Endometrial stromal proliferation
Elongation of spiral arteries

**What are the hormonal levels during the proliferative phase?**

Estradiol level increases and peaks just before the LH surge and ovulation.
Progesterone level remains low.
FSH peaks at mid-cycle with LH but produces a smaller surge.
LH rapidly peaks at mid-cycle and triggers ovulation.

**What is the secretory phase?**

Endometrial phase that begins on day 14 and lasts until day 28, approximately

**What uterine changes occur during the secretory phase?**

Progesterone stimulates the glands to secrete mucus and glycogen.
Glands become tortuous and dilated.
Convoluted spiral arteries extend to the superficial layer of the endometrium.
Stroma becomes edematous.

**What is the luteal phase?**

Ovarian phase that begins after ovulation
The corpus luteum forms from the granulosa cells of the ruptured follicle.

**What is the function of the corpus luteum?**

Produces progesterone and estradiol

**What are the normal hormonal levels during the secretory phase?**

**Estradiol** level decreases after ovulation, then begins to rise with production from the corpus luteum, and peaks on day 20 to 21.
**Progesterone** level begins to rise after ovulation to peak at approximately days 20–21 with production by the corpus luteum.
**LH and FSH** are at low levels because of negative feedback of the high progesterone and estradiol levels.

**Does estradiol or progesterone have a higher peak in the secretory phase?**

Progesterone

**What happens to the following if pregnancy does not occur:**

**Corpus luteum?**

Degenerates into a scar called the corpus albicans

**Progesterone level?**

Declines as corpus luteum regresses

**Estradiol level?**

Decreases as corpus luteum regresses

**FSH level?**

Increases slowly as corpus luteum regresses

**Endometrium?**

If pregnancy does not occur by day 23, the endometrium begins to degenerate.

**What is PMS?**

Premenstrual syndrome
Also known as luteal phase dysphoric disorder
Cyclic recurrence of physical, psychological, and behavioral changes that cause distress and interfere with normal daily activities or relationships

**When during the menstrual cycle does PMS occur?**

Signs and symptoms occur during the luteal phase of the menstrual cycle and remit after the onset of menses.

**In whom does it occur?**

Most common in women age 25 to 44 years

**What is its incidence?**

An estimated 5% of women of reproductive age can be diagnosed with PMS by the American Psychiatric Association and National Institute of Mental Health criteria.
About 40% of women report significant problems related to their menstrual cycles, with 2%–10% reporting an impact on work or lifestyle.

**What are the American Psychiatric Association criteria for PMS/luteal phase dysphoric disorder?**

Symptoms are temporally related to the menstrual cycle, starting during the last week of the luteal phase and ending after the onset of menses.

At least five of the following, including one of the first four symptoms:

1. Affective lability (e.g., sudden onset of irritability, anger, sadness)
2. Persistent and marked anger or irritability
3. Marked anxiety or tension
4. Markedly depressed mood, feeling of hopelessness
5. Decreased interest in usual activities
6. Easy fatigability or marked lack of energy
7. Subjective sense of difficulty in concentrating
8. Marked change in appetite, overeating, or food craving
9. Hypersomnia or insomnia
10. Physical symptoms such as breast tenderness, headaches, edema, joint or muscle pain, weight gain

Symptoms interfere with work or usual activities or relationships.

Symptoms are **not** an exacerbation of another psychiatric disorder.

**What is the evaluation for PMS?**

Examination of patient's daily diary of symptoms over a period of 2–3 months

History and physical examination to rule out other illness (e.g., depression)

**What is the treatment of PMS?**

Supportive:
  Counseling and education
  Goal is to provide the patient with greater control over her life.
  May include lifestyle changes such as exercise and dietary modifications

Medications:
    Fluoxetine (Prozac) and alprazolam (Xanax) have been shown to be effective in treating PMS in randomized trials.
    Nonsteroidal anti-inflammatory drugs (NSAIDs) such as mefenamic acid may also be of benefit.
    Gonadotropin-releasing hormone agonists have been used to treat severe PMS, but have significant side effects associated with the resultant low estrogen level.

**What is dysmenorrhea?**

Painful menstruation

**What is its incidence?**

About 50%–75% of women report dysmenorrhea.

**What are the two main categories of dysmenorrhea?**

**Primary dysmenorrhea:** Painful menstruation without associated pelvic disease

**Secondary dysmenorrhea:** Painful menstruation caused by pelvic pathology

**Describe the typical pattern of pain in primary dysmenorrhea.**
    **When?**

Usually begins with the onset of menstruation, then gradually decreases.

    **How long?**

Twelve to seventy-two hours

    **Where?**

Lower abdomen; most intense in midline

    **What type?**

Often crampy and colicky

**Other symptoms?**

Back pain
Nausea
Diarrhea
Fatigue
Headache
Malaise

**What is thought to be the cause of primary dysmenorrhea?**

Increased prostaglandin release from endometrial cells at the time of menstruation causes uterine smooth muscle contraction, increased intrauterine pressure, and some degree of uterine ischemia.

**What is the treatment of primary dysmenorrhea?**

NSAIDs are the mainstay of treatment:
  Propionic acid derivatives—ibuprofen, naproxen, ketoprofen
  Fenamates—mefenamic acid, meclofenamate, flufenamic acid
  Oral contraceptives: If NSAIDs are not effective or are contraindicated and contraception is desired; not as effective as NSAIDs
  Follow-up: Consider pathologic cause and secondary dysmenorrhea if there is no improvement with therapy.

**What is the pharmacologic mechanism that is responsible for relieving dysmenorrhea for the following drugs:**
  **NSAIDs?**

Inhibit prostaglandin production
The fenamates also have an antagonistic action at the prostaglandin receptors.

**Oral contraceptives?**

Decrease prostaglandins through suppression of ovulation and the normal sequence of hormones

**What are the side effects of NSAIDs?**

Gastric irritation
Nausea
Gastrointestinal ulcer
Increased bleeding time
Nephrotoxicity
Fenamates also associated with blurred vision, headaches, and dizziness.

**What is the effectiveness of NSAIDs in treating dysmenorrhea?**

Relieve dysmenorrhea in about 80% of women

**What are the common causes of secondary dysmenorrhea?**

Chronic pelvic inflammatory disease
Endometriosis
Adhesions
Müllerian duct abnormalities

| | |
|---|---|
| **What characteristics of secondary dysmenorrhea can help distinguish from primary dysmenorrhea?** | Difficult distinction to make<br>Must look for other signs and symptoms to indicate pathology, such as an increased white blood cell count<br>Secondary dysmenorrhea usually begins after age 20 years.<br>Pelvic pain is often present at times other than menstruation.<br>Patients may have an abnormal pelvic exam, although a normal pelvic exam does **not** rule out disease. |
| **What other illness is commonly associated with menstruation?** | Headache: Tension or vascular type<br>Migraine headaches may occur only at menses or may increase in frequency or severity at time of menstruation. |

## ABNORMAL UTERINE BLEEDING

| | |
|---|---|
| **What is considered excessive blood loss?** | > 80 ml |
| **Describe the patterns of abnormal bleeding.**<br>   **Oligomenorrhea?** | Infrequent, irregular bleeding usually at intervals > 40 days |
| **Polymenorrhea?** | Frequent but regular bleeding usually occurring at intervals of 21 days or less |
| **Menorrhagia (or hypermenorrhea)?** | Excessive bleeding in amount and duration at regular intervals |
| **Metrorrhagia?** | Irregular but not excessive uterine bleeding |
| **Menometrorrhagia?** | Frequent bleeding that is excessive in amount and duration and occurs at irregular intervals |
| **Hypomenorrhea?** | Regular bleeding that is decreased in amount |
| **What is the differential diagnosis for abnormal uterine bleeding?** | Blood dyscrasia<br>Inflammatory: Cervicitis, endometritis<br>Malignancy: Uterine, cervical, fallopian tube, ovarian, gestational trophoblastic disease<br>Benign growth: Leiomyomas, cervical polyps, endometrial polyps |

Dysfunctional uterine bleeding
Pregnancy related: Subinvolution of
    uterus, ectopic pregnancy,
    spontaneous abortion, postpartum
    hemorrhage, retained products of
    conception
Iatrogenic: Intrauterine device,
    anticoagulants, progestational agents
Other sites: Vaginal cancer, vaginal
    laceration, atrophic vaginitis, urethral
    or gastrointestinal source, external
    genitalia lesions

**What are the two main causes of abnormal bleeding in an adolescent?**

1. Dysfunctional uterine bleeding
2. Blood dyscrasia

**What is Halban disease?**

Increased bleeding due to persistent
    corpus luteum
Usually self-limited and not recurrent

**What must always be considered in a perimenopausal or postmenopausal woman with abnormal uterine bleeding?**

Cancer

**What should always be suspected in an ovulatory patient with abnormal bleeding?**

A pathologic abnormality such as a polyp

**What diagnostic procedures aid in this diagnosis?**

Hysteroscopy
Hysterosalpingogram
Biopsy

**What features help differentiate ovulatory from anovulatory cycles?**

Ovulatory cycles tend to be consistent in
    cycle length, duration of menses, and
    amount of bleeding.
Also look for associated mid-cycle pain,
    vaginal discharge, premenstrual breast
    tenderness, and dysmenorrhea.

**What is "dysfunctional uterine bleeding"?**

Abnormal uterine bleeding associated
with an anovulatory menstrual cycle
without the presence of organic disease;
a diagnosis of exclusion

**What are two theoretical causes?**

1. **Hormonal theory:** The normal hormonal controls are defective, and therefore the endometrial changes are not synchronous and universal as in normal menstrual cycles. The structural stability of the endometrium is compromised and the fragile tissue is subject to random breakdown. The usual rhythmic vasoconstriction that initiates normal ischemia and endometrial sloughing and the prolonged vasoconstriction that encourages stasis are also defective.

2. **Tissue theory:** The endometrial regeneration is thought to be triggered by endometrial tissue loss, not hormonal changes. Loss of tissue in the presence of excess estrogen is insufficient to restore endometrial structural stability. Curettage may be an effective treatment.

**What age-groups are typically affected?**

About 50% of patients are 40 years of age or older (perimenopausal).

Twenty percent are adolescents, about one or two years past menarche.

Both populations tend to be anovulatory.

**What is a commonly associated physical finding?**

Obesity

**What does the workup include?**

History and physical examination
Pap smear
Laboratory studies based on clinical suspicion:
    Complete blood count
    Human chorionic gonadotropin
    Prolactin
    Thyroid panel
    Serum androgen levels if clinical evidence indicates androgen excess
    Head magnetic resonance imaging if hyperprolactinemia or clinical evidence of hypopituitarism

Biopsy and hysteroscopy can be helpful, especially if patient is older or has history of unopposed estrogens.

**What are the four main categories of dysfunctional uterine bleeding?**

1. **Estrogen withdrawal bleeding:** Low estrogen level
2. **Estrogen breakthrough bleeding:** Chronic estrogen stimulates endometrial proliferation, which outgrows the structural support and leads to endometrial breakdown.
3. **Progesterone withdrawal bleeding:** Low progesterone level; **only** occurs if the endometrium is first primed to proliferate by estrogen
4. **Progesterone breakthrough bleeding:** High progesterone-to-estrogen ratio

**What are the etiologic factors for estrogen withdrawal bleeding?**

Bilateral oophorectomy
Radiation of mature follicles
Cessation of exogenous estrogen therapy

**What type of bleeding pattern is typically seen in estrogen breakthrough bleeding?**

Can only be predicted generally
Relatively **low** levels of estrogen lead to intermittent spotting that is low in flow but prolonged in duration.
**High** levels of estrogen allow the endometrium to build up beyond the limits of endometrial structural support, leading to prolonged periods of amenorrhea followed by profuse bleeds (oligomenorrhea with bouts of heavy bleeding).

**What are two conditions in which estrogen breakthrough bleeding can occur?**

Polycystic ovary syndrome and obesity

**What is the typical bleeding pattern in progesterone breakthrough bleeding?**

Intermittent, low-flow bleeding of variable duration (similar to low estrogen breakthrough bleeding)

**What is a common cause of progesterone breakthrough bleeding?**

Long-acting progestin-only contraceptives, such as Norplant and Depo-Provera

| | |
|---|---|
| **When does progesterone withdrawal bleeding occur?** | Usually after discontinuation of a progestin, such as a contraceptive |
| **What is the usual therapy for dysfunctional uterine bleeding?** | Intense estrogen–progestin therapy for 7 days (one low-dose combination monophasic oral contraceptive pill twice a day)<br>Cyclic low-dose oral contraceptive pill for 3 months (one pill once a day for 3 weeks, then 1 week of withdrawal bleeding)<br>**Contraception wanted:** Continue oral contraceptives<br>**Contraception not desired:** Medroxyprogesterone acetate 10 mg once a day for 10 days every month<br>Follow-up: Always needed because recurrent hemorrhage accompanies persistent anovulation and endometrial atypia may occur with unopposed estrogen exposure. |
| **What should you always tell the patient about oral contraceptive therapy for abnormal bleeding?** | Expect severe cramping and heavy bleeding for 2–4 days after stopping therapy. |
| **What circumstances warrant initial treatment with estrogens rather than the estrogen–progestin therapy above?** | Bleeding has been heavy for several days (need estrogen-stimulated endometrial proliferation).<br>Biopsy produces minimal tissue.<br>Patient has been on progestins (endometrium is atrophic).<br>When follow-up is uncertain: Estrogen therapy stops all types of dysfunctional bleeding temporarily. |
| **What is the estrogen therapy?** | Conjugated estrogens (1.25 mg) or estradiol (2.0 mg) daily for 7–10 days; then combine with 10 mg of medroxyprogesterone acetate for 7 days.<br>If bleeding is acute and moderately heavy, the oral estrogen can be given every 4 hours during the first 24 hours. |

If the acute bleeding is very heavy, then conjugated estrogens can be give intravenously every 4 hours until the bleeding stops, followed by estrogen-progestin therapy. If there is no response in 12–24 hours, reevaluate. Patient will likely need dilation and curettage.

**What is an alternative therapy if heavy bleeding is thought to be due to estrogen-stimulated proliferation?**

Medroxyprogesterone acetate 5 mg for 1 week in each cycle

# 31

# Infertility: The Infertile Couple

**What is the definition of infertility?**

Inability of a couple of reproductive age to achieve conception after 1 year of sexual intercourse without contraception

**What is primary infertility?**

Infertility that occurs without any prior pregnancies

**What is secondary infertility?**

Infertility that occurs after a previous conception

**What is the incidence of infertility?**

In the United States, occurs in about 28 million couples, or 14% of couples

**What are some contributing factors and their incidence in infertility?**

Male fertility factor: 35%
Ovulatory factors: 25%
Peritoneal factors: 25%
Cervical factors: 5%
Uterine factors: 5%
Idiopathic: 5%

**How are these factors used in evaluation and management of infertility?**

Each factor should be considered in the initial evaluation of the infertile couple.
Factors should serve as a guide for further evaluation and management.

**What percentage of couples have more than one reason for infertility?**

15%

## HISTORY

**What general questions should be asked during an initial infertility evaluation to elicit information about specific contributing factors?**

Age of each partner?
Previous pregnancies?
Length of time conception has been attempted?
Frequency of intercourse?
Lubricants used? (spermicidal?)
History of impotence or dyspareunia?

**What questions should be asked of the male partner during an initial infertility evaluation?**

Fathered a previous child?
Testicular surgery or injury?
Genitourinary infections (including sexually transmitted diseases)?
Postpubertal mumps?
Genital radiation or chemotherapy?
Hypospadias?
Neuropathy associated with nerve damage or medical conditions, such as diabetes mellitus?
Use of chemotherapeutic drugs, Furadantin, or sulfasalazine?
Excessive exposure to heat (hot tubs), pesticides, toxins, marijuana, nicotine, or alcohol?

**What questions should be asked of the female partner during an initial infertility evaluation to elicit information about possible ovulatory factors?**

Detailed menstrual history. Irregularities are frequently seen in chronic anovulation or oligo-ovulation.
Headaches, visual changes, and galactorrhea? Suggests pituitary adenoma and resultant hyperprolactinemia.
If amenorrhea, primary or secondary?
Excessive exercise? Suggests hypothalamic–pituitary failure.
Extreme emotional stress? Suggests hypothalamic–pituitary failure.
Excessive hair growth?
Changes in hair texture, weight gain or loss, palpitations, heat/cold intolerance? Suggest thyroid dysfunction.
Hot flashes and vaginal dryness? Suggest menopause, perimenopause, or premature ovarian failure.
Cycle lengths < 25 days or > 35 days, or that vary by > 7 days from cycle to cycle? Suggest ovulatory irregularity, especially if patient has premenstrual symptoms, dysmenorrhea, variation in amount/duration of flow.

**Peritoneal factors?**

Pelvic/adnexal surgery (including bilateral tube ligation)?
Pelvic infection [salpingitis/pelvic inflammatory disease (PID)]? PID doubles the incidence of infertility.

Previous ectopic pregnancies?
History of appendicitis, especially
  ruptured?
Septic abortion?
Previous intrauterine device (IUD) use?
  IUD use is associated with a fourfold
  increase in risk for development of
  pelvic adhesions.
Premenstrual spotting; dysmenorrhea;
  dyspareunia; and cyclic abdominal or
  pelvic pain? Suggest endometriosis,
  which doubles the incidence of
  infection.

**Cervical factors?**

A history of the following can cause
problems with cervical mucus
production or quality, leading to
infertility:
Cone biopsy?
Cautery (LEEP)?
Cryosurgery?
Obstetric trauma?
Cervicitis?

**Uterine factors?**

Leiomyomas?
Diethylstilbestrol (DES) exposure in
  utero? Can lead to a T-shaped uterus.
Previous dilation and curettage (D & C)?

**What are the rates of
infertility (percentage)
associated with the age of
the woman?**

20–24 years:7%
25–29 years: 9%
30–35 years: 15%
35–40 years: 22%
40–44 years: 29%

**What is the normal rate of
conception with
unprotected intercourse?**

After 1 month: 15%–20%
After 6 months: 50%–75%
After 1 year: 80%–90%

**What is the optimal coital
interval for conception?**

24–48 hours

## PHYSICAL EXAMINATION

**What findings in the male
physical examination
suggest a male infertility
factor?**

Evidence of congenital abnormalities
associated with male infertility, such
as lack of body hair; gynecomastia;
tall, thin, gynecoid appearance

Abnormalities in testicular descent, size, and consistency; presence of varicoceles

Varicoceles are compressible globular scrotal distentions that cannot be transilluminated and are caused by a venous abnormality.

Associated with increased male infertility

Evidence of infection (orchitis, epididymitis)

Penile abnormalities

**What findings in the female physical examination suggest ovulatory factors?**

Signs of androgen excess (as seen in polycystic ovary) including:

Clitorimegaly

Enlarged ovaries on pelvic examination

Hirsutism

Acne

Balding

Male escutcheon

Signs/symptoms of hyperthyroidism:

Goiter

Tremor

Very fine hair

Nervousness

Exophthalmos

Palpitations

Signs/symptoms of hypothyroidism

Goiter

Bradycardia

Sluggishness

Dry skin

Coarse hair

Myxedema

Obesity

Excess adipose tissue increases extragonadal steroid production.

Increased estrogen production inhibits follicle-stimulating hormone (FSH) secretion from the anterior pituitary and can cause anovulation.

Emaciation leads to hypothalamic dysfunction with loss of pulsatile gonadotropin-releasing hormone (GnRH) secretion.

334 Obstetrics and Gynecology Recall

Galactorrhea

Seen in hyperprolactinemia

High levels of prolactin suppress the
pulsatile secretion of GnRH from
the hypothalamus, thus preventing
cyclic gonadotropin release.

**Peritoneal and uterine
factors?**

Evidence of current infection: Pelvic
tenderness or mass or cervical
discharge

Nodularity felt on palpation of the
uterosacral ligaments suggests
endometriosis; best felt on
rectovaginal examination.

Fixation of the uterus or ovaries suggests
pelvic adhesions or fibrosis from
previous pelvic or abdominal
infection, surgery, or endometriosis.

Irregularly shaped uterus suggests the
presence of leiomyomas or congenital
malformation.

**Cervical factors?**

Discharge, cervical friability, and motion
tenderness suggest cervicitis.

Copious amount of cervical mucus
suggests impending ovulation or
estrogen excess.

Evidence of past surgical procedure or
trauma

Signs of DES exposure including:
Vaginal adenosis (glandular
appearance of vaginal wall mucosa)
Cervical "hood" or "coxcomb"

Atrophy consistent with estrogen
deficiency

## BASIC INFERTILITY WORKUP

**What is the first test that
should be ordered in the
workup?**

Varies; an infertility workup is unique to
the couple and should be guided by the
information obtained from the history
and physical examination.

**What is the basic workup
to evaluate male factors?**

Semen analysis

| | |
|---|---|
| **Procedure?** | Semen sample should be collected after 48 hours of abstinence and examined within 2 to 3 hours of collection. |
| **Normal values?** | Ejaculate volume between 2 and 8 ml<br>Sperm concentration > 20 million/ml<br>> 50% motility at 6 hours<br>> 60% sperm normal morphology |
| **Repeat testing?** | If any of the values are abnormal, two additional samples should be evaluated at 2-week intervals.<br>Urologic examination if abnormalities persist |
| **What is the basic workup to evaluate ovulatory factors?** | Documentation of ovulation by:<br>Basal body temperature (BBT)<br>Endometrial biopsy<br>Serum progesterone measurement |
| **What is the procedure for BBT?** | Patient measures her temperature before arising in the morning and records results on chart. |
| **Normal results?** | A biphasic chart characterized by a sustained rise in body temperature of at least 0.4°F (thermogenic effect of progesterone) is typical of ovulation.<br>Ovulation is thought to occur on the day of lowest temperature; however, ovulation can vary by as much as 2 days, making BBTs a poor method. |
| **What is the procedure for endometrial biopsy?** | Biopsy and microscopic examination of endometrial tissue |
| **Why is endometrial biopsy performed in the infertility workup during the luteal phase?** | Microscopic examination of the endometrium can be used to "date" the endometrium based on histology.<br>An endometrial biopsy performed in the luteal phase provides indirect evidence of the presence or absence of ovulation. |
| **Normal results?** | No more than a 2-day discrepancy between the date of the endometrium based on histologic findings and the date based on clinical calculation of the menstrual cycle |

A discrepancy of 3 or more days suggests a luteal phase defect.

**What is the procedure for serum progesterone measurement?**

Measurement of progesterone level in serum

**Normal values?**

A serum progesterone level of 4 ng/ml or three samples (drawn on separate days during the luteal phase) totaling 15 ng/ml indicates that ovulation has occurred.
Because progesterone levels can vary, this test is not as useful as biopsy.

**What is a luteal phase defect?**

A group of hormonal alterations clinically linked to recurrent abortions and infertility

**Diagnosis?**

BBT elevations last 10 days or less (short luteal phase) or endometrial biopsy is histologically more than 2 days out of phase with the clinically calculated menstrual cycle.

**Incidence in women without infertility?**

Found in up to 30% of isolated cycles in normal women

**Role in infertility?**

Controversial; should be considered as a cause of infertility only if it is documented in at least two consecutive cycles

**What is the basic workup to evaluate peritoneal and uterine factors?**

Hysterosalpingography (HSG)
Laparoscopy

**What is the procedure for HSG?**

Oil or water-soluble contrast material is slowly injected through the cervix and into the fallopian tubes to produce fluoroscopic x-ray images of the uterus and fallopian tubes.
Images outline the size, shape, and position of the uterus and also reveal obstruction of the fallopian tubes.
Best performed in the early proliferative phase, after menses, to avoid disturbing a possible pregnancy and to prevent reflux of endometrial tissue (may be a cause of endometriosis).

| | |
|---|---|
| **What abnormalities can be revealed with HSG?** | Congenital uterine malformations<br>T-shaped or hypoplastic uterine cavities associated with in utero DES exposure<br>Submucous leiomyomas<br>Intrauterine polyps<br>Salpingitis isthmica nodosa (SIN)<br>   Defined as the presence of localized numerous diverticula along the interstitial segment or isthmus of the fallopian tube<br>   Associated with "healthy" fallopian tubes as well as chronic or healing salpingitis<br>   Associated with a significantly increased incidence of tubal pregnancy<br>Proximal or distal fallopian tube occlusion<br>Pelvic adhesions or hydrosalpinx, as suggested by retained dye on a delayed abdominal flat-plate radiograph<br>Asherman syndrome |
| **Why does HSG have a high false-positive rate?** | Thought to be because of transient tubal blockages caused by smooth muscle spasm |
| **What are the contraindications to HSG?** | Pelvic mass or tenderness (to avoid exacerbation of an ongoing process)<br>Allergy to iodine or contrast dye (relative) |
| **What are the risks of HSG?** | Dye embolization (rare)<br>Salpingitis (1%–3%) |
| **What is the procedure for laparoscopy?** | Visualization of peritoneal cavity with a rigid scope |
| **When should laparoscopy be performed?** | In general, after the basic minimum workup is completed<br>Considered a valuable test for detecting endometriosis or pelvic adhesions, which are difficult to evaluate with HSG alone |

| | |
|---|---|
| **What percentage of patients undergoing laparoscopy for infertility have pelvic pathology?** | Approximately 50% |
| **What conditions can be surgically managed with laparoscopy?** | Adhesions and endometriosis |
| **What does the basic workup to evaluate cervical factors consist of?** | Postcoital test |
| **What is the procedure for postcoital test?** | Couple is instructed to have intercourse after 24 to 48 hours of abstinence and 2 days before ovulation<br>Cervical mucus and semen interaction are analyzed within 12 hours of intercourse. |
| **How is the cervical mucus analyzed?** | For impending ovulation, by spinnbarkeit (ability to be pulled into a string between two surfaces)<br>Glass coverslip is placed on the mucus and slowly drawn from the slide. |
| **Normal results?** | Cervical mucus suggesting impending ovulation will stretch 6 to 10 cm |
| **How is semen interaction analyzed?** | For the degree of cellularity and the number of sperm |
| **Normal results?** | More than 20 sperm/high-power field has been correlated with a statistically significant increase in the percentage of pregnancies. |
| **Abnormal results?** | Absence of sperm suggests faulty sperm production or poor coital technique.<br>"Shaking" sperm suggests immunologic infertility. |

## EVALUATION OF RESULTS AND MANAGEMENT

### MALE FACTORS

| | |
|---|---|
| **What is the treatment for low sperm count?** | Referral to a urologist for a thorough evaluation, including a complete physical examination, repeat semen analysis, |

postejaculate urine sample (to look for retrograde ejaculation), and measurement of serum gonadotropin levels

**What is the treatment for varicocele?**

Varicocele's role in infertility is controversial.

Most believe that surgical ligation improves semen quantity in the majority of men.

Associated with a 30%–50% pregnancy rate

The improved semen quantity is thought to be due to improved blood flow or temperature regulation.

**What is intrauterine insemination?**

Method by which washed sperm are injected through the cervix around the time of ovulation

**Why are sperm washed?**

Washing isolates a population of sperm with a higher percentage of motile forms and removes proteins, prostaglandins, and bacteria commonly associated with adverse reactions.

**What is the procedure for sperm washing?**

Techniques vary. General:
Dilution with 7–10 ml of buffer
Sample is gently centrifuged.
Resultant sperm pellet is resuspended in 0.5-ml buffered solution.

**Indications?**

Retrograde ejaculation
Neurologic impotence
High semen volume
Isolation of the motile sperm
Donor insemination
Infertility due to cervical factors

## FEMALE FACTORS

### Ovulatory factors

**What is the rate of conception after treatment in women with anovulation as the cause of infertility?**

Women with anovulation alone as the cause of infertility have the highest rate of conception with treatment (~ 70%).

**What factors should therapeutic decisions be based on?**

Whether the dysfunction lies within the ovary or elsewhere in the hypothalamic–pituitary–ovarian axis

**What are the categories of ovarian dysfunction?**

It is helpful to diagnose and manage patients according to the World Health Organization's classification of ovulatory deficiencies.

Group I: Hypothalamic–pituitary failure
  Patients have hypogonadotropic hypogonadism with low FSH and estrogen levels, normal prolactin concentrations, and failure to bleed after a progesterone challenge.
  Includes hypothalamic amenorrhea, anorexia nervosa, and stress-related amenorrhea
Group II: Hypothalamic–pituitary dysfunction
  Patients have anovulation and oligomenorrhea with normal gonadotropin and estrogen levels.
  Includes idiopathic anovulation and the classic polycystic ovary syndrome
Group III: Ovarian failure
  Patients are hypergonadotropic and hypogonadal with low estrogen levels.
  Includes ovarian failure and ovarian resistance
A separate, but important, clinical entity is the hyperprolactinemic patient with ovulatory dysfunction.

**What tests should be performed after ovulatory dysfunction is documented?**

Measurement of serum thyroid-stimulating hormone (TSH) level
Measurement of serum prolactin level
Progesterone challenge to assess estrogen levels
If the patient fails to bleed after the progesterone challenge, measurement of serum FSH and luteinizing hormone (LH) to rule out ovarian failure

**Why should TSH be measured?**

Both hypothyroidism and hyperthyroidism can cause anovulation by altering estrogen metabolism and clearance.

Thyroid disease leads to increased estrogen levels, thus inhibiting FSH secretion and follicular development.

**What can the progesterone challenge test reveal?**

The presence of estrogen production (the absence of ovarian failure), because only endometrium that has been primed to thicken by the influence of estrogen sloughs when challenged by progesterone withdrawal. Proves hypothalamic–pituitary–ovarian axis is intact.

**What is the procedure for progesterone challenge test?**

Patient is given medroxyprogesterone acetate 10 mg orally daily for 7 days

**Normal result?**

Withdrawal bleeding after medroxyprogesterone acetate is discontinued indicates that the hypothalamic–pituitary–ovarian axis is intact

**Abnormal result?**

Withdrawal bleeding may be delayed in cases of androgen excess (e.g., polycystic ovary syndrome).

**What are additional tests for androgen excess?**

Measurement of serum dehydroepiandrosterone sulfate (DHEAS) and testosterone levels

**What is DHEAS?**

An adrenal androgen that may be overproduced in cases of adrenal hyperplasia (or in some cases of hyperprolactinemia) and can cause an anovulatory hypoestrogenic state by direct inhibition of follicular maturation (as in polycystic ovary syndrome)

**What is the treatment for hypothalamic–pituitary failure?**

When failure is due to lack of LH and FSH production (hypogonadotropic hypogonadism), ovulation can be induced by replacement of the necessary hormones using human menopausal gonadotropin (hMG).

**What is hMG?**

A mixture of LH and FSH derived from postmenopausal women

**Rate of pregnancy with hMG in patients with hypogonadotropic hypogonadism?**

Sixty to 80% of patients achieve pregnancy, most within six cycles.

**Risks of hMG therapy?**

Increased risks of multiple gestation (10%–15%) and ovarian hyperstimulation syndrome
Because of risks, should be used selectively

**What is ovarian hyperstimulation syndrome?**

Can be life-threatening if severe
Mild cases: Ovarian enlargement, weight gain, and abdominal distention
Severe cases:
Ovaries > 10 cm
Weight gain of > 20 pounds due to peritoneal, pleural, and pericardial (extravascular) fluid accumulation
Loss of fluid from the intravascular space results in low blood pressure and poor perfusion of tissues, and can cause permanent organ damage or even death.

**How is ovarian hyperstimulation syndrome prevented?**

Periodic measurement of serum estradiol levels and ultrasonic monitoring of size and number of follicles

**What is polycystic ovary syndrome (PCO)?**

A hypothalamic–pituitary dysfunction
"Vicious cycle" of hormonal dysfunction:
Increased production of androgens by ovaries, some of which are peripherally converted to estrogen, causes hyperestrogenic and virilizing state.
The high estrogen level increases pituitary production of LH ("pituitary hypersensitivity") but suppresses FSH production by normal feedback inhibition.
The low level of FSH is enough to allow follicle formation, but not maturity and ovulation.

The high LH level stimulates the follicular cells to secrete androgens, and the resulting high ovarian androgen levels further inhibit full maturation of the multiple follicles, and provide substrate for peripheral conversion to estrogen. The anovulatory cycle thus continues.

**What is the treatment of PCO?**

Patients with PCO have functional ovaries that produce estrogen and are good candidates for treatment with clomiphene citrate.

**What is clomiphene citrate and how does it work?**

A nonsteroidal "antiestrogen agent" that causes enhanced release of pituitary gonadotropins by an unknown mechanism

**What are the indications for treatment with clomiphene citrate?**

PCO (generates follicular maturation and ovulation in anovulatory women who can produce estrogen)
Oligo-ovulation (creates regular cycles)
Luteal phase defect (stimulates follicular development)
Assisted reproduction techniques (produces multiple follicles)
Overproduction of DHEAS by adrenals (stimulates follicular growth and suppresses adrenal DHEAS production when combined with glucocorticoid treatment)

**What is the ovulation rate after treatment with clomiphene citrate?**

Induces ovulation in 70% of patients

**What is the pregnancy rate after treatment with clomiphene citrate?**

40% in anovulatory patients

**What is the increase in incidence of twin pregnancy after treatment with clomiphene citrate?**

5% to 10% increase

**What are the side effects of treatment with clomiphene citrate?**

Hot flashes
Visual disturbances
Headaches
Nausea
Abdominal bloating
Mood lability
Ovarian enlargement (should be screened for by frequent pelvic examinations)

**What is the treatment of ovarian failure?**

Anovulation due to menopausal or premature ovarian failure cannot be treated with ovulation induction.
Treatment options include egg donation and adoption.

**What is the incidence of elevated prolactin level in ovulation disturbances?**

Occurs in about 15% of ovulation disturbances

**What conditions should be ruled out in patients with an elevated prolactin level?**

Pituitary tumor (macroadenoma) by magnetic resonance imaging
Primary hypothyroidism
Results in a low level of dopamine, which normally inhibits prolactin production
Lack of inhibition leads to hyperprolactinemia.
Dopamine depletion due to antihypertensive or neuroleptic drugs

**What is the treatment of patients with an elevated prolactin level?**

Initial treatment: Bromocriptine
Depending on symptoms, surgical removal of a pituitary tumor may be required after maximal treatment/ tumor shrinkage with bromocriptine.

## Peritoneal factors

**What factors influence the success of tubal disease treatment?**

Success varies widely, and depends on:
The extent of original inflammatory damage
Location of blockage (distal occlusion with hydrosalpinx has a worse prognosis than isthmic block)
The pathogen (surgery is contraindicated if tuberculosis is involved)
Postoperative tube length

**What is the treatment of tubal disease?**

Endoscopic surgery:
  Has largely replaced laparotomy and microsurgery for most cases of obstructive tubal disease.
  Laparoscopic salpingostomy is usually performed for distal obstruction.
  Tubal cannulation by hysteroscopy is performed for proximal obstruction.
Microsurgery
In vitro fertilization and adoption

**What are the goals of microsurgery?**

Restore anatomy to its normal appearance
Avoid serosal insults (trauma, ischemia, hemorrhage, infection, foreign body exposure, exposure of raw surfaces), which may lead to adhesions

**What techniques are involved in microsurgery?**

Removal of talc from gloves
Minimal use of sponges
Bipolar coagulation of bleeding vessels
Use of fine, minimally antigenic sutures to approximate closely tissue planes with minimal tension.
Surgery usually is performed under an operating microscope.
Perioperative antibiotics (usually doxycycline 100 mg twice daily from the night before surgery to 5 days postoperatively) and systemic glucocorticoids may play a role in improved outcome.

**What are the risks of microsurgery?**

Increased postoperative risk of ectopic pregnancies

**Can tubal ligation be reversed?**

Yes, but success rates largely depend on the type of sterilization procedure used as well as on the tubal segments anastomosed, postoperative tubal length, and surgical technique.
Banding or ligation procedures create fairly localized damage.
Unipolar electrocautery is associated with the destruction of a large segment of tube.

**What is the incidence of endometriosis in infertility?**

Generally estimated to be between 10% and 25%

Infertility rates are twice those of women without endometriosis.

**What is the treatment of endometriosis?**

Most forms can be treated at the time of laparoscopic exploration by electrocoagulation and laser ablation.

Medical treatment

Most successful in mild to moderate disease;

includes leuprolide, danocrine, and low-dose monophasic oral contraceptive pills (OCPs)

**What is leuprolide?**

A GnRH analog administered in a nonpulsatile manner

**How does it work?**

Constant level of leuprolide → GnRH inhibition of gonadotropin release → hypoestrogenic state similar to menopause → atrophy of the endometrial implants

**What is Danocrine and how does it work?**

A drug with a direct androgenic effect that is used to cause an anovulatory, hypoestrogenic state that can result in atrophy of endometrial implants

**How do low-dose OCPs work?**

Can suppress endometrial implants when used continuously for 6–12 months

**What is the pregnancy rate after stopping OCPs in infertile women?**

Between 40% and 50%

**What are the postoperative pregnancy rates?**

Relate directly to stage:

60% for mild to moderate disease

35% for severe disease

**Cervical factors**

**What follow-up is indicated for each of the following abnormal results of the postcoital test?**

**Few or absent sperm**

Repeat test

Evaluate mucus

Reevaluate male factor

Review coital technique (lubricants, etc.)

| | |
|---|---|
| **Thick, tenacious mucus, with spinnbarkeit < 8 cm** | Exclude: <br> Inaccurate timing of intercourse with ovulation <br> Inadequate estrogen production <br> Cervicitis (if lymphocyte count is high) with culture for bacteria, *Ureaplasma urealyticum,* and *Chlamydia trachomatis* <br> Cervical trauma, surgery <br> DES syndrome |
| **Nonprogressive ("shaking") sperm** | Suggests anti-sperm antibodies in either partner <br> Treatment involves steroid suppression or intrauterine insemination. |

## Uterine factors

| | |
|---|---|
| **What kinds of leiomyomas are more commonly associated with infertility?** | Submucous or intramural |
| **What is the treatment of leiomyomas?** | Surgical removal with or without leuprolide therapy for 3 months before surgery |
| **What is Asherman syndrome?** | Partial or complete obliteration of the uterine cavity by intrauterine synechiae (adhesive bands of tissue between opposing uterine walls) <br> Often associated with menstrual abnormalities (amenorrhea, hypomenorrhea, and dysmenorrhea); recurrent abortion; and infertility |
| **What are its etiologic factors?** | Complication of endometritis followed by surgical instrumentation of the uterus (e.g., D & C after term pregnancies or spontaneous or elective abortions) |
| **On what is a diagnosis based?** | Filling defect on HSG |
| **What is the treatment for Asherman syndrome?** | Hysteroscopically guided lysis of adhesions followed by 14 days of antibiotics and 2 months of oral high-dose estrogen |

| | |
|---|---|
| **What are the pregnancy rates after treatment?** | As high as 70% |
| **What are the risks of treatment?** | Increased risks of spontaneous abortion, placenta previa, placenta accreta, and abruptio placentae |
| **What is DES and how does it cause infertility?** | DES is a synthetic estrogen used in the 1950s and 1960s for recurrent abortion.<br>Exposure to DES in utero causes müllerian defects, including:<br>Vaginal adenosis<br>Irregular uterine cavities with adhesions<br>T-shaped uterus with hypoplastic cavity<br>These defects are associated with increased infertility, ectopic pregnancy, spontaneous abortion, and premature labor.<br>Poor outcome is associated with an abnormal HSG. |
| **What is the treatment?** | The only treatment available is cervical cerclage for incompetent cervix or drugs for preterm labor. |

## ASSISTED REPRODUCTIVE TECHNOLOGIES

| | |
|---|---|
| **What are assisted reproductive technologies (ART)?** | Techniques involving the direct retrieval of eggs from the ovary<br>Most of these procedures require ovarian stimulation with timed retrieval of oocytes. |
| **What factors influence the success of ART?** | Underlying disorder<br>Number of oocytes/zygotes transferred<br>Institutional experience |
| **What is in vitro fertilization (IVF)?** | Extraction of oocytes (through the vaginal wall under ultrasound guidance), fertilization in the laboratory, and transcervical transfer of the embryos into the uterus 2 days later<br>Usually requires 100,000 to 200,000 sperm per egg |

| | |
|---|---|
| **What are the indications for IVF?** | Previously damaged tubes<br>Immunologic infertility (antisperm antibodies)<br>Unexplained infertility |
| **What is gamete intrafallopian transfer (GIFT)?** | Extraction of oocytes (laparoscopically or through the vaginal wall with ultrasound guidance) and the placement of oocytes and sperm into the fallopian tube laparoscopically<br>Fertilization occurs in the fallopian tube. |
| **Contraindications to GIFT?** | Tubal disease |
| **Indications for GIFT?** | Healthy fallopian tubes<br>Endometriosis<br>Previous evidence of embryo formation with IVF or zygote intrafallopian transfer (ZIFT)<br>Unexplained infertility |
| **What is ZIFT?** | Extraction of oocytes (through the vaginal wall with ultrasound guidance) and placement of zygotes into the fallopian tube laparoscopically<br>Fertilization occurs in the laboratory. |
| **Contraindications to ZIFT?** | Tubal disease |
| **Indications for ZIFT?** | Same as for GIFT |
| **What is subzonal insertion (SUZI)?** | Subzonal insertion of sperm by microinjection into the perivitelline space of the oocyte<br>After oocyte retrieval, 5 to 10 sperm are injected into the perivitelline space, and the embryos are transferred to the uterus or fallopian tubes. |
| **Risks of SUZI?** | Increased risk of triploid embryos |
| **Indications for SUZI?** | Oligospermia<br>Sperm motility disorders |

**What is intracytoplasmic sperm injection (ICSI)?**

Retrieval of oocytes followed by the injection of a *single* spermatozoon into the egg with a micropipette; embryos are then transferred to the uterus or fallopian tube 2 days later.

**Indications for ICSI?**

Same as for SUZI

# 32

# Amenorrhea

**What are the two types of amenorrhea?**

Primary and secondary

**What are the criteria for primary amenorrhea?**

1. No period by age 14 years and no growth or development of secondary sexual characteristics
2. No period by age 16 years regardless of presence of normal development and secondary sexual characteristics

**What is secondary amenorrhea?**

Cessation of regular menstruation for > 3 cycle intervals or > 6 months total

**How are the disorders divided into axes?**

Menstrual function involves a four-step interrelated system.

Disorders are divided into four axes, depending on the step that fails to function properly.

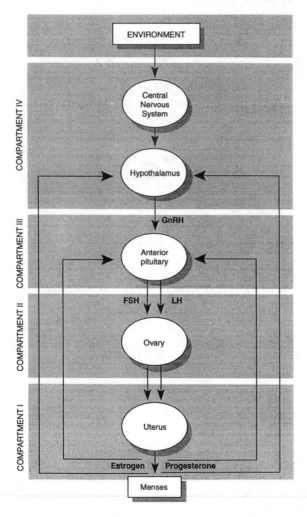

**What are the four axes?**

I. Disorders of the outflow tract—patency and continuity
II. Disorders of the ovary
III. Disorders of the anterior pituitary
IV. Disorders of the central nervous system/hypothalamus

**For each axis, what is the corresponding physiologic step in normal menstrual function?**

I. Intact outflow tract (vaginal orifice and canal, endocervix, and endometrium)

II. Development of endometrium through influence of estrogen and progesterone; follicle development, ovulation, and corpus luteum function

III. Follicle maturation through gonadotropins from the anterior pituitary [follicle-stimulating hormone (FSH) and luteinizing hormone (LH)]

IV. Anterior pituitary production of FSH and LH through gonadotropin-releasing hormone (GnRH) from the hypothalamus and central nervous system

## EVALUATION OF THE AMENORRHEIC PATIENT

**What is the first step in evaluating an amenorrheic patient?**

History and physical examination:
  Discuss psychological dysfunction, emotional stress, eating habits, exercise, and the like, all of which can cause hypothalamic amenorrhea by unknown mechanisms.
  Obtain a personal and family history of genetic and endocrine anomalies and whether any other family member has or had similar problems.
  Review growth and development if amenorrhea is primary.
  Determine pattern of menses before cessation if secondary.
  Discuss use of tampons and intercourse activity to delineate anatomic problems.
Laboratory tests:
  Pregnancy test
  Thyroid-stimulating hormone: Both hypothyroidism and hyperthyroidism can lead to amenorrhea.
  Prolactin: Excess prolactin inhibits gonadotropin secretion.
  Progesterone challenge test

| | |
|---|---|
| **What is the procedure for a progesterone challenge test?** | Ten milligrams progesterone daily for 5 days<br>Patient will then either bleed or not bleed. |
| **What does it assess?** | Endogenous estrogen and competency of outflow tract |
| **What is the significance of the result if patient bleeds?** | Outflow tract is intact and the endometrium has responded to endogenous estrogen.<br>Anovulation, an axis II disorder, is established.<br>　Because ovulation has not occurred, no progesterone has been made.<br>　Menses cannot occur until exogenous progesterone is provided. |
| **What is the significance of the result if patient does not bleed?** | Outflow tract or endometrium is inoperative (axis I).<br>Estrogen proliferation of endometrium did not occur (axis II, III, or IV).<br>Go to step 2 of evaluation. |
| **What is the second step in evaluating an amenorrheic patient?** | Necessary if tests administered in first step are negative<br>Estrogen and progesterone challenge test |
| **What is the procedure for an estrogen and progesterone challenge test?** | 1.25 mg estrogen daily for 21 days with the addition of 10 mg progesterone during last 5 days |
| **What is the significance of the result if patient does not bleed?** | Axis I disorder: problem with outflow tract |
| **What is the significance of the result if patient bleeds?** | Disorder may be axis II, III, or IV.<br>Go to step 3. |
| **What is the third step in evaluating an amenorrheic patient?** | Determine reason for lack of estrogen production. |

**What are the possible etiologic factors for lack of estrogen production?**

Follicle problem (axis II)
Gonadotropin problem (axis III or IV)

**What diagnostic procedure is administered to determine the cause of lack of estrogen production?**

Serum assay of gonadotropin levels: measure FSH and LH

**What are the normal values of FSH and LH?**

FSH: 5–30 international units per liter (IU/L)
LH: 5–20 IU/L

**What are abnormal values and their significance?**

Hypogonadotropic state (axis III or IV):
    FSH < 5 IU/L, LH < 5 IU/L
    Prepubertal state
    Hypothalamic disorder
    Pituitary dysfunction
Hypergonadotropic state (axis II):
    FSH > 30 IU/L, LH > 40 IU/L
    Postmenopausal
    Ovarian failure
**Key point:** When gonadotropins are low, the problem is at the higher centers (hypothalamus or pituitary). When gonadotropins are high, the problem is at the ovary/follicle (no estrogen = no negative feedback).
Go to Step 4.

**What is the fourth step in evaluating an amenorrheic patient?**

Determine cause of hypogonadotropic or hypergonadotropic state.

**What axes must be differentiated if the patient is hypogonadotropic?**

Axis III (pituitary) and axis IV (hypothalamus)

**What diagnostic procedure is used to differentiate between the axes?**

Imaging of sella turcica (computed tomography or magnetic resonance imaging)

**What is the significance of abnormal imaging?**

Pituitary tumor (axis III)

| | |
|---|---|
| **What is the significance of normal imaging?** | Assume axis IV problem by exclusion. |
| **For a hypergonadotropic patient with primary amenorrhea younger than 30 years of age, what diagnostic procedure should be performed, and why?** | Karyotype determination<br>Mosaicism with a Y chromosome requires gonadal excision to eliminate the risk of the testicular component becoming malignant.<br>Thirty percent of women with a Y chromosome do not have virilization, so normal appearance does not preclude karyotyping. |

## SPECIFIC DISORDERS

| | |
|---|---|
| **What axis I disorders (disorders of the outflow tract) cause primary amenorrhea?** | Müllerian anomalies: Imperforate hymen, lack of vaginal orifice, discontinuity by segmental disruptions<br>Müllerian agenesis (Mayer-Rokitansky-Küster-Hauser syndrome): Karyotype is 46XX with normal female phenotype (axillary and pubic hair) but reproductive tract does not develop (see Chapter 29, Sexual Differentiation and Development).<br>Androgen insensitivity (testicular feminization): Patient is phenotypically female with XY karyotype, testes, and normal or slightly elevated male testosterone levels; caused by a defect in testosterone end-organ receptor (see Chapter 29, Sexual Differentiation and Development). |
| **What axis I disorder (disorders of the outflow tract) causes secondary amenorrhea?** | Asherman syndrome:<br>  Caused by destruction of the endometrium from scarring via IUD, dilation and curettage, and the like<br>  Diagnosed by hysterogram or hysteroscopy<br>  Treatment involves dilation and curettage to remove adhesions and supplemental estrogen. |
| **What axis II disorders (disorders of the ovary) cause primary amenorrhea?** | Disorders under the broad term "gonadal dysgenesis"<br>Genetic or enzymatic problem that results in abnormal ovarian function |

**What are some conditions that cause gonadal dysgenesis?**

Turner syndrome (see Chapter 29, Sexual Differentiation and Development)

Mosaicism (see Chapter 29, Sexual Differentiation and Development)

17 Hydroxylase deficiency or 17,20 desmolase deficiency: Enzyme deficiency that prevents synthesis of steroid hormones (i.e., estrogen and progesterone); hypertension and hypokalemia are also present in mineralocorticoid deficiencies.

Gonadal agenesis: Ovaries fail to develop; often of unknown etiology

**What axis II disorder causes secondary amenorrhea?**

Premature ovarian failure: Early menopause (before age 40 years); idiopathic

**What axis III disorders (disorders of the pituitary) cause amenorrhea?**

Pituitary tumor: May cause additional problems such as prolactinemia, visual changes, acromegaly, hyperthyroidism

Empty sella syndrome: Congenital incompleteness of the sellar diaphragm, which deforms both the pituitary fossa and gland

Sheehan syndrome: Acute necrosis of the pituitary gland due to shock, often from postpartum hemorrhage

**What is the most common pituitary tumor?**

Prolactin-secreting adenoma (50%)

**How do pituitary tumors cause amenorrhea?**

If tumor secretes FSH and LH, it is a continuous release, without regulation by GnRH from the hypothalamus.

Pulsatile release of hormones from both the hypothalamus and pituitary is required for a normal menstrual cycle.

**What axis IV disorder (disorders of the central nervous system) causes amenorrhea?**

Hypothalamic amenorrhea/ hypogonadotropic hypogonadism: Defect in the pulsatile secretion of GnRH from the hypothalamus; diagnosed by exclusion

**What are the etiologic factors of hypothalamic amenorrhea/ hypogonadotropic hypogonadism?**

Stress

Weight loss/low body weight: Anorexia

Excessive exercise

Kallmann syndrome: Congenital defect characterized by hypothalamic amenorrhea and anosmia

# 33

## Menopause

### INTRODUCTION

**What is menopause?**

Cessation of menses corresponding to the loss of ovarian activity

**What is the climacteric?**

Transitional period leading to menopause, in which ovarian activity decreases

Includes the perimenopausal and menopausal periods

**What percentage of the female population in the United States is currently postmenopausal?**

Twenty percent

**Why is this percentage increasing?**

Life expectancy is also increasing

**What is the median age of the onset of menopause?**

Age 50–52 years

**What is the age range of the onset of menopause?**

Age 48–55 years

**What is the approximate length of the perimenopausal period?**

Four years

**What factors influence the age at which menopause occurs?**

Family history, race, parity, or age of menarche **do not** influence the age at which menopause occurs.

Smoking and low weight may decrease the age at which menopause occurs.

### EFFECTS OF MENOPAUSE

**What hormonal changes occur in perimenopause?**

The number of anovulatory cycles increases and cycle length increases.

The level of follicle-stimulating hormone (FSH) increases; the levels of luteinizing hormone (LH) and estradiol remain normal until follicular growth ceases.

The level of LH eventually increases; however, the increase is only 3-fold, compared to a 10- to 20-fold increase in the level of FSH.

With the increased levels of gonadotropins (FSH and LH), the ovarian stroma produces increased levels of testosterone.

**Describe sex steroid production.**

Estrogen production persists from fat conversion of androstenedione and testosterone to estrogen

**What is the correlation between peripheral conversion of estrogen and body weight?**

The percentage of peripheral conversion is proportional to body weight—that is, obesity correlates with increased peripheral conversion.

**What are the vasomotor symptoms of perimenopause?**

So-called "hot flashes"
Typified by a sensation of warmth in the head, neck, and chest with associated sweating
May last from seconds to minutes
Occur more frequently at night, during episodes of stress, and in increased temperatures

**How many women experience vasomotor symptoms of perimenopause?**

10% to 25%

**For how long do vasomotor symptoms continue?**

Usually only 1–2 years; at most 5 years

**How can vasomotor symptoms be relieved?**

Vasomotor symptoms are associated with decreased estrogen levels and may be relieved with hormone (estrogen) replacement therapy (HRT), progesterone, or clonidine.

**What atrophic changes occur in perimenopause?**

Genitourinary atrophy, which may cause vaginitis, pruritus, urethritis, vaginal stenosis, and dyspareunia

**What is the cause of atrophic changes?**

Decreased estrogen levels

**How can atrophic changes be relieved?**

HRT

**What is osteoporosis?**

Reduction of the quantity of bone or atrophy of the skeletal tissue

**When does bone loss typically begin in women?**

In the spine, which is composed of trabecular bone, the onset of bone loss begins at age 20 years.
In the femur, composed of cortical bone, density peaks in the late third decade.

**When does bone loss accelerate?**

After menopause

**What are the rates of bone loss before and after menopause?**

After age 40 years, the rate of bone loss is 0.5% per year.
After menopause, the rate of trabecular bone loss is 5% per year; the rate of total bone loss is 1%.

**Why does the rate of bone loss accelerate after menopause?**

Because of decreased estrogen levels; trabecular bone is the most sensitive to changes in estrogen levels.

**What are the risk factors for osteoporosis?**

The risk is increased in thin, white, or Asian women; smokers; and women with sedentary lifestyles. All of these factors decrease peak bone density.

**What is the incidence of fractures?**

Twenty-five percent of women older than age 70 years experience spinal fractures, usually compression fractures.
Twenty percent of all white women experience hip fractures.

**Treatment and prevention of osteoporosis?**

Estrogen at a dosage 0.625 mg/day, especially when coupled with calcium supplements, can help decrease the rate of bone loss.
Progestins may also decrease the rate of bone reabsorption.
Annual intramuscular injections of vitamin D may decrease the number

of hip fractures. Oral vitamin D
supplements may also be taken.
Etidronate may be used in women in
whom estrogens are contraindicated,
such as women with a history of
estrogen-dependent malignancies or
venous thrombosis. It reduces bone
loss by decreasing osteoclastic activity.
Alendronate (Fosamax) is the newest
medication for the prevention and
treatment of osteoporosis. Alendronate
is related to etidronate, and it also
decreases osteoclastic activity.
Parenteral calcitonin prevents bone loss
by inhibiting bone resorption.
High doses of fluoride stabilize bone
and stimulate the osteoblast to form
new bone, primarily in trabecular
bone. Potential side effects of fluoride
treatment include gastrointestinal
irritability and joint tenderness.

**What are the mechanisms by which estrogen prevents bone loss?**

Increases calcium absorption
Increases calcitonin, which decreases
bone absorption
Increases vitamin D receptors

**What effects does estrogen have on the cardiovascular system?**

Increases low-density lipoprotein (LDL)
cholesterol catabolism, increases
triglyceride levels, and decreases
atherosclerotic plaque formation
Estrogen also has a poorly understood
protective effect on the arterial walls
independent of the aforementioned
benefits. This effect may occur through
vasodilatation and antiplatelet activity.
Estrogen has a direct inotropic effect on
the heart and increases left ventricular
diastolic filling.
Men have a three to four times greater
risk for coronary artery disease than
premenopausal women; this difference
in risk may be related to estrogen.

**In general, what is the ratio of HDL cholesterol to low-density lipoprotein (LDL) cholesterol in premenopausal women?**

In premenopausal women, HDL
cholesterol levels are higher than those
of LDL cholesterol; this difference is
probably secondary to estrogen.

| | |
|---|---|
| **What happens to the HDL/ LDL ratio in postmenopausal women?** | The HDL cholesterol level decreases and the LDL cholesterol level increases. |
| **What are the risk factors for cardiovascular disease?** | Obesity, hypertension, smoking, diabetes, and hypercholesterolemia |
| **What do studies show about the cardioprotective effects of HRT during menopause?** | Most studies show a cardioprotective effect from estrogen supplementation during menopause, with decreased morbidity and mortality from strokes and myocardial infarctions.<br>Progestins do not diminish the cardioprotective effect of estrogen. |

## HORMONE REPLACEMENT THERAPY

| | |
|---|---|
| **Does the type of estrogen prescribed for HRT matter?** | No. The dosage and method of estrogen replacement are the key factors, not the specific type of estrogen. |
| **What are the various estrogen regimens?** | The standard oral estrogen dosage is 0.625 mg of conjugated estrogens daily.<br>This dosage has been shown to have a beneficial effect on bone density and lipid profile.<br>Dosage can be adjusted depending on a particular patient's menopausal symptoms.<br>Estradiol in a transdermal system at a dosage of 50 µg twice a week has been shown to be as effective as the standard dosage of conjugated estrogens. Currently, there is no consensus about the long-term effects of bypassing the liver with a transdermal regimen compared with the oral regimen.<br>Estradiol implants and estrogen ointment are also available.<br>Studies of these regimens are not as extensive as those of the previously mentioned methods.<br>Estradiol levels need to be monitored because blood levels increase over time. |

**What are the combined HRT regimens?**

There are two types, sequential and continuous.

Sequential therapy: Estrogen plus a progestational agent such as 10 mg medroxyprogesterone daily for either the first 14 days of the month or the last 10 days (days 16–25) of estrogen therapy

Continuous therapy: estrogen plus 2.5 mg medroxyprogesterone acetate or 0.35 mg norethindrone daily

**What percentage of women taking combined sequential HRT experience withdrawal bleeding?**

80% to 90%

**What percentage of women taking combined continuous HRT experience breakthrough bleeding?**

40% to 60%
This incidence decreases to 25% with prolonged use.

**For what conditions should a woman taking combined continuous HRT who continues to have breakthrough bleeding be evaluated?**

Polyps, fibroids, and hyperplasia

**For what population of women is combined HRT strongly recommended, and why?**

Because of the risk of endometrial hyperplasia, a combined regimen is strongly recommended in women who have **not** undergone a hysterectomy.

**What are the arguments for using a combined regimen in women who have undergone a hysterectomy?**

Adenocarcinoma has been described in women with a history of endometriosis who take estrogen alone. Therefore, in women with endometriosis, combination therapy should be advocated.
The combined regimen has been shown to be more beneficial in decreasing the rate of bone loss.

**What is an advantage of combined continuous HRT therapy over combined sequential HRT?**

Continuous HRT allows the use of lower doses of progestins; therefore, the risk of progestin side effects such as fluid retention, breast tenderness, and depression may decrease.

| | |
|---|---|
| **How should women on HRT be followed?** | An endometrial biopsy should be performed before starting HRT if a woman has a history of irregular bleeding, unopposed estrogen use, or endometrial hyperplasia.<br><br>The endometrial cavity and the endometrium should be evaluated if a woman experiences breakthrough bleeding once stable on a particular regimen.<br><br>Postmenopausal women should have annual pelvic examinations, including Papanicolaou smears.<br><br>An annual mammogram should be performed after age 50 years, as recommended by the American Cancer Society. |
| **What are the risks of HRT?** | Increased risk of endometrial neoplasia<br><br>Increased risk of thromboembolic disease in patients with a history of venous thrombosis with pregnancy or with the use of oral contraceptives |
| **What is endometrial neoplasia?** | Abnormal proliferation of the endometrium, ranging from simple hyperplasia to carcinoma |
| **What is the increase in risk of endometrial neoplasia attributable to HRT?** | A 2- to 10-fold increase in risk |
| **What can decrease the risk of endometrial neoplasia in women taking HRT?** | Adding progestins to the HRT regimen obviates the increased risk of endometrial neoplasia.<br><br>Progestins inhibit the growth of the endometrium; estrogens promote endometrial proliferation. |
| **What dosage of progestin has been shown to decrease the risk of endometrial neoplasia?** | Studies have shown that progestins should be given for at least 10 days each month.<br><br>Either 10 mg of medroxyprogesterone acetate for days 16–25 each month, or 2.5 mg of medroxyprogesterone acetate every day of the month can reduce the risk of endometrial neoplasia. |

366 Obstetrics and Gynecology Recall

**Does HRT increase the risk of breast cancer?**

Controversy remains about the possibility of increased risk of breast cancer with long-term HRT.

A large study conducted by the Centers for Disease Control and Prevention did not find an increased risk of breast cancer in women using HRT over a 20-year study period.

However, other large studies have shown a small but statistically significant increase in risk in women on doses of estrogen greater than 1.25 mg/day or in women with a history of benign breast disease or a family history of breast cancer.

The dose most commonly used, 0.625 mg of conjugated estrogen, is not associated with an increased risk of breast cancer.

It is not known how combined HRT affects the risk of breast cancer.

**Do women taking HRT have an increased risk of thromboembolic disease?**

No. However, the risk is increased in women with a history of venous thrombosis with pregnancy or with the use of oral contraceptives.

**Do women taking HRT have an increased risk of gallbladder disease?**

No

**Do women taking HRT have an increased risk of recurrence of endometriosis?**

No

**How does HRT affect fibroid tumors of the uterus?**

Rarely do fibroid tumors of the uterus increase in size in response to HRT.

**When is HRT contraindicated?**

Contraindications include liver disease, acute vascular thrombosis, migraine headaches, and possibly seizure disorders.

**Can women with a history of endometrial or breast cancer take HRT?**

Patients with a history of endometrial or breast cancer must be evaluated on an individual basis.

HRT is contraindicated in patients with a history of endometrial cancer and endometrioid cancer of the ovary. Combination therapy may be instituted 5 years after the cancer has been treated if there is no evidence of recurrent disease.

No long-term studies have been completed that evaluate HRT after breast cancer.

# 34

# Preventive Care: Cancer Screening

**Not every disease should be screened for in a population. What are the criteria for screening a disease?**

The disease should have significant morbidity and mortality.
The disease should be treatable.
The disease should have an identifiable preclinical stage.
Treatment of the disease during the asymptomatic period should be more effective than treatment during the symptomatic period.
The disease should be sufficiently prevalent in the screened population.

**What are the criteria for screening tests?**

The test should be simple and inexpensive.
The test should be painless, safe, and accurate (i.e., the test must be sufficiently sensitive and specific).

**What is sensitivity?**

The percentage of positive test results among individuals who have the disease

**What is specificity?**

The percentage of negative test results among individuals who do not have the disease

**What is positive predictive value (PPV)?**

The probability that a person with a positive test result will have the disease; for example, a PPV of 10% means that there will be nine false-positive test results for each cancer detected.

**What are the potential biases of screening tests?**

Selection bias: The screened population does not correspond to the general population.
Lead time bias: Early diagnosis of the disease does not extend the patient's life; only the length of time that the patient has the diagnosis is increased.

Length time bias: The apparent prolongation of life is related more to the intrinsic nature of the disease rather than to its early diagnosis.

**What are the American College of Obstetrics and Gynecology (ACOG) guidelines for cervical cancer screening?**

Should begin at age 18 years or at onset of sexual activity

Annual examinations throughout a woman's life

**What are the National Cancer Institute (NCI) guidelines for cervical cancer screening?**

Should begin at age 20 years or at onset of sexual activity

Ages 18–35 years: Annual screening until two negative results; thereafter, every 3 years

Ages 36–60 years: Screening at least every 3 years; more frequent screening if high risk; annual pelvic examination

Age > 60 years: Same as for ages 36–60 years

**What are the National Cancer Society (NCS) guidelines for cervical cancer screening?**

Should begin at onset of sexual activity

Ages 18–35 years: Annual screening until two negative results; thereafter, every 3 years

Ages 36–60 years: Every 1–3 years

Age > 60 years: After two negative tests, testing may be stopped.

**What test is used to screen for cervical cancer?**

The Papanicolaou smear test (Pap test)

**Is the Pap test simple, safe, inexpensive, and acceptable to patient and provider?**

Yes

**What is the sensitivity of a Pap test?**

Sixty-seven percent

**What is the specificity?**

Sixty percent

**What are the implications of the Pap test's overall low specificity?**

The Pap test has a high false-positive rate and a low PPV. However, because of the characteristics of this screening test and the consequences of undiagnosed cervical cancer, the low PPV is acceptable.

**What are the guidelines for breast cancer screening?**

Some controversy exists, but the general guidelines are as follows:
A baseline examination between ages 35 and 39 years [National Cancer Institute (NCI), baseline examination at age 40 years]
Examination every 1–2 years between ages 40 and 49 years
Annual examination after age 50 years

**What test is used to screen for breast cancer?**

Mammogram

**Is the mammogram simple, safe, inexpensive, and acceptable to patient and provider?**

In general, yes. However, the test is only relatively inexpensive. Annual mammograms of 0.5 rad carry a small risk of radiation exposure, but the clinical significance of this risk is not known.

**What is the sensitivity of a mammogram?**

Eighty-five percent

**What is the specificity?**

Eighty percent

**What are the guidelines for colorectal cancer screening?**

The ACS and NCI recommend an annual digital rectal examination after age 40 years.
Annual fecal occult blood sampling after age 50 years
ACS only: After age 50 years, sigmoidoscopy every 3–5 years after two negative test results performed 1 year apart
All individuals considered high risk (strong family history, familial polyposis, and ulcerative colitis) should have periodic screening with colonoscopy.

**What test is used to screen for colorectal cancer?**

Fecal occult blood sampling (FOBS; not a stool guaiac in the office). In this test, patients are given six stool guaiac cards. The patient must follow dietary restrictions, such as no meat and vegetables, for 1–2 days prior to the test. The patient then takes consecutive stool samples, places them on the cards, and mails them to the physician.

**Is FOBS simple, safe, inexpensive, and acceptable to patient and provider?**

The test is safe and relatively inexpensive. However, patients comply poorly with this test, indicating that most patients find the test unacceptable.

**What is the sensitivity of FOBS?**

Fifty percent

**What is the specificity of FOBS?**

Unknown; in general, 2% of the test results are positive, and the PPV is 30%. The positive test results also include polyps as well as carcinomas. Of all individuals with positive test results, only 20%–25% have cancer.

**What are the guidelines for endometrial cancer screening?**

The ACS recommends that women have a pelvic examination at the onset of menopause and that high-risk women have an endometrial biopsy when identified as high risk.
There is currently no indication to biopsy asymptomatic women.
Endometrial cancer is the most common genital cancer in women in the United States.

**Which women are considered at high risk for endometrial cancer?**

Women with a history of infertility, obesity, failure to ovulate, abnormal uterine bleeding, diabetes, tamoxifen use, or unopposed estrogen use

**What test is used to screen for endometrial cancer?**

Endometrial biopsy. In this test, a small catheter is placed through the cervical os into the uterine cavity. The endometrium is then aspirated into the catheter for sampling.

**What are the guidelines for lung cancer screening?**

Although lung cancer is the most lethal cancer in men and women, there is no benefit at this time from screening for lung cancer, even in high-risk populations. Several large studies have shown no benefit in screening chest radiographs or sputum cytologies. The mortality rate from lung cancer is the same in screened populations as in unscreened populations.

# 35

# Thyroid Disease and Pregnancy

## NORMAL PREGNANCY

**What is the thyroid state of a healthy pregnant woman?**

Euthyroid, but changes in thyroid function test values occur.

**What is the significance of an enlarged thyroid (goiter) in pregnancy?**

Mild thyroid enlargement is normal and results from glandular hyperplasia and increased vascularity. Development of a true goiter during pregnancy signifies thyroid disease.

**Should pregnant women in the United States take iodine supplements during pregnancy?**

No. The renal clearance of iodine almost doubles during pregnancy secondary to a rise in cardiac output and the ensuing rise in glomerular filtration rate. Although this increased iodine loss can lead to deficiency in areas of the world with borderline iodine intake, in the United States the average iodine intake is substantially above the minimum requirement (150 $\mu$g/day).

**What are the changes in thyroxine-binding globulin (TBG), thyroid-stimulating hormone (TSH), and free thyroxine (T$_4$) and triiodothyronine (T$_3$) levels during pregnancy?**

TBG levels rise in response to elevated estrogen levels.
Rise in TBG levels is associated with a parallel but smaller increase in total T$_4$ and T$_3$ levels; therefore, free (i.e., functional) T$_4$ and T$_3$ levels are slightly reduced but remain within the normal range.
TSH remains normal.

**What is a normal result of a thyroid uptake test administered during pregnancy?**

Low, which reflects the increase in thyroid hormone binding capacity

**What effect does human chorionic gonadotropin (hCG) have on thyroid function?**

Because hCG and TSH have the same α-subunit, hCG can stimulate thyroid hormone production in a manner similar to TSH. As hCG levels increase early in pregnancy, the level of $T_4$ increases and the level of TSH decreases. However, because hCG is a less potent stimulator of thyroid hormone production than TSH, thyrotoxic $T_4$ levels are unusual in normal pregnancy. Thyrotoxic levels may occur in gestational trophoblastic disease, which is associated with very high hCG levels.

**Do thyroid hormones cross the placenta?**

Currently, the answer is thought to be "no." It is believed that the development and function of the fetal thyroid gland are unrelated to maternal thyroid function. However, it is known that the fetus depends on the mother for its supply of iodine.

**Which thyroid-active drugs cross the placenta?**

Iodine
Thionamides
β-blockers
Somatostatin
Thyrotropin-releasing hormone
Dopamine agonists and antagonists

## THYROID DYSFUNCTION AND INFERTILITY

**How does hypothyroidism affect fertility?**

In hypothyroidism, libido and fertility are decreased. The mechanism is unclear. It has been hypothesized that decreased activity of the central dopaminergic system may be responsible for the increased prolactin and luteinizing hormone levels associated with hypothyroidism. The increased levels of these hormones cause amenorrhea, anovulation, and, in rare cases, galactorrhea, which may be associated with hypothyroidism.

**What is the relationship between spontaneous abortion and hypothyroidism?**

Women with hypothyroidism have been shown to have a higher incidence of recurrent spontaneous abortions than euthyroid women. Early $T_4$ replacement therapy improves fetal outcome in this setting.

**Does hyperthyroidism affect fertility?**

Mild hyperthyroidism does not seem to affect fertility. Thyrotoxicosis is rare in early pregnancy, implying a negative effect on fertility. The exact mechanism is unknown but probably involves alterations in sex hormone levels. Most women with mild to moderate thyrotoxicosis do ovulate, and the evaluation of amenorrhea in such patients should include a pregnancy test.

## HYPERTHYROIDISM AND PREGNANCY

**What is the incidence of hyperthyroidism in pregnancy?**

Occurs in 1 in every 1000 pregnant women

**What signs and symptoms are common to both pregnancy and thyrotoxicosis?**

Signs and symptoms of hyperthyroidism include:
Heat intolerance
Diaphoresis and warm skin
Fatigue
Anxiety and emotional lability
Tremulousness
Tachycardia

**What signs and symptoms differentiate thyrotoxicosis from normal pregnancy?**

Signs seen in thyrotoxicosis but usually not in pregnancy include:
Weight loss
Onycholysis
Diarrhea
Proximal myopathy
Tachycardia that is unresponsive to Valsalva maneuver
Thyromegaly and ophthalmopathy may also be present, but do not necessarily indicate active disease.

**What thyroid function test results indicate hyperthyroidism?**

Suppressed TSH levels in the absence of pituitary disease are diagnostic.
Increased free $T_4$ levels are frequently seen.

Occasionally, $T_4$ levels may be normal; in this case, an isolated elevation of $T_3$ levels should be sought.

**What other laboratory abnormalities may be seen in hyperthyroidism?**

All of the following abnormalities may be associated with thyrotoxicosis, especially Graves' disease:
Normochromic normocytic anemia
Mild neutropenia
Elevated liver function test results
    (alkaline phosphatase, transaminases, and bilirubin)
Mild hypercalcemia
Hypomagnesemia

**What is the most common cause of hyperthyroidism during pregnancy?**

Graves' disease (90% of cases)

**What are other causes of hyperthyroidism during pregnancy?**

Less frequent causes include:
Toxic multinodular goiter
Toxic adenoma
Gestational trophoblastic disease
Pituitary adenoma
Metastatic follicular cell carcinoma
de Quervain's thyroiditis
Struma ovarii

**What physical findings are commonly associated with Graves' disease?**

Some or all of the following may be seen in Graves' disease:
Nontender goiter that is diffusely enlarged and firm
Exophthalmos, which is associated with retraction of the upper eyelids, widened palpebral fissures, lid-lag on downward gaze, and infrequent blinking
Pretibial myxedema or clubbing, or both

**What tests support the diagnosis of Graves' disease?**

Increased level of free $T_4$
Decreased level of TSH
Increased level of thyroid-stimulating immunoglobulin (TSI)
Radioactive thyroid scan normally shows increased uptake by the thyroid gland; however, this study is contraindicated during pregnancy.

| | |
|---|---|
| **What is the cause of Graves' disease?** | Production of autoimmune antibodies against the TSH receptor<br>These antibodies usually have a stimulatory effect; however, inhibitory action has also been reported. |
| **Describe the course of Graves' disease during pregnancy.** | The same poorly understood mechanisms responsible for immunotolerance of the mother to the fetoplacental unit are thought to play a role in the improvement of the course of Graves' disease during pregnancy.<br>Initially, as the hCG levels rise, thyrotoxicosis may worsen, but as the pregnancy progresses, TSI levels fall and signs and symptoms improve. |
| **When should Graves' disease be treated?** | Best fetal outcome is achieved when thyrotoxicosis is treated before conception.<br>If treatment is not an option before conception, thyrotoxicosis should be treated during pregnancy. |
| **Why should Graves' disease be treated?** | Hyperthyroid women have a higher risk of complications during labor and delivery.<br>Hyperthyroidism is associated with an increased incidence of minor fetal anomalies.<br>The risks of preterm delivery, perinatal mortality, and maternal heart failure are significantly increased among inadequately treated or untreated thyrotoxic pregnant women. |
| **What is the goal of treatment of hyperthyroidism in pregnancy?** | Control the maternal hyperthyroidism while avoiding fetal or neonatal hypothyroidism (because drugs used in treatment of hyperthyroidism cross the placenta).<br>The maternal $T_4$ level should be maintained in the high normal to slightly elevated range normally seen in pregnancy. |
| **What drugs are available for the treatment of hyperthyroidism?** | Usual agents are the thionamides: Propylthiouracil (PTU) and carbimazole (metabolized to methimazole). |

**Mechanism of action of thionamides?**

Inhibits iodination of thyroglobulin and thyroglobulin synthesis by competitively inhibiting the enzyme peroxidase
PTU also inhibits the conversion of $T_4$ to $T_3$; methimazole does not.

**Risk to fetus with methimazole?**

Methimazole has been reported to cause fetal aplasia cutis of the scalp.

**How soon after initiating thionamide therapy does the patient's condition improve?**

Because thionamides work by inhibiting new hormone synthesis, response is seen after thyroid follicle stores are depleted. Most patients begin to show improvement after about 1 week of therapy.

**How should patients taking thionamides be monitored?**

Free $T_4$, free $T_3$, and TSH levels should be monitored monthly to maintain a euthyroid state using the smallest dose of thionamide.

**What are the main maternal side effects of thionamides?**

Uncommon and include:
Pruritus
Rash
Drug fever
Metallic taste
Nausea
Oral ulcerations
Hepatitis
Agranulocytosis (rare)

**In what percentage of patients taking thionamides does agranulocytosis occur?**

0.1%

**How should patients be monitored for agranulocytosis?**

A baseline white blood cell count should be obtained in all patients at the onset of therapy and repeated periodically.

**What are the fetal effects of thionamide therapy and how can they be prevented?**

Most important fetal effect is hypothyroidism, because antithyroid drugs cross the placenta (methimazole crosses four times more efficiently than PTU). Hypothyroidism can lead to development of neurologic impairment.

The fetus should be closely monitored for signs of hypothyroidism (goiter, bradycardia, and intrauterine growth retardation).

**When is additional therapy necessary for the treatment of hyperthyroidism?**

Because thionamides do not have an immediate onset of action, additional agents may be necessary for treating severe thyrotoxicosis. In this setting, labor and delivery, cesarean section, infection, or eclampsia can precipitate thyroid storm.

**What drugs are used to treat severe thyrotoxicosis?**

**β-blockers** are useful for treating the sympathetic symptoms of thyrotoxicosis such as tachycardia, although they have no effect on hormone production.

**Iodides** (e.g., potassium iodide) can be used in conjunction with β-blockers in cases of severe hyperthyroidism, although not during pregnancy. They decrease serum $T_4$ and $T_3$ levels by inhibiting the release of stored thyroid hormone.

**What is the goal of therapy with β-blockers and iodides?**

Short-term control of severe hyperthyroidism while awaiting the effects of thionamide therapy

**For what condition is it necessary to be cautious when prescribing β-blockers?**

Heart failure

**Can radioactive iodine be used to treat thyrotoxicosis during pregnancy?**

No; contraindicated in pregnancy because it crosses the placenta and is concentrated in the fetal thyroid gland

## HYPOTHYROIDISM AND PREGNANCY

**What is the incidence of hypothyroidism during pregnancy in the United States?**

Occurs in about 1 in every 170 pregnancies
Severe hypothyroidism is rare because of its association with infertility.

**What risks are associated with hypothyroidism during pregnancy?**

Increased risks of preeclampsia, placental abruption, and low-birth weight and stillborn infants. These outcomes improve with early thyroxine replacement therapy.

**What signs and symptoms are associated with hypothyroidism?**

Most are insidious in onset and may be masked by signs and symptoms associated with pregnancy:
Modest weight gain or inability to lose weight while dieting
Decreased exercise ability
General lethargy
Cold intolerance
Menorrhagia
Hoarseness
Constipation
Bradycardia
Goiter
Hair loss

**What information in the history can alert the physician to the possibility of hypothyroidism?**

Personal or family history of thyroid disease
History of head and neck irradiation
Past or present treatment with lithium- or iodine-containing drugs

**How is hypothyroidism diagnosed?**

History
Physical examination
Measurement of serum TSH and free $T_4$ levels

**What is primary hypothyroidism and what abnormalities are seen in the thyroid function tests?**

The thyroid gland is not producing enough thyroid hormone to maintain a euthyroid state.
TSH level is elevated and $T_4$ level is usually low.

**What is subclinical hypothyroidism and in what patients is it prevalent?**

Form of primary hypothyroidism
Elevated TSH level in the presence of $T_4$ levels within the normal range
Prevalent in pregnant women and is thought to be autoimmune in nature

**What is secondary hypothyroidism and what thyroid function test abnormalities are associated with it?**

Also called pituitary hypothyroidism
Inadequate TSH secretion by the pituitary gland
Low $T_4$ levels

| | |
|---|---|
| **What other laboratory abnormalities may be associated with hypothyroidism?** | Elevated serum creatine phosphokinase, serum glutamic oxaloacetic transaminase, lactic dehydrogenase, cholesterol, and prolactin levels<br>Anemia secondary to menorrhagia and other, poorly understood causes |
| **What group of patients is at particular risk for development of hypothyroidism during pregnancy?** | Women with insulin-dependent diabetes mellitus (type I) |
| **What is the most common cause of hypothyroidism during pregnancy in the United States?** | Hashimoto's (chronic lymphocytic) thyroiditis |
| **What is the second leading cause of hypothyroidism during pregnancy in the United States?** | Prior treatment of Graves' disease with radioactive iodine or thyroidectomy |
| **What are other, less frequent causes of hypothyroidism during pregnancy in the United States?** | Acute (suppurative) thyroiditis<br>Subacute (viral) thyroiditis<br>Iatrogenic causes: Thionamide, iodide, and lithium therapy |
| **Is iodine deficiency a cause of hypothyroidism in the United States?** | No |
| **What is the typical presentation of a patient with Hashimoto's thyroiditis?** | Firm, diffusely enlarged, usually painless goiter<br>Histology reveals infiltration of the gland with lymphocytes, although a biopsy is seldom necessary. |
| **What are the characteristic immunologic findings associated with Hashimoto's thyroiditis?** | Antimicrosomal antibodies: Almost all patients<br>Antithyroglobulin antibodies: 70% of patients |
| **How does pregnancy affect the course of Hashimoto's thyroiditis?** | As in Graves' disease, the immunotolerance associated with pregnancy improves the course of Hashimoto's thyroiditis. During the course of pregnancy, antimicrosomal and |

antithyroglobulin antibody titers and the size the goiter decrease. However, relapse frequently occurs after delivery.

**What are the signs and symptoms of acute (suppurative) thyroiditis?**

Severe pain and swelling in the neck; fever

**In what patient population is acute thyroiditis common?**

Terminally ill patients

**What is the cause of acute thyroiditis?**

Bacteria such as *Staphylococcus aureus* and group A streptococci
*Aspergillus fumigatus*

**What is the treatment of acute thyroiditis?**

Antibiotics directed against the appropriate organism

**What are the signs and symptoms of subacute thyroiditis?**

May present in the setting of an ongoing viral illness as a firm, mildly tender goiter
This illness tends to have a variable clinical course, starting with a hyperthyroid state which gradually becomes euthyroid and progresses to a hypothyroid state in 20% of patients.

**What is the cause of subacute thyroiditis?**

Thought to be viral

**What is the treatment of subacute thyroiditis?**

The duration of illness is 6 weeks to 6 months, and it tends to be self-limited.

**What is the treatment of hypothyroidism during pregnancy?**

Replacement with levothyroxine should be initiated promptly. Initial dosage is 0.1–0.15 mg/day; dosage should be increased every 4 weeks until TSH level decreases to the low-normal range.

## POSTPARTUM THYROIDITIS

**What is the course of postpartum thyroiditis?**

Starts with a brief hyperthyroid state about 3 months postpartum, which lasts a few weeks and evolves into a hypothyroid state
The hypothyroid phase persists for a few months.
Most patients return to euthyroid state by about 12 months after the delivery.

**In what percentage of patients with postpartum hypothyroidism does permanent hypothyroidism develop?**

10% to 30%

**What is a hallmark of this disease?**

Transient nature of thyroid dysfunction associated with it

**What are its signs and symptoms?**

Thyrotoxic phase: Fatigue, palpitations, dizziness, and weight loss; patients may assume that these signs and symptoms are normal in the postpartum period.

Hypothyroid phase: Weight gain, constipation, cold intolerance, and dry skin. A goiter develops in 50% of the patients; an increased incidence of depressive symptoms is associated with this phase.

**What is the cause of postpartum thyroiditis?**

Postpartum thyroiditis is a lymphocytic thyroiditis involving antimicrosomal antibodies, similar to Hashimoto's disease. The cause is poorly understood, but it is thought to involve both genetic and environmental factors.

**How is postpartum thyroiditis diagnosed?**

Increased TSH and decreased free $T_4$ levels with positive antimicrosomal antibody titers in the postpartum period

**Is it possible to predict the development of this condition?**

Elevated levels of antimicrosomal antibodies in the first trimester and on the second postpartum day have been shown to be predictive of the development of postpartum thyroiditis.

# 36

## Preinvasive Neoplastic Disease of the Cervix, Vagina, and Vulva

### CERVICAL NEOPLASTIC DISEASE

| | |
|---|---|
| **What are the two histologic regions of the cervix?** | Endocervix and ectocervix, based on epithelial type |
| **What is the ectocervix?** | The portion of the cervix that is continuous with the vagina |
| **What type of epithelium covers the ectocervix?** | Squamous epithelium that is continuous with the squamous epithelium lining the vagina |
| **What is the endocervix?** | The portion of the cervix that is adjacent to the external cervical os and extends into the endocervical canal |
| **What type of epithelium covers the endocervix?** | Mucin-secreting columnar epithelium that is continuous with the cuboidal cells of the endometrial lining |
| **What is the original squamocolumnar junction (OSCJ)?** | The histologic boundary in the fetus that separates the squamous epithelium of the vagina from the columnar epithelium of the endocervix |
| **Where is the OSCJ located?** | Its position varies, lying on the ectocervix in 66% of fetuses, within the canal in 30%, and on the vaginal fornices in 4%. |
| **What is the new squamocolumnar junction (NSCJ)?** | During a woman's life, the OSCJ moves closer to the endocervical canal by a process called metaplasia; the NSCJ represents the boundary between mature and immature squamous metaplasia. |

**What is the significance of the NSCJ in the diagnosis of dysplasia?**

The NSCJ is the upper limit of squamous intraepithelial neoplasia and the lower limit of any adenocarcinoma in situ for the following reasons:

The NSCJ defines the upper border of any histologically definable dysplasia in women who have not undergone previous therapy.

It does not, however, define the upper limit of squamous metaplasia (ULSM). ULSM extends up into the endocervical canal, above the NSCJ

Figure 36-1. OCSJ = old squamocolumnar junction; NSCJ = new squamocolumnar junction; ULSM = upper limit of squamous metaplasia.

**What is the transformation zone?**

One to three centimeter (cm) area of squamous metaplasia between the old and new squamocolumnar junctions that separates the ectocervix and endocervix.

**What is the significance of this zone in cervical cancer?**

Location is most susceptible to the development of both preinvasive and invasive cervical neoplastic disease.

**Why is this zone susceptible to malignant transformation?**

The metaplastic process occurring in this region appears to predispose the area to malignant transformation.

**What is metaplasia?**

A reversible change in which one type of fully differentiated cell type is replaced by another fully differentiated cell type.

**Is metaplasia a malignancy?**

No

**What is dysplasia?**

The abnormal growth or development of organs, tissues, or cells; characterized by an increased mitotic rate and atypical cytologic features (size, shape, organization)
Potentially reversible

**What is the relationship of dysplasia to cancer?**

Dysplastic changes may be found adjacent to foci of cancer.
Dysplasia may progress to cancer.

**What are the different types and frequencies of the various forms of cervical cancer?**

Squamous cell neoplasias: 80%–90%
Adenocarcinoma and adenosquamous carcinomas: approximately 20%; incidence of these forms seems to be increasing in a relative sense.
Other types (e.g., melanomas, sarcomas, lymphomas): approximately 1%

**What are the causative factors of squamous cell neoplasia?**

Cervical squamous cancer and its precursors appear to follow a pattern typical of a sexually transmitted disease. Risk factors are consistent with this pattern and include:
Early age at first coitus (under 20 years)
Multiple sexual partners
Venereal infection
Young age at marriage
Young age at first pregnancy
High parity
Divorce
Lower socioeconomic status
Coitus with high-risk males (sexual partner with multiple sexual partners)
Other factors include cigarette smoking, pelvic radiation, immunodeficiency, and vitamin A and C deficiency.

**What is currently thought to be the principal causative agent of cervical squamous cell neoplasia?**

Human papilloma virus (HPV)

**For what other neoplasias is HPV thought to be the principal causative agent?**

Cervical intraepithelial neoplasia (CIN), vaginal intraepithelial neoplasia (VAIN), vulvar intraepithelial neoplasia (VIN), and penile neoplasia HPV is also a likely inciting agent in some invasive vulvar and vaginal malignancies.

**What percentage of cervical condylomata contain HPV DNA?**

Over 90%

**What percentage of cervical cancers contain HPV DNA?**

Over 60%

**Does a type-specific association between HPV subtype and severity of cervical cancer exist?**

Yes

**How many subtypes of HPV exist?**

More than 55

**What are the most common subtypes found in genital lesions?**

6, 11, 16, 18, 31, and 33

**What subtypes are associated with malignant transformation (i.e., commonly seen in high-grade CIN as well as invasive cervical malignancies)?**

16, 18, 31, 33, 35, 45, 51, 52, 56, and 58

**Of the two main HPV subtypes associated with malignant transformation, which subtype also appears to influence the progressive potential of a precursor lesion?**

HPV 18 is reported to be a more progressive subtype than HPV 16 (i.e., it is associated with poor prognostic features and frequently occurs in younger patients with adenocarcinomas and in tumors that tend to recur).

In contrast, HPV 16 DNA has been found in almost all large-cell keratinizing tumors, which tend to recur infrequently.

**Is herpesvirus infection a causative factor in genital cancers?**

A cause-and-effect relationship with genital cancer has not been proved although it is suspected.

**What is the definitive predisposing factor of adenomatous and adenosquamous neoplasia of the cervix?**

Transplacental exposure to diethylstilbestrol (DES)

**Is HPV associated with adenocarcinomas of the cervix?**

Recent data show that many adenocarcinomas are associated with HPV.

**What are the predisposing factors of the other types of cervical cancer?**

Little is known about predisposing factors for other types of cervical cancer.

**List the systems that are used in the classification of cervical neoplasia.**

Papanicolaou system
Cervical intraepithelial system (CIN)
Bethesda system

**Table 36.1    Comparison of Cytology Classification Systems**

| Bethesda System | Dysplasia/CIN System | Papanicolaou System |
|---|---|---|
| Within normal limits | Normal | I |
| Infection (organism should be specified) | Inflammatory atypia (organism) | II |
| Reactive and reparative changes | | |
| Squamous cell abnormalities | | |
| Atypical squamous cells of undetermined significance | Squamous atypia | IIR |
| Low-grade squamous intraepithelial lesion (LSIL) | HPV atypia | |
| | Mild dysplasia    CIN 1 | |
| High-grade squamous intraepithelial lesion (HSIL) | Moderate dysplasia    CIN 2 | III |
| | Severe dysplasia | |
| | CIN 3 | IV |
| | Carcinoma in situ | |
| Squamous cell carcinoma | Squamous cell carcinoma | V |

CIN = cervical intraepithelial neoplasia.

**What is the Papanicolaou system?**

A numerical grading system that defines lesions based on the degree of atypia:
  Class I: normal
  Class II: inflammatory atypia
  Class III: dysplasia
  Class IV: carcinoma in situ
  Class V: invasive carcinoma

**What is the CIN system?**

Grades cervical dysplasia as mild (1), moderate (2), or severe (3); still used frequently

**What is the Bethesda system?**

The most recent classification system; intended to replace the Papanicolaou system
Reports in this system contain:
  A statement on adequacy of the specimen for interpretation
  Diagnostic category (normal or other)
  A descriptive diagnosis
Introduced the terms "low-grade" and "high-grade" squamous intraepithelial lesions (LSIL and HSIL). LSILs include condylomata and CIN 1, and HSILs include CIN 2 and CIN 3.
The new cytologic classification is not meant to replace the histologic terms "dysplasia" and "CIN."

**Is cervical cancer rapidly or slowly progressive?**

Slowly progressive

**In what Bethesda classes does spontaneous regression occur frequently? Rarely?**

Frequently: CIN 1
Rarely: CIN 2 or 3

**What is the estimated duration of disease in women with CIN 3 who progress to invasive cancer?**

Three to ten years

**What percentage of untreated CIN 3 disease will progress to invasive disease?**

Thirty-six percent

**What procedure is used to screen for cervical cancer?**

Cervical cytology [Papanicolaou (Pap) smear]

**How is a Pap smear performed?**

Samples of cervical epithelial cells are taken from the ectocervix using a wooden spatula, and samples of endocervical cells are obtained with a cytobrush which is inserted into the external os and rotated.

**Since the introduction of Pap smear screening, how has the mortality rate from cervical cancer changed?**

Prior to the widespread use of the Pap smear, cervical cancer was the leading cause of cancer death among American women.

Mortality rate has declined by more than 50% to 9 deaths per 100,000 women per year.

Five-year survival after diagnosis of cancer has also increased.

**What is the major benefit of the Pap smear?**

Its ability to detect preinvasive disease

**What are some problems with Pap smear screening?**

It is not possible to screen all high-risk patients before they develop invasive disease; many high-risk patients do not have access to screening services.

The Pap smear is not as successful in identifying adenocarcinoma; therefore, the rates of this type of cervical carcinoma have not declined.

The Pap smear false-negative rate can approach 20%–30% for preinvasive squamous lesions and may be as high as 40% for adenocarcinoma. Invasive cancer may have a false-negative rate as high as 50% due to accompanying ulceration and infection (in which inflammation may make the smear difficult to interpret).

Patients do not always obtain follow-up after an abnormal Pap smear.

It is often difficult to evaluate the transformation zone in postmenopausal women because of its location high in the endocervical canal.

**What are the current American College of Obstetricians and Gynecologists recommendations for Pap smear screening?**

Screening and pelvic examinations should begin at age 18 or at onset of sexual activity

Annual screening and pelvic examination until three negative results; thereafter less frequent screening and examinations at discretion of physician

An annual physical and pelvic examination and an annual Pap smear for patients at high or unknown level of risk

**What constitutes high risk?**

American Cancer Society's criteria are intercourse by age 20 or more than two lifetime sexual partners.

When defining the high-risk patient, it is important to remember that the majority of women are considered high-risk by this definition.

In addition, it is impossible to determine a woman's level of risk without knowing the sexual history of each of her previous partners.

**How should a patient with an abnormal Pap smear be managed?**

Complete history and physical examination to look for grossly abnormal lesions or discoloration within the vulva, vagina, or perianal region that may identify a likely source of the abnormal cytology; all three areas must be examined because of the prevalence of multicentric disease.

Colposcopy: examination by microscopy

Mandatory in patients with a persistent class II Pap smear (inflammatory atypia) or class III (dysplasia) or above

When no gross invasive lesion is visible, a colposcopic exam may help identify subclinical disease that may be the source of the abnormal cells.

**Why is colposcopy necessary in diagnosis?**

Because the lesions of CIN are located in the transformation zone and because early lesions are located primarily on the ectocervix, many of the more subtle lesions can be visualized by colposcopy.

| | |
|---|---|
| **Visualization of what structure constitutes a satisfactory colposcopic examination?** | Visualization of the NSCJ |
| **What is the follow-up if the colposcopic exam is normal after an abnormal Pap smear?** | Exfoliation from other sites must be considered (e.g., endometrial, ovarian, or metastatic breast cancer).<br>Cellular contamination from a vulvar or urinary tract lesion should also be considered.<br>If a CIN smear is not explained after examination by an experienced colposcopist, the smear itself should be sent for expert review. If the presence of a high-grade cytologic abnormality is confirmed, diagnostic conization is mandatory. |
| **What are the indications for colposcopically directed biopsy?** | Biopsy is used as an adjunct to colposcopy.<br>Carefully directed punch biopsies taken of the most abnormal appearing areas of epithelium can adequately sample a CIN lesion that is visible in its entirety. |
| **What is the main problem with colposcopically directed biopsy?** | Risk of not selecting the most abnormal sites for target biopsy, as the most prominent areas of colposcopic change do not always coincide with the areas of greatest histologic abnormality. |
| **How can this problem be overcome?** | Representative biopsy specimens should be taken from all significant acetowhite areas including the most prominent area of epithelial opacity and the most prominent area of vascular atypia.<br>Any area suspected of occult invasion must also be sampled carefully. |
| **What kind of lesions can endocervical curettage (ECC) identify?** | Lesions in the endocervical canal that are invisible to the colposcope |

**When is ECC used in the diagnosis of cervical cancer?**

Experts vary as to when to perform an ECC.

Some advocate mandatory ECC to rule out an extension of a lesion into the endocervix. Others feel that if the entire NSCJ is visualized and a surrounding rim of normal columnar epithelium is seen within the lower canal, ECC can be omitted (in previously untreated patients).

ECC is not performed in pregnant patients because it may cause labor or bleeding.

**How is a final outpatient evaluation performed?**

All three parameters of the study [cytology, colposcopy, and tissue samples (cervical biopsies and ECC)] should be reviewed.

All "diagnoses" should be compatible before definitive outpatient therapy is begun (e.g., cytology, colposcopy, and biopsies should indicate similar degrees of CIN).

**How are treatment decisions made based on results of all three parameters of study?**

If all parameters agree, the area may be treated locally.

If significant correlation is lacking, additional evaluation, usually with a cold knife cone (a large cervical biopsy including all of the transformation zone and the canal) is mandatory.

**When is conservative (also known as local or superficial ablative) therapy indicated?**

Invasive cancer must be excluded.

Patients with squamous lesions are suitable for superficial ablative therapies provided that:

The entire transformation zone can be visualized colposcopically.

The biopsy is consistent with the Pap smear.

The ECC is negative.

Occult invasion after cytologic or colposcopic evaluation is not suspected.

**What therapeutic modalities are used in conservative therapy?**

Cone biopsy or superficial ablative techniques such as electrocoagulation diathermy, cryosurgery, or $CO_2$ laser

**Is hysterectomy beneficial as a treatment of uncomplicated CIN?**

No. It is no longer considered appropriate treatment of uncomplicated CIN.

**What is excisional conization?**

Surgical excision of a cone of tissue containing the abnormal area of epithelium with a cold knife or a tightly focused beam of superpulsed $CO_2$ laser energy

**What are the indications?**

Inability to visualize the NSCJ on colposcopy
CIN 2–3 on ECC
Colposcopic suspicion of occult invasion, even if target biopsies show only CIN 3
Significant discrepancies (2 grades) between cytology and histology
Cytologic suspicion of adenocarcinoma in situ
Microinvasion on the punch biopsy
When colposcopic expertise is unavailable

**What are the complications?**

Complication rate is about 12% and seems to depend on the configuration of the excised cone (i.e., the rate of cervical incompetence increases with larger excisions due to removal of a greater portion of fibromuscular cervix).
Possible complications include hemorrhage, sepsis, infertility, cervical stenosis, and cervical incompetence.

**What is loop electrosurgical excision procedure (LEEP)?**

Surgical excision of the transformation zone and the distal cervical canal under anesthesia using an electrosurgical wire loop; the loop can also be used for fulguration and electrocoagulation.

**What are the complications?**

Similar to those of continuous wave laser ablation, including hemorrhage (1%–8%), postoperative pelvic cellulitis or abscess formation, cervical stenosis (1%), cervical deformity, and midtrimester abortion

**What is electrocoagulation diathermy (not commonly used in the United States)?**

Ablation of abnormal epithelium using high-voltage electricity in two different processes, fulguration and electrocoagulation.

**What is fulguration?**

An electrode is held just above the surface of the epithelium which produces an arc of electricity from the energy source (electrode) to the ground (the epithelial surface). The heat produced rapidly desiccates the tissue at the site of the spark.

**What is electrocoagulation?**

Deeper and more widespread tissue destruction is caused by insertion of the electrode below the epithelial surface. Energy is conducted along tissue planes, resulting in heat denaturation and enzymatic degradation of structural proteins within large volumes of tissue.

**How is electrocoagulation diathermy different from radial electrocautery?**

Electrocautery produces a simple conduction burn at the epithelial surface with a red-hot wire. It does not destroy the epithelium of the cervical crypts, and therefore will not adequately treat cervical dysplasia.

**What is cryosurgery?**

Application of liquid refrigerants, such as $N_2O$ to the epithelial surface by use of a metal probe. Evaporation of the substances induces hypothermia accompanied by cryonecrosis of the tissue.

**What are the benefits of cryosurgery?**

It is a cost-effective, well-tolerated means of outpatient treatment of cervical dysplasia.
Large studies have reported a primary success rate of about 84% in the treatment of CIN 3.
Anesthesia is not necessary (although premedication with nonsteroidal anti-inflammatory drugs may help relieve discomfort associated with prostaglandin release from dying cells).

**What problems are associated with cryosurgery?**

Cryonecrosis is not uniform. Adequately treated areas of epithelium are surrounded by a wide margin of sublethal tissue injury.

Success rate also appears to be dependent on both the extent of the lesion and the volume of tissue that must be destroyed.

**How can the cryosurgery treatment failure rate be reduced?**

By using a freeze-thaw-refreeze cycle, which increases the reliability of cell death

**When is $CO_2$ laser ablation used?**

Due to its short wavelength, the $CO_2$ laser may be used for superficial ablation of abnormal epithelium as well as for conization.

**What are the indications for more radical therapy (i.e., hysterectomy)?**

If gynecologic indications exist that would be well-treated by hysterectomy, or if a permanent means of sterilization is desired

In these circumstances, invasive cancer must be excluded prior to hysterectomy.

**Why is follow-up important after conservative therapy?**

Cervical epithelial abnormalities probably increase the risk of vaginal and vulvar lesions.

**When should Pap smears be evaluated following conservative therapy? Why?**

Pap smears should not be evaluated for 3 months after treatment (especially after cryotherapy) because of the reparative process.

**Why is follow-up important after hysterectomy?**

Recurrences (on the vaginal mucosa) have occurred up to 10 years after therapy.

## PREINVASIVE NEOPLASTIC DISEASE OF THE VAGINA

**What is the frequency of vaginal cancer?**

Carcinoma of the vagina is rare, accounting for 1%–2% of all gynecologic malignancies.

**What is the incidence of vaginal cancer?**

Age-adjusted incidence is 0.6 per 100,000.

**Between what ages does peak incidence occur?**

Between ages 60 and 70

**What is the most common type of vaginal cancer?**

Squamous cell carcinoma
Multicentric disease (i.e., neoplasia involving several different anatomic sites within the lower genital tract)

**What is the cause of vaginal cancer?**

Risk factors commonly associated with carcinoma of the cervix and vulva have not shown the same degree of significance in patients who develop vaginal carcinomas.
Long-term pessary use and long-standing uterine procidentia (prolapse of the uterus which causes the cervix to protrude from the vaginal opening) or both may predispose to vaginal cancer by causing chronic local irritation of the vaginal mucosa; however no causal link has been proved.
Whereas the role of a sexually transmitted infectious agent has not been proved in vaginal cancer, the multicentric nature of the disease has led the search for a common agent to which the mucosa of the cervix, vagina, and vulva is exposed, e.g., HPV.

**How is vaginal cancer screened for?**

Due to the low incidence of vaginal carcinoma, it is not cost-effective to screen all women.
However, most physicians screen with a vaginal Pap as part of periodic check-ups.

**What is a predisposing factor to adenocarcinoma of the vagina?**

DES exposure *in utero*

**What is the incidence of clear cell adenocarcinoma in women exposed to DES?**

Estimated to be 1 in 1000 or less

| | |
|---|---|
| **At what stage are most of these adenocarcinomas diagnosed?** | Approximately 70% of these vaginal adenocarcinomas are diagnosed at Stage I |
| **What percentage of women with vaginal intraepithelial neoplasia (VAIN) 3 and vulvar intraepithelial neoplasia (VIN) 3 have preexisting or synchronous cervical neoplasia (preinvasive or invasive)?** | VAIN 3: about 60%<br>VIN 3: about 30% |
| **What percentage of women with primary vaginal carcinoma have a history of in situ or invasive cervical cancer treated at least 5 years earlier?** | Up to 30% |
| **What percentage of women who have vaginal cancer have had a hysterectomy?** | Sixty percent |
| **What is benign condyloma acuminatum?** | Focal capillary and epithelial proliferation that results in formation of a local papilloma or "wart"<br>Condylomata are the result of HPV infection.<br>Condylomata often involve vulva as well as vagina. |
| **What are the most common subtypes of HPV found in benign condylomata, and do these subtypes have neoplastic potential?** | HPV types 6 and 11; they have no neoplastic potential (excluding verrucous carcinoma) |
| **What HPV subtypes are associated with malignant transformation and in what percent of benign condylomata are they found?** | HPV 16 or 18; 7% of histologically benign condylomata |

**In what percentage of VAIN lesions can HPV DNA be isolated?**

Seventy percent

**Is the prevalence increasing or decreasing?**

Increasing

**Is the mean age at diagnosis increasing or decreasing?**

Decreasing

**What is the malignant potential of VAIN?**

Unknown

**How is VAIN diagnosed?**

By colposcopy

**What are the clinical features of VAIN?**

VAIN usually involves the posterior upper third of the vagina.
Two clinical patterns can be distinguished:
  Keratotic plaques, often visible with the naked eye
  Flat patches of acetowhite epithelium that are often completely invisible before vinegar application

**What is the treatment of VAIN?**

Often difficult to treat
Historically treated by surgical excision or vaginal irradiation; however, current therapy is generally more conservative and consists of photovaporization or topical 5-FU application.

**What are the requirements for conservative therapy?**

Physician with expert training in colposcopy
Directed biopsies consistent with the abnormality seen on the Pap smear
No cytologic or colposcopic suspicion of occult invasion
Choice of conservative versus radical therapy also depends on the amount of tissue involved and clinical circumstances.

## PREINVASIVE NEOPLASTIC DISEASE OF THE VULVA

**What is the frequency of vulvar malignancies?**

Vulvar cancer is rare, representing about 4% of gynecologic malignancies.

**What are the relative frequencies of the various forms of vulvar cancer?**

Squamous cell carcinoma in situ: most common intraepithelial lesion of the vulva; accounts for about 90% of all vulvar cancers

Malignant melanoma: 2% of vulvar cancers

Basal cell carcinomas: 2% of vulvar cancers

Vulvar sarcomas: 1%–2%

Lymphomas, plasmacytomas, endodermal sinus tumors, and Paget's disease: extremely rare

**What is the cause of vulvar cancer?**

No specific cause has been identified for vulvar cancer.

The association between cervical neoplasia and vulvar cancer, however, has led to speculation that a common pathogen may be involved.

**What is the relationship between vulvar carcinoma in situ and sexually transmitted disease?**

Patients with vulvar carcinoma in situ have an increased frequency of sexually transmitted disease.

**What is the relationship between vulvar cancer and condylomata acuminata or herpes simplex vulvitis?**

At least 5% of vulvar cancers have been estimated to develop within preexisting genital condylomata.

Antecedent or concurrent condylomata acuminata or herpes simplex vulvitis is age-associated; patients are usually age 40 or younger.

**What is the relationship between vulvar cancer and HSV?**

Remains to be determined

**What other sexually transmitted diseases are associated with vulvar cancer?**

Syphilis (approximately 5% of patients with vulvar cancer have a positive serologic test for syphilis)

Lymphogranuloma venereum
Granuloma inguinale

**What other factors are associated with vulvar cancer?**

Obesity
Hypertension
Diabetes mellitus
Arteriosclerosis
Menopause at an early age
Nulliparity
Immunosuppression: Progression from vulvar intraepithelial neoplasia (VIN) to invasive cancer is most often seen in elderly and immunosuppressed patients.

**What is the malignant potential of vulvar dystrophies?**

Recent studies suggest that the malignant potential of vulvar dystrophies is small.
Adequately treated, a vulvar dystrophy should not significantly predispose a patient to the development of vulvar cancer.
Less than 5% of such patients followed for periods of up to 25 years develop vulvar cancer.

**What factors increase the risk of vulvar cancer in patients with vulvar dystrophy?**

Cellular atypia on the initial biopsy; occurs in less than 10% of cases

**What is vulvar intraepithelial neoplasia (VIN)?**

Preinvasive neoplastic disease of the vulva

**Is the prevalence of VIN increasing or decreasing?**

Substantially increasing; largest increases have been of the multifocal variety, especially in young women.

**What are the risk factors for VIN?**

Patients with preinvasive and invasive squamous lesions of the cervix and vagina have an increased risk of developing VIN.
Patients with vulvar intraepithelial neoplasia have a 15%–30% chance of having synchronous or metachronous cervical or vaginal squamous neoplasia or both.

**Where are VIN lesions typically located?**

Hairless areas of the vulva; the skin of the interlabial folds, posterior fourchette, and perineum are most frequently affected.

Twenty-five percent of cases have perianal involvement.

Multifocal disease is common, especially in younger patients.

**What are the signs and symptoms of VIN?**

Fifty percent of patients are asymptomatic at diagnosis.

Pruritus is the most common symptom.

There is no characteristic appearance of the lesions.

Lesions may be macular or papular in shape.

Discoloration is usual. The color may be white, red, pink, gray, or brown.

**What does each color signify?**

White: hyperkeratosis and epithelial thickening

Red: hypervascularity and parakeratosis

Gray or brown: melanocyte overactivity and pigment incontinence (premalignant keratinocytes are unable to retain melanin, which is then deposited within macrophages.)

**What histologic changes are characteristic of VIN?**

Disorganization of the epithelial architecture

Giant cells with abnormal nuclei

Multinucleated cells

Disorders of cytoplasmic and nuclear maturation

Changes usually but not always extend the full thickness of the epithelium.

**List and describe the three histologic patterns of VIN.**

Bowenoid type VIN

Accounts for the majority of intraepithelial lesions of the vulva

Consists of dyskaryotic cells showing partial but disordered maturation

Keratinization is common and lesions have elevated, sharp borders.

Can closely resemble condyloma acuminatum

Characterized by parakeratosis, hyperkeratosis, and acanthosis

Basaloid VIN
  The epithelium is composed
    completely of atypical immature
    parabasal cells that extend
    throughout the thickness of the
    epithelium.
  Lesions have minimal or no
    abnormality of the surface
    epithelium but atypical maturation
    and pearl formation at the base of
    the rete pegs.

**What histologic type of**
**VIN is most common?**

A mixture of histologic patterns is most
  commonly seen.
Two-thirds of cases have confluent or
  multicentric lesions.

**What procedures are used**
**in diagnosis of VIN?**

Toluidine blue
Colposcopy with application of 3% acetic
  acid
Pap smears of the cervix or vagina to
  exclude concurrent disease in these
  areas

**What is the mainstay**
**treatment used in VIN?**

Surgical excision
Methods for excising the lesions include
  vulvectomy, superficial "skinning"
  vulvectomy, or wide local excision.

**What is the relationship**
**between the amount of**
**tissue removed and**
**recurrence rate?**

The amount of tissue removed has not
  been shown to significantly influence
  recurrence rate (which is
  approximately 30% for all three
  modalities).
Emphasis should be placed on retaining
  vulvar tissue for both aesthetic and
  functional reasons.

**When is total/radical**
**vulvectomy indicated?**

It is no longer indicated in the
  management of this disease.

**What is skinning**
**vulvectomy?**

Removal of vulvar skin and replacement
  with a split-thickness skin graft

**What are the benefits?**

Effective in treating multifocal or
  extensive disease which may be
  difficult to treat by excision alone
Subcutaneous tissues of the vulva are
  preserved, allowing for an increased

probability of an excellent functional and cosmetic result.

**What are the drawbacks?** Cosmetic and functional results are still unpredictable.

**What is wide excision?** Surgical excision of a vulvar lesion and a disease-free margin of approximately 5 millimeters (mm) with primary reapproximation of the skin edges

**What are the indications?** Discrete lesions less than 2 cm in diameter

**What are the benefits?** It produces excellent, nonmutilating results in the treatment of small foci.

**What is $CO_2$ laser evaporation?** Use of a short wavelength laser to ablate tissue

**What are the indications?** It is an acceptable treatment alternative to local excision provided patients are carefully evaluated and undergo biopsy prior to treatment to exclude microinvasive or invasive carcinoma. It may be used to treat the Bowenoid (warty) variety of VIN.

**What are the benefits?** Treatment is nonmutilating. It is very effective, particularly for multiple, small lesions.

**What are the drawbacks?** Because occult invasion > 1 mm carries a risk of lymph node metastases, there is little room for error. It cannot be used to treat the basaloid (undifferentiated) variety of VIN, which has a different natural history from the bowenoid type; premalignant foci occurring in association with lichen sclerosis or lichen simplex chronicus always require excision. Unlike excisional techniques, this method does not allow for proper histologic evaluation.

| | |
|---|---|
| **What is the benefit of topical 5-FU in the treatment of vulvar carcinoma in situ?** | It is effective in 50% to 75% of cases of vulvar carcinoma in situ. |
| **What are the drawbacks?** | Application causes painful ulceration. It does not allow proper histologic evaluation. |
| **What is a drawback of topical immunotherapy with dinitrochlorobenzene in the treatment of VIN?** | It does not allow for proper histologic evaluation. |
| **What is observation?** | Patients are followed closely for a period of 6 months to 1 year. |
| **What are the indications?** | Young patients who are pregnant or recovering from recent herpetic vulvitis may be observed closely, as spontaneous regression has been reported in this population. |
| **What is the prognosis for patients with VIN?** | Clinical course cannot be predicted on the basis of histopathology or DNA analysis. Lesions rarely progress. The rate of invasive vulvar cancer associated with VIN is about 8%, and four-fifths of this number are superficially invasive (< 1 mm). |
| **What is Paget's Disease?** | A disease of abnormal differentiation of cells derived from the germinal layer of the epidermis |
| **What is the histologic appearance?** | Pathognomonic abnormal cells, called "Paget's cells," are rich in mucopolysaccharide, a diastase-resistant, periodic acid-Schiff (PAS)-positive substance |
| **Histochemical staining can be used to differentiate Paget's disease from what other diseases?** | Carcinoma in situ, amelanotic melanoma, and junctional nevi |

**What is the relationship between Paget's disease and vulvar cancer?**

In about 20% of cases, Paget's disease is associated with an underlying adenocarcinoma.

In about 29% of patients, it may herald synchronous or metachronous invasive cancer at other sites.

**What is the treatment of Paget's disease?**

Because histologically demonstrable disease extends farther than the visible lesion, very wide local excision is required to decrease the likelihood of recurrence.

A wide superficial vulvectomy is often necessary with extensive disease.

**What is the treatment of recurrences?**

Recurrences are almost always in situ and may be treated by minor local excision or laser therapy if detected early.

# 37

## Breast Cancer

**What is the incidence of breast cancer?**

One in every 14 women will have breast cancer in her lifetime.

Leading cause of cancer death among American women ages 44–55 years

Second most common cause of cancer death in women overall after lung cancer

**What percentage of women with breast cancer die of the disease?**

Fifty percent

**What age-group is affected?**

Less than 2% of cases occur in women younger than age 30 years.

The incidence increases rapidly in the fourth decade.

After menopause, the rate of increase slows.

**Risk factors?**

Breast cancer in a first-degree relative: Increases the risk two- to threefold

Relative with premenopausal breast cancer: Increase is threefold.

With bilateral breast cancer: Increase is 5.5-fold.

With premenopausal bilateral breast cancer: Increase is ninefold.

Personal history of contralateral breast cancer: Increases the risk twofold

Nulliparity

Late pregnancy: First full-term pregnancy after age 30 years poses greater risk than nulliparity.

Late menopause: Women who reach menopause after age 55 years have twice the risk of women who reach menopause before age 45 years.

Early menarche: Weak risk factor

Ionizing radiation

Atypical hyperplasia: Increases risk
  fourfold; with positive family history
  of breast cancer, increases risk
  ninefold

**Is obesity a risk factor?**

In postmenopausal women: Weak risk
  factor
In premenopausal women: Protective

**Do oral contraceptive pills
increase the risk of breast
cancer?**

No

**Is long-term estrogen
replacement therapy a risk
factor?**

Controversial
One study found that long-term estrogen
  replacement therapy increases the risk
  of breast cancer by 40%. The
  increased risk may be related to the
  proliferative effect of estrogen on
  undiagnosed microscopic breast
  cancer.
Other studies have found no increased
  risk.

## DIFFERENTIAL DIAGNOSES

**What benign diseases
should be included in the
differential diagnosis?**

Fibrocystic disease
Fibroadenoma
Cystosarcoma phylloides
Intraductal papilloma
Fat necrosis
Mammary duct ectasia
Galactocele
Gynecomastia
Granular cell myoblastoma (rare)
Breast abscess
Mastitis

**What is fibrocystic disease
of the breast?**

Denotes a variety of noninflammatory
  histopathologic changes in the breast,
  including epithelial, stromal, and duct
  proliferation

**What is the cause of
fibrocystic disease?**

Multifactorial, including genetic and
  hormonal factors (estrogen)

| | |
|---|---|
| **What are the signs and symptoms of fibrocystic disease?** | Diffuse breast fullness<br>Fibronodularity<br>Cysts may or may not be present.<br>In general, pain and fullness are noticed immediately before menses; symptoms gradually decrease over 10 to 14 days. |
| **How is the diagnosis of fibrocystic disease confirmed?** | Clinically by palpation<br>Fine-needle aspiration of single cysts<br>Aspirate should be straw-colored or greenish. Bloody fluid or lesions that do not resolve with aspiration raise suspicion of malignancy. |
| **What is the treatment of fibrocystic disease?** | Mild analgesia<br>Reduction in caffeine intake<br>Oral contraceptive pills in refractory cases |
| **What is the most common tumor in women younger than 30 years of age?** | Fibroadenoma |
| **What is fibroadenoma?** | Benign tumor consisting of stromal and epithelial elements |
| **How is the tumor characterized?** | Most are solitary, solid, well encapsulated, well circumscribed, rubbery, firm, nontender, lobulated, mobile breast masses 1–4 cm in size.<br>Hormonally dependent, so may fluctuate in size<br>Giant fibroadenoma is typically > 5 cm. |
| **What is the treatment of fibroadenoma?** | Excisional biopsy for definitive diagnosis and treatment |
| **What is cystosarcoma phylloides?** | A rare variant of fibroadenoma that has greater cellularity and pleomorphism and a tendency to recur after simple excision<br>Some undergo malignant transformation with 10% metastasizing, usually to the lungs |

| | |
|---|---|
| **What are the signs and symptoms of cystosarcoma phyllodes?** | Large, often teardrop mass with microscopic penetration<br>Overlying skin may be warm and erythematous.<br>Mass is not well encapsulated |
| **What is the treatment of cystosarcoma phyllodes?** | Smaller lesions: Wide local excision with at least 1-cm margin<br>Larger, breast-occupying lesions: Simple mastectomy (without axillary node dissection) |
| **What is the most common breast mass after trauma to the breast?** | Fat necrosis |
| **Why is fat necrosis easily confused with carcinoma?** | The mass of fat necrosis is firm and tender with ill-defined borders and is often surrounded by ecchymosis, skin retraction, and other skin changes. |
| **What is the most common cause of bloody nipple discharge in premenopausal women?** | Intraductal papilloma |
| **What is the treatment of intraductal papilloma?** | Wedge resection of ductal lesion |
| **What is mammary duct ectasia?** | A benign, **painful** mass due to duct dilatation and plasma cell infiltration |
| **What are the signs and symptoms of duct ectasia?** | Breast edema, dermal fixation, inflammatory changes; nipple inversion may or may not be present. |
| **What diagnostic/ therapeutic procedures *must* be performed in mammary ectasia?** | Multiple biopsies to rule out malignancy and local excision |

## TYPES OF BREAST CANCER

| | |
|---|---|
| **What is the most common type of breast cancer?** | Infiltrating ductal carcinoma<br>Represents 70%–80% of all breast cancers |

**What are the two types of noninvasive breast cancer?**

Ductal carcinoma in situ (DCIS)
Lobular carcinoma in situ (LCIS)

**Which type is commonly characterized by multicentricity and a significant risk of progressing to invasive cancer?**

DCIS; 25%–30% of patients progress to invasive breast cancer.

**What percentage of patients with LCIS have bilateral disease?**

25% to 40%

**What percentage of patients with LCIS will have recurrent LCIS in the ipsilateral or contralateral breast?**

25% to 40%

**What are some types of invasive carcinoma that have a low risk of metastasis?**

Colloid carcinoma, medullary carcinoma, tubular carcinoma, comedocarcinoma, and papillary carcinoma

**Which type is known to enlarge rapidly because of hemorrhage and necrosis?**

Medullary carcinoma, which represents 3%–5% of all breast cancers, is typically a mobile, deeply set encapsulated tumor that is otherwise slow growing.

**Which of these breast cancers has the best 5-year survival rate?**

Papillary carcinoma has the lowest frequency of axillary nodal spread. It is typically bulky and centrally located. It is usually seen in younger patients and is not derived from intraductal papilloma.

**Which of the moderately metastasizing carcinomas is characterized by numerous microcalcifications?**

Infiltrating ductal carcinoma has microcalcifications and significant fibrosis, whereas infiltrating lobular carcinoma extensively infiltrates and does not have microcalcifications.

**What is inflammatory carcinoma?**

A rare, highly aggressive form of carcinoma of any histologic type that causes skin changes such as erythema and peau d'orange and other local inflammatory changes
Represents 1.5%–3% of all breast cancers

Poor prognosis, with a 5-year survival
rate of 3%–5%
Seventy-five percent of patients present
with palpable axillary metastasis.

**What is Paget's disease of the nipple?**

DCIS or infiltrating ductal carcinoma
involving the epidermis causing
inflammatory, eczematous dermatitis
of the nipple and areola
Represents 1%–3% of all breast cancers
One-third of patients present with
axillary node metastasis.
Usually a favorable prognosis secondary
to early diagnosis

## DIAGNOSIS OF BREAST CANCER

**What are typical presenting signs and symptoms of breast cancer?**

Palpable breast mass that is firm, ill
defined, not freely mobile, and usually
nontender
Unilateral bloody nipple discharge
Nipple retraction, flattening, or
thickening
Skin changes, including dimpling, peau
d'orange, crusting
Palpable lymph nodes
Diffuse breast pain (rare)
Constitutional symptoms such as weight
loss, anorexia, bone pain (advanced
disease)
Abnormal mammogram

**Where are most breast cancers located?**

Upper outer quadrant (tail of Spence)

**What is peau d'orange?**

Swollen, pitted skin overlying carcinoma
of the breast; resembles orange peel
Caused by stromal infiltration and
edema due to lymphatic obstruction

**What are the common sites for metastasis?**

Bone, lungs, liver, and brain

**What procedures are used for breast cancer screening?**

Breast self-examination monthly,
preferably 1 week after menses
Physical examination:
Every 3 years for women ages 20–40
years and annually for women age
40 years or older

Known breast lesions should not be followed for more than two menstrual cycles without a diagnosis.

Mammogram:

The recommended schedule for screening mammogram is continually being reevaluated and revised.

Some current guidelines include first screening mammogram at age 40 years, every 2 years until age 50, and yearly after age 50 years.

**What size mass can a mammogram detect?**

Masses ≥ 0.5 cm

**What are the false-negative and false-positive rates of mammography?**

False-negative rate: 5%–15%
False-positive rate: < 5%

**Why is it more difficult to evaluate young women by mammography?**

The breasts of young women contain more fibrous tissue than those of older women.

**What findings on mammography require further evaluation?**

Spiculated, stellate, clustered microcalcifications (< 1 mm)

**What diagnostic tests are helpful in evaluating a breast mass?**

Ultrasound can differentiate between cystic and solid masses.

Fine-needle aspiration biopsy
Hemocult-positive fluid should be examined cytologically.
Cysts that do not resolve with two aspirations should be evaluated with needle or excisional biopsy.

Needle biopsy for superficial, fairly well circumscribed lesions > 1 cm; establishes diagnosis in 80% of patients

Open biopsy: definitive diagnostic method
Excisional biopsy (i.e., total removal) for benign tumors and for lesions < 3 cm
Incisional biopsy (or needle biopsy) for suspect lesions ≥ 3 cm

immediately before planned
mastectomy
Estrogen/progesterone receptor studies
and flow cytometry of tissue biopsy
samples can aid in formulating
treatment plan in some cases.

## STAGING AND TREATMENT OF BREAST CANCER

**What tests are necessary
for staging and treatment
planning of breast cancer?**

Essential: Examination, bilateral
mammogram, complete blood count,
chemistry panel including liver
function tests, chest radiograph
Selected studies based on results of
tests: Radionuclide bone scan, liver
computed tomography scan

**What classification is used
in breast cancer staging?**

TNM classification: T (primary tumor),
N (regional nodes), M (metastasis)

**What are the TNM stages
of breast cancer?**

Tumor size
   Tx: Cannot assess
   T0: No evidence of primary tumor
   Tis: In situ
   T1: ≤ 2 cm
   T2: > 2 cm but < 5 cm
   T3: > 5 cm
   T4: Extension onto chest wall/skin
Regional node status
   Nx: Cannot assess
   N0: No regional lymph node spread
   N1: Mobile ipsilateral axillary nodes
   N2: Fixed ipsilateral axillary nodes
   N3: Ipsilateral internal mammary
      nodes
Metastasis
   Mx: Cannot assess
   M0: No distant metastasis
   M1: Distant metastasis; includes
      ipsilateral supraclavicular lymph
      nodes

**What are the available
treatment options for
breast cancer?**

Surgical:
   Lumpectomy with axillary dissection
      and radiation
   Simple mastectomy
   Modified radical mastectomy

Systemic treatment:
  Radiation therapy
  Chemotherapy
  Hormonal treatment: Tamoxifen, an
    antiestrogen; oophorectomy in
    premenopausal women; and
    adrenalectomy or hypophysectomy
    (rarely)

**What is the difference between simple mastectomy and modified radical mastectomy?**

Modified radical mastectomy includes axillary node dissection.

**What are the complications of mastectomy/axillary dissection?**

Injury to the thoracodorsal nerve to the
  latissimus dorsi
Injury to the long thoracic nerve to the
  serratus anterior, causing "winging of
  the scapula"
Lymphedema of the ipsilateral upper
  extremity
Loss of sensation due to injury of
  intercostobrachial nerves
Injury to the medial and lateral thoracic
  nerves to the pectoralis muscles

**For what pathologic type is radiation therapy most effective?**

Local chest wall lesions, regional lymph node metastasis, and bony and brain metastasis

**What are the side effects of tamoxifen?**

Mild nausea
Hot flashes, particularly in
  premenopausal women
Transient thrombocytopenia or
  leukopenia

**For each of the following stages of breast cancer, list the current recommended treatment options and prognosis.**
  **Clinically local disease, stage I–II**

Treatment options:
  Lumpectomy ± axillary dissection ±
    radiation therapy
  Modified radical mastectomy
  Add adjuvant chemotherapy for
    positive lymph nodes

Prognosis:
  Overall 5-year survival rate for stage I
    is 85%.
  Overall 5-year survival rate for stage
    II is 66%.

**Clinically advanced local disease, stage III**

Treatment: Simple mastectomy +
  radiation therapy + chemotherapy
Prognosis: Overall 5-year survival rate
  for stage III is 41%.

**Systemic disease, Stage IV**

Treatment: Systemic therapy
Prognosis: Overall 5-year survival rate
  for stage IV is 10%.

# 38

# Cervical Cancer

**What is the incidence of cervical cancer?**

Approximately 15,000 new cases occur per year.

Second most common gynecologic malignancy following uterine malignancies

**What are the signs and symptoms of cervical cancer?**

The most common symptom is vaginal bleeding, which may be postcoital, postmenopausal, or intermenstrual.

Later in the disease, vaginal discharge, pelvic pain, or back pain secondary to ureteral obstruction may develop.

Ten percent to twenty percent of patients complain of pain radiating to the back or legs.

**How is cervical cancer diagnosed?**

Cervical biopsy provides definitive diagnosis and is easily performed if the patient has a visible cervical tumor.

If an abnormal PAP smear or routine examination raises suspicion of cervical cancer, colposcopically directed biopsy may be helpful.

**What colposcopic findings are suggestive of cervical cancer?**

Abnormally branched, looped, or punctate blood vessels (secondary to neovascularization of the tumor and distortion of the blood vessels by the growing mass)

Abnormal appearance of the surface of the cervix

**What procedures are used in the staging of cervical cancer?**

Cervical cancer is clinically staged, based on careful pelvic examination and general physical examination with particular attention to inguinal and supraclavicular lymph nodes.

Other procedures that may be used for clinical staging include chest x-ray, intravenous pyelogram, barium enema, cystoscopy, proctoscopy, and cervical conization and examination under anesthesia.

**What procedures are useful in treatment planning, but not in staging?**

Computed tomography (CT) scan, magnetic resonance imaging (MRI), ultrasound, and lymphangiogram

**What are the stages of cervical cancer?**

Stage 0: Carcinoma in situ
Stage I: Carcinoma is limited to the cervix.
  Ia: Microscopic diagnosis only
    Ia1: Minimal invasion
    Ia2: Lesions not exceeding 5 mm in depth from the surface epithelium or 7 mm in horizontal spread
    Ib: Lesions larger than Ia2 lesions, but still limited to the cervix
Stage II: Carcinoma extends beyond the cervix, but has not extended to the pelvic sidewall or to the lower third of the vagina.
  IIa: No obvious parametrial involvement
  IIb: Obvious parametrial involvement
Stage III: Carcinoma extends to the pelvic sidewall or lower third of the vagina or there is evidence of hydronephrosis.
  IIIa: No extension to the pelvic sidewall but the lower third of the vagina is involved
  IIIb: Pelvic sidewall involvement or hydronephrosis
Stage IV: Carcinoma extends outside the true pelvis or clinically involves the mucosa of the bladder or rectum.
  IVa: Spread to adjacent organs
  IVb: Distant spread

**What are the histologic types of cervical cancer and their frequency?**

Squamous cell carcinoma: 80%
Undifferentiated: 10%
Adenocarcinoma: 5%
Sarcoma:3%
Primary melanoma, small cell, lymphoma: rare

## SQUAMOUS CELL CARCINOMA

| | |
|---|---|
| **Describe the demographics of squamous cell carcinoma.** | Mean age is 50 to 55 years with a bimodal distribution (peaks occur at 35 to 39 years and at 60 to 64 years). |
| **What are the risk factors for squamous cell carcinoma?** | Early age at first coitus, multiple sexual partners, human papillomavirus (HPV) infection, smoking, multiparity |
| **What are the treatment options for squamous cell carcinoma?** | Radiation therapy can be used for **all** stages of cervical cancer. Surgery, however, is limited to stages I and IIa disease. Chemotherapy is occasionally an option. |
| **What is the treatment of stage Ia1?** | No involvement of lymphovascular space: cervical conization, if patient wants to preserve fertility, or a type I hysterectomy Nonsurgical candidates: intracavitary radiotherapy |
| **What is the treatment of stage Ia2?** | No involvement of lymphovascular space; invasion less than 3 mm: type I hysterectomy or cervical conization Involvement of lymphovascular space; invasion less than 3 mm: type I or type II hysterectomy with a pelvic node dissection Invasion of 3 to 5 mm: type II hysterectomy with a pelvic node dissection Intracavitary radiotherapy is an option. |
| **What is the treatment of stages Ib and IIa?** | Surgery and radiotherapy offer the same cure rates for these stages. Surgery: Surgical candidates have lesions less than 4 to 5 centimeters (cm). Type III or radical hysterectomy with pelvic node dissection and para-aortic node sampling Radiotherapy: 4500 cGy external beam and intracavitary radiation External beam radiotherapy may be followed with type I hysterectomy in patients whose lesions respond poorly to radiation. |

| | |
|---|---|
| **What is the treatment of stages IIb through IVa?** | Radiotherapy using external beam and intracavitary radiation |
| **What is the treatment of stage IVb?** | Chemotherapy is the primary treatment modality for metastatic disease. The most effective chemotherapeutic agent is cisplatin.<br>Radiotherapy may be used to control local disease and relieve bleeding, edema, or pain. |
| **What are the complications of surgery?** | Immediate postoperative complications: hemorrhage, ureterovaginal or vesicovaginal fistulas, fever, sepsis, pulmonary embolus, and wound infection<br>Long-term complications: lymphocyst formation, bladder dysfunction, ureteral strictures, and fistula formation |
| **What are the complications of radiotherapy?** | Acute: nausea, diarrhea, and superficial skin damage<br>Long-term: fistula formation involving the bladder, bowel, and vagina; vaginal stenosis and sexual dysfunction; rectal bleeding from radiation proctitis; and ureteral stenosis |
| **What is the treatment of recurrent disease?** | Generally, patients who were initially treated surgically are candidates for radiotherapy, and patients initially treated with radiotherapy may be candidates for surgical excision of recurrent disease.<br>Surgical options include local excision or pelvic exenteration [anterior, posterior, or total]. |
| **What is the overall 5-year survival rate for squamous cell carcinoma?** | Sixty percent |
| **What is the 5-year survival rate for each stage of squamous cell carcinoma?** | Stage I: 85% to 90%<br>Stage II: 60% to 80%<br>Stage III: 30%<br>Stage IV: 10% |

## UNDIFFERENTIATED CARCINOMAS

**Describe the demographics of undifferentiated carcinomas.**

The patient demographics are not like those of squamous cell carcinoma; however, these carcinomas tend to occur in a similar age-group.

**What are the risk factors for undifferentiated carcinomas?**

No specific risk factors

**What is the treatment?**

The treatment of each stage is the same as the treatment of each stage of squamous cell carcinoma.

**What is the prognosis?**

The numbers are too small to assign percentages; however, overall prognosis is worse than that of squamous cell carcinomas because of the more aggressive or poorly differentiated histopathologic component of these carcinomas.

## ADENOCARCINOMAS

**Describe the demographics of adenocarcinomas.**

The frequency of this type of cancer is increasing; however, this increase may be due to improvement in the early detection of squamous cell carcinomas. The average age is 56 years.
Eighty percent of patients have stage I or II disease at the time of diagnosis.

**What are the risk factors?**

Same as squamous cell carcinomas

**In general, what are the treatment options for adenocarcinoma?**

Generally, the treatment is the same as that of squamous cell carcinoma.
These tumors may occasionally be "bulkier" than squamous cell carcinomas. Therefore, radiotherapy may be advocated, even with early stage disease, because it is technically difficult to achieve negative margins with surgery.
In some cases, radiation plus type I hysterectomy is proposed for bulky stage I and stage II tumors.

**What is the prognosis?**   Adenocarcinoma and squamous cell carcinoma have similar patterns of lymphatic dissemination; however, adenocarcinoma is more aggressive in both lymphatic spread and local extension. Therefore, the survival rates are lower in adenocarcinoma compared with squamous cell carcinoma.

**What is the overall 5-year survival rate for adenocarcinoma?**   Fifty percent

**What is the 5-year survival rate for each stage of adenocarcinoma?**   Stage I: 70% to 75%
Stage II: 30% to 40%
Stage III: 20% to 30%
Stage IV: < 15%

# 39

# Ovarian Neoplasms

**What is the incidence of ovarian cancer in the United States?**

About 1 in 70 women will develop ovarian cancer.

Incidence begins to rise around the fifth decade of life and is highest in postmenopausal women.

Ovarian cancer is the leading cause of death from gynecologic cancer in the United States.

**How are ovarian neoplasms classified?**

According to the tissue type from which they originate:

Coelomic epithelium

Sex cord–ovarian stroma

Germ cell

Nonspecialized stroma

Metastatic tumors

## EPITHELIAL OVARIAN NEOPLASMS

### GENERAL FEATURES AND GENETICS

**What is the embryologic origin of epithelial neoplasms?**

Arise from coelomic epithelium (i.e., the mesothelium), which covers and is incorporated into the ovary during embryonic development

This epithelium also gives rise to peritoneum and the paramesonephric (müllerian duct), which explains the histologic similarities between lesions of ovaries, peritoneum, and urogenital tract.

**In what age-group do most epithelial ovarian cancers occur?**

Greater than 80% of epithelial ovarian cancers occur in postmenopausal women, with a peak incidence at age 62.

Approximately 30% of ovarian epithelial neoplasms in postmenopausal women are malignant, compared with only 7% in premenopausal women.

**Is there a hereditary pattern of development for ovarian cancers?**

Hereditary or familial cases are seen, but account for < 5% of all ovarian malignancies.

**What is a feature that distinguishes hereditary cases of epithelial ovarian cancers?**

Tend to present about 10 years earlier than nonfamilial cases

**How can patients at risk for hereditary epithelial ovarian cancer be identified?**

A specific genetic marker is not available.

A pedigree analysis is useful and may reveal an autosomal dominant pattern of transmission.

**How are patients with familial risk of ovarian cancer managed?**

Management is controversial because of the lack of reliable screening methods.

In general, women who have a significant family history of ovarian cancer and wish to preserve their fertility should be followed by transvaginal ultrasonography every 6 months.

Women who no longer wish to maintain their fertility should be offered prophylactic bilateral salpingo-oophorectomy; they should be informed that peritoneal carcinomas occasionally occur after this operation.

**What specific inheritance patterns for ovarian cancer have been identified?**
   **Site-specific familial ovarian cancer**

Patients with two first-degree relatives with epithelial ovarian cancer: risk of developing ovarian cancer is as high as 50%, representing an autosomal dominant mode of transmission.

Patients with a single first-degree relative with epithelial ovarian cancer: risk is increased three- to ten-fold over those without a family history.

**Breast/ovarian familial cancer syndrome**

May exist if there is familial history of epithelial ovarian and breast cancers.

Recently, this syndrome has been associated with the BRCA1 gene, a locus on the 17q chromosome.

**Lynch II syndrome**
Syndrome of multiple adenocarcinomas involving familial colon cancer (Lynch I syndrome) and ovarian, endometrial, breast, and other cancers
Women with this syndrome appear to have at least three times the risk of the general population for development of epithelial ovarian cancer.

**What are the signs and symptoms of ovarian cancer?**
Majority of patients are either asymptomatic or present with symptoms that are nonspecific and usually ignored
Early stage disease: urinary symptoms and/or constipation (secondary to a growing pelvic mass), irregular menses, and pelvic pain or pressure
Advanced disease: abdominal distention, bloating, constipation, anorexia, nausea, and early satiety secondary to ascites and intestinal spread

**What is the most important sign that should raise suspicion of ovarian cancer?**
Presence of a pelvic mass on physical examination

**What is postmenopausal palpable ovary syndrome?**
Women who are more than 1 year past menopause should have atrophic, nonpalpable ovaries. Any palpable mass in a woman more than 1 year postmenopause must be viewed as suspicious of a neoplasm and necessitates further investigation.

**What is the role of screening in the diagnosis of this disease?**
Currently, no tests are available that are specific and sensitive enough to serve as a valuable screening tool for ovarian cancer.

**How is ovarian cancer diagnosed?**
An ovarian mass requires definitive diagnosis, which usually entails exploratory laparotomy/laparoscopy.
In premenopausal patients, observation and hormonal suppression with oral contraceptives to check for regression of the mass before proceeding with laparotomy are reasonable.

Ultrasound may be helpful in
characterizing the nature of the mass.
Young women with sonographic
findings suggestive of a benign
process may be followed. Persistent
masses require definitive diagnosis by
tissue sample.

**What are the differential diagnoses for an ovarian mass?**

Gynecologic causes:
Functional cysts of the ovaries
Pelvic inflammatory disease (PID)
Endometriosis
Massive edema of the ovary (secondary
    to torsion)
Pedunculated uterine leiomyomas
Ectopic pregnancy
Nongynecologic causes:
Inflammatory or neoplastic colonic mass
Lymphoma
Metastasis from distant primary tumors
    (e.g., breast)

**What is the role of tumor markers in the diagnosis and treatment of epithelial cancers?**

CA 125
Elevated in about 80% of patients with
    epithelial ovarian cancers, but it is not
    specific
Positive values are highly predictive of
    recurrence of disease; however,
    negative values are not sensitive in
    predicting the absence of disease.
Carcinoembryonic antigen (CEA)
Elevated in the majority of patients with
    mucinous ovarian cancer
However, it is neither sensitive nor
    specific enough to be useful in patient
    screening.

**How do epithelial ovarian cancers spread?**

Primarily by "surface implantation"
throughout the peritoneal cavity,
lymphatic dissemination involving pelvic
and para-aortic nodes, and less
commonly, hematogenous dissemination

**Describe the general staging system for ovarian cancers.**

Stage I: growth limited to the ovaries
Stage II: growth involving one or both
    ovaries with pelvic extension
Stage III: tumor involving one or both
    ovaries with peritoneal implants

outside the pelvis, positive retroperitoneal or inguinal nodes, or superficial liver metastasis

Stage IV: growth involving one or both ovaries with distant metastasis; includes pleural effusion with positive cytology and parenchymal liver metastasis

**What histologic features are used to determine the grade of an ovarian tumor?**

Pattern of differentiation, extent of cellular anaplasia, and proportion of undifferentiated cells are used for grading lesions on a scale of 1 (few changes from normal morphology) to 3 (poorly differentiated and rapidly dividing).

**Name the different histologic types of epithelial ovarian neoplasms.**

Serous
Mucinous
Endometrioid
Clear cell
Brenner
Mixed epithelial
Undifferentiated

**What classification system is used to describe the likelihood of metastasis of epithelial neoplasms?**

Each histologic type (except for undifferentiated) is further subclassified as:
A: benign
B: low malignant potential (LMP), also called borderline
C: malignant based on the extent of proliferation, nuclear features, mitotic activity, and stromal invasion

## TYPES OF EPITHELIAL NEOPLASMS

### Serous neoplasms

**What is the most common type of epithelial neoplasm?**

Serous histology is seen in both the majority of benign and malignant epithelial ovarian tumors (75% of all epithelial cancers).

**What percentage of serous neoplasms are benign? Malignant? LMP?**

Benign: 70%
LMP: 5% to 10%
Malignant: 20% to 25%

**How frequently do bilateral serous tumors occur?**

Overall, serous tumors are bilateral 10% of the time. Malignant tumors are more frequently bilateral (35%–50%).

**What are psammoma bodies and what is their significance?**

Concentric calcifications that occur occasionally in benign serous neoplasms and frequently in serous cystadenocarcinomas

## Mucinous neoplasms

**What percentage of mucinous tumors are benign?**

Eighty percent

**What is the bilateral occurrence rate of malignant mucinous tumors?**

Ten percent to twenty percent

**What is pseudomyxoma peritonei?**

Secretion of large amounts of gelatinous mucinous material into the peritoneal cavity by the neoplastic epithelium

Most commonly associated with appendiceal adenocarcinomas; well-differentiated colorectal adenocarcinomas; and less frequently, ovarian mucinous adenocarcinomas

## Endometrioid neoplasms

**What are some examples of LMP endometrioid epithelial neoplasms?**

LMP tumors can have various morphologic presentations (e.g., tumors with a prominent fibrous component are sometimes referred to as "adenofibromas")

**What histologic features alter the prognosis of malignant endometrioid tumors?**

Good prognosis if histology shows benign squamous metaplasia
Poor prognosis if histology shows mixed adenosquamous carcinoma

**What is the relationship between ovarian endometrioid lesions and similar lesions in the endometrium?**

Ovarian endometrioid tumors are associated with similar lesions in the endometrium.

| | |
|---|---|
| **What is the management of cases with associated ovarian and endometrial tumors?** | It is important to differentiate multifocal disease (i.e., separate primaries) from disease that has metastasized from the uterus because of the much better prognosis associated with the former. |

### Clear cell neoplasms

| | |
|---|---|
| **Which type of epithelial ovarian tumor is most frequently associated with hypercalcemia and hyperpyrexia?** | Clear cell tumors |
| **What histologic features are characteristic of clear cell tumors?** | Clear cells with vacuolated or clear cytoplasm<br>Hobnail cells in which the nuclei are projected to an apical cytoplasm<br>Sometimes associated with focal areas of endometriosis or endometrioid carcinoma |

### Brenner tumors

| | |
|---|---|
| **Do Brenner tumors tend to be benign or malignant?** | Less than 2% of these tumors are malignant. |
| **What are the gross and histologic features of Brenner tumors?** | Gross features: resemble ovarian fibromas due to their solid consistency and white or yellow-white color<br>Histologic features:<br>Stromal proliferation around nests of epithelial cells resembling transitional epithelium of the urinary tract<br>These tumors are associated with mucinous cystadenomas or dermoid cysts in the same or contralateral ovary. |

## TREATMENT OF EPITHELIAL NEOPLASMS

| | |
|---|---|
| **What are the main principles in the treatment of ovarian cancers?** | Three concepts:<br>1. Importance of meticulous and extensive surgical staging in disease that on inspection appears to be limited to the ovaries<br>2. Importance of "adequate" cytoreduction [macroscopic disease should be reduced to ≤ 1 cm] |

3. Importance of platinum-based combination chemotherapy in all stages

**What is the treatment of choice of stage Ia and Ib (tumor limited to one or both ovaries with no evidence of extra-ovarian spread), grade 1 lesions?**

If no evidence of spread beyond the ovary: abdominal hysterectomy and bilateral salpingo-oophorectomy (TAH-BSO)

The uterus and the contralateral ovary may be preserved if patient wants to preserve fertility.

**What is the treatment of stages Ia and Ib, grades 2 and 3, and stage Ic?**

No single optimal treatment exists; however, surgery alone is not sufficient.

Options:

Chemotherapy with a single agent (e.g., cisplatin, carboplatin, or taxol)

Combination chemotherapy (cisplatin and taxol or cyclophosphamide with or without adriamycin)

Radiation (intraperitoneal $^{32}$P or whole abdominal radiation)

**What is the treatment of stages II, III, and IV lesions?**

Surgery followed by chemotherapy/radiation

Initial surgery: maximal removal of disease including metastases (cytoreductive or debulking procedure)

Upon the completion of surgery plus chemotherapy/radiation, patients with no clinical evidence of disease and negative tumor markers may undergo a reassessment laparotomy or a "second look surgery." If disease is still present, second-line or salvage therapy may be recommended.

**What clinical factors negatively affect the prognosis?**

Advanced age, residual tumor after primary surgery, volume of ascites

**What is the 5-year survival rate for ovarian cancers?**

Great variability exists in survival of patients with same-stage ovarian cancer because survival is highly dependent on tumor grade, sensitivity to chemotherapeutic agents, success of debulking procedure, and many

other factors. Thus, the 5-year survival
rate is not a practical concept in
ovarian cancer.
In general, for properly staged patients,
5-year survival rates are:
Stages I and II: 80% to 100%
Stage IIIa: 30% to 40%
Stage IIIb: 20%
Stage IIIc and IV: 5%

## NONEPITHELIAL OVARIAN NEOPLASMS

**What is the prevalence of
nonepithelial ovarian
cancers?**

Nonepithelial ovarian cancers comprise
only 10% of all ovarian cancers.

**What are the three main
types of nonepithelial
tumors?**

1. Germ cell tumors
2. Sex cord–stromal tumors
3. Tumors metastatic to the ovary

**How are these tumors
staged?**

They are surgically staged in the same
manner as epithelial cancers.

## GERM CELL TUMORS

**Germ cell tumors comprise
what percentage of all
ovarian neoplasms?**

Neoplasms: 20% to 25%
  **Of ovarian malignancies?**
  Malignancies: < 5% (in western
    countries)

**What percentage of germ
cell neoplasms are
malignant?**

About 33% (one-third)

**In what age-group are
most germ cell tumors
seen?**

Third and fourth decade of life

**What is the embryologic
origin of germ cell
neoplasms?**

Arise from primitive germ cells and may
  occur within, or more commonly,
  outside the gonads
Extragonadal involvement may occur
  from the pineal gland to the
  retroperitoneum. This widespread
  involvement is due to the embryonic
  migration of germ cells from the
  caudal portion of the yolk sac to the
  posterior mesentery before they are
  incorporated into the developing

gonads. These cells are often multipotent cells and may present as embryonic, extraembryonic, or mixed structures.

**Name the main histologic types of germ cell neoplasms.**

Dysgerminoma (also called germinoma)
Teratoma
Endodermal sinus tumor (EST)
Embryonal carcinoma
Polyembryoma
Choriocarcinoma
Gonadoblastoma
Mixed germ cell tumors

**What are the benign types of germ cell neoplasms?**

Gonadoblastomas and mature cystic teratomas

**Name the secretory markers for different pure malignant germ cell tumors.**

Placental alkaline phosphatase (PLAP) and lactate dehydrogenase (LDH) are commonly produced by dysgerminomas.
Human chorionic gonadotropin (hCG) and alpha fetoprotein (AFP) are secreted by many different tumors (see Table 39-1).
Mixed germ cell tumors may secrete more than one marker.

Table 39–1.

| Tumor type | hCG produced | AFP produced |
| --- | --- | --- |
| Dysgerminoma | no | no |
| Embryonal carcinoma | yes | yes |
| Teratoma | no | no |
| Endodermal sinus tumor | no | yes |
| Choriocarcinoma | yes | no |

**What are the signs and symptoms of germ cell tumors?**

Subacute pelvic pain (secondary to characteristic rapid growth rate of these tumors)
Bladder and rectal symptoms
Menstrual irregularities (may be confused with pregnancy)
Torsion or rupture of the adnexa may be confused with appendicitis.

| | |
|---|---|
| **What is the diagnostic workup for germ cell tumors?** | In the presence of a pelvic mass on physical examination, preliminary evaluation includes ultrasound and serum hCG, AFP, PLAP, and LDH measurements. Chest x-ray is important because germ cell tumors can metastasize to lungs or mediastinum. |
| **When and why is karyotyping indicated?** | A karyotype should be obtained on all premenarchal girls with germ cell tumors because of the association between these lesions and gonadal dysgenesis. |
| **Which germ cell tumors tend to be associated with gonadal dysgenesis?** | Gonadoblastomas, dysgerminomas, and ESTs |
| **When should surgical exploration be considered?** | Premenarchal patients: adnexal mass ≥ 2 cm<br>Postmenarchal premenopausal patient: adnexal mass > 8 cm |

## DYSGERMINOMAS

| | |
|---|---|
| **What percentage of germ cell tumors are dysgerminomas?** | Thirty percent to forty percent |
| **In what age-group are most dysgerminomas seen?** | Between ages 10 and 30 |
| **What percentage of ovarian malignancies associated with pregnancy are dysgerminomas?** | Twenty percent to thirty percent |
| **What is the association between dysgerminomas and gonadal dysgenesis?** | Five percent of dysgerminomas are discovered in phenotypic females with abnormal gonads, hence the need for karyotyping. |
| **How common is the involvement of the contralateral ovary?** | Dysgerminomas are the only malignant germ cell tumor with a **significant rate of bilateral occurrence** (about 10%–15%) |

**What is the treatment of dysgerminomas?**

Unilateral oophorectomy in order to preserve fertility

Surgery may be followed with chemotherapy; contralateral ovary, fallopian tube, and the uterus can therefore be preserved even in the presence of metastatic disease because the tumor is sensitive to chemotherapy.

**What is the treatment if karyotyping reveals a Y chromosome?**

Bilateral gonadectomy

**Should the contralateral ovary be biopsied?**

Yes, because not all bilateral lesions have obvious ovarian enlargement

**When is chemotherapy used in treatment?**

For advanced or incompletely resected tumors

**What chemotherapy regimen is prescribed in these cases?**

Combination chemotherapy using bleomycin, etoposide, and cisplatin (BEP)

**Can radiation be used in the treatment of dysgerminomas?**

Although dysgerminomas are very sensitive to radiation, loss of fertility limits its use to recurrent or chemoresistant cases.

**What is the prognosis after treatment of dysgerminomas?**

Cure rates of 85% to 90%, even for patients with advanced disease, with the use of BEP chemotherapy

## TERATOMAS

**What are teratomas?**

Tumors composed of totipotent cells capable of differentiating into derivatives of more than a single germ layer

**In what age-group are most teratomas seen?**

First two decades of life

**How are teratomas classified?**

Classified as mature or immature based on histologic appearance of nervous tissue elements of the tumor and the malignant behavior observed in immature teratomas

**What is the prevalence of immature teratomas?**

Represent < 1% of all teratomas

**What is the incidence of bilateral presentation in teratomas?**

Bilateral incidence of mature teratomas is 15% to 20%.
Immature teratomas are almost always unilateral, although metastasis to the contralateral ovary may occur.

**Do mature teratomas transform into immature teratomas?**

Mature and immature teratomas are thought to represent related but separate neoplastic processes, and the mature form does not transform into the immature form.
Malignant degeneration of mature cystic teratomas is thought to occur in only 1% to 2% of cases; in this situation, the most frequent malignancy developed is squamous carcinoma.

**What is Rokitansky's protuberance and what is its significance?**

Definition: protuberance on the inner wall of the cyst containing a wide variety of tissue present in the tumor
Significance: must be sectioned thoroughly because it often contains populations of immature cells important to the accurate grading of the lesion

**What are the possible complications of mature cystic teratomas?**

Other than malignant transformation, they include torsion, rupture and hemorrhage, infection, and gliomatosis peritonei.
Rupture is uncommon, but becomes more common in pregnant patients and may occur during labor.

**What is gliomatosis peritonei?**

Implantation of benign, mature glia in the peritoneal cavity; may occur following the rupture of a mature cystic teratoma

**What are the three specialized forms of teratoma?**

Dermoid cyst: consists entirely of skin and appendages (i.e., ectodermal derivatives).
Struma ovarii: consists primarily of thyroid tissue
Carcinoid: composed of gut neuroendocrine cells which secrete serotonin and/or other catecholamines

**What is the treatment of mature teratomas?**

Ovarian cystectomy with preservation of remaining normal ovarian tissue, if possible

**What is the treatment of immature teratomas?**

Premenopausal patients who want to preserve fertility: unilateral oophorectomy if the tumor is limited to a single ovary

Postmenopausal patients: TAH-BSO

Chemotherapy (BEP) for all patients except those with stage Ia grade 1 tumors; chemotherapy is also indicated if ascites is present, regardless of the tumor grade.

**What is the most important prognostic factor for survival following treatment of teratomas?**

Grade of the lesion

**What other factors influence survival?**

Patients with incompletely resected tumors prior to chemotherapy have a lower probability of cure compared to those with complete tumor resection.

**What are the 5-year survival rates for patients with grades 1, 2, and 3 lesions?**

Grade 1: 82%
Grade 2: 62%
Grade 3: 40%

## ENDODERMAL SINUS TUMORS

**What is the epidemiology of endodermal sinus tumors (ESTs)?**

Also known as yolk sac tumor
Represents the third most common germ cell malignancy
This aggressive malignancy tends to occur in young females (median age is 18) and is almost always unilateral.

**What are Schiller-Duval bodies?**

Cystic spaces lined by a flattened endothelium that contain a tuft with a vascular core resembling a glomerulus; they are characteristic of EST histology.

| | |
|---|---|
| **Is there a useful marker for ESTs?** | Most lesions secrete AFP.<br>However, AFP is not useful as a screening tool but can be used to monitor response to therapy and recurrence. |
| **What is the treatment of ESTs?** | Surgical exploration and unilateral salpingo-oophorectomy<br>Gross metastases should be removed, but thorough debulking is not indicated because all patients must receive chemotherapy.<br>Chemotherapy currently consists of cisplatin-containing combination regimens. |

## EMBRYONAL CARCINOMA

| | |
|---|---|
| **How common are embryonal carcinomas?** | Rare tumor of young females (median age is 14) |
| **What feature of embryonal carcinoma distinguishes it from choriocarcinoma?** | Histologic absence of trophoblastic cells |
| **What are the characteristic tumor markers for embryonal carcinoma?** | Frequently secrete hCG and AFP<br>May secrete estrogen<br>May lead to precocious pseudopuberty or irregular bleeding at presentation |
| **What is the treatment of embryonal carcinoma?** | Same as that of endodermal sinus tumors (i.e., unilateral oophorectomy followed by cisplatin-based combination chemotherapy) |

## CHORIOCARCINOMA OF THE OVARY

| | |
|---|---|
| **What is choriocarcinoma of the ovary?** | A tumor composed of trophoblastic tissue |
| **How frequently does choriocarcinoma occur in nonpregnant patients?** | Purely nongestational occurrence in the ovary is extremely rare. These patients tend to be younger than 20 years old, and the majority have metastases at the time of presentation. |

| | |
|---|---|
| **What tumor markers are associated with this disease?** | hCG secretion is common. AFP elevation indicates an endodermal sinus component. |
| **What is the treatment of choriocarcinoma?** | Combination chemotherapy has been employed in these rare cases using methotrexate, actinomycin D, and cyclophosphamide (same as treatment of gestational trophoblastic disease), or alternatively, BEP |
| **What is the prognosis after treatment?** | Poor |

## POLYEMBRYOMA

| | |
|---|---|
| **In what age-group do polyembryomas occur?** | Very young patients |
| **How common is this tumor?** | Extremely rare |
| **What is the characteristic histology of this tumor?** | The tumor is composed of embryoid bodies that reflect the histology of early embryonic differentiation (ectoderm, endoderm, mesoderm). |
| **What tumor markers are associated with this tumor?** | Elevated hCG, AFP |
| **Can polyembryoma be associated with precocious puberty?** | Yes |

## GONADOBLASTOMA

| | |
|---|---|
| **What is gonadoblastoma?** | Benign neoplasm composed of a mixture of germ cells and sex cord derivatives; found in patients with gonadal dysgenesis |
| **Are gonadoblastomas ever malignant?** | No; however, they are associated with the development of malignant germ cell tumors in up to 50% of cases. |
| **What is the characteristic genetic abnormality seen in gonadoblastomas?** | The karyotype commonly reveals a Y chromosome or a fragment of it. |

| | |
|---|---|
| **What is the significance of the presence of a Y chromosome in a female patient?** | Prompt bilateral gonadectomy is required because of the risk of malignancy. The exception is patients with androgen insensitivity syndrome in whom this procedure can be delayed until age 30 (before this age, the risk of developing cancer is not significant). |

## MIXED GERM CELL TUMORS

| | |
|---|---|
| **What are mixed germ cell tumors composed of?** | Contain two or more of the above tumor elements |
| **What is the incidence of dysgerminoma, EST, immature teratoma, and choriocarcinoma in mixed germ cell tumors?** | Dysgerminoma: 80% <br> EST: 70% <br> Immature teratoma: 53% <br> Choriocarcinoma: 20% |
| **What factors determine the prognosis in these tumors?** | Tumor size and the relative amounts of the most malignant component |

## SEX CORD–STROMAL TUMORS

| | |
|---|---|
| **How common are sex cord–stromal tumors?** | Account for 5% to 8% of all ovarian malignancies |
| **What is the origin of these neoplasms?** | Derived from sex cords and ovarian mesenchyme |
| **What differentiation patterns are seen in these tumors?** | Because the primitive stromal cells can differentiate into either male or female, these tumors can have predominantly male or female characteristics. |
| **What are the three general groups of sex chord–stromal tumors?** | 1. Granulosa–stromal (including granulosa and thecoma–fibroma tumors) <br> 2. Androblastomas (Sertoli-Leydig cell tumors) <br> 3. Gynandroblastomas |

## GRANULOSA–STROMAL CELL TUMORS

| | |
|---|---|
| **What is a granulosa–stromal cell tumor?** | Tumor defined by the presence of granulosa cells, with or without thecal elements |

**In what age-groups are these tumors usually seen?**

Occur in women of all ages

**What are the signs and symptoms?**

Granulosa-stromal cell tumors typically secrete estrogen. Depending on the reproductive age of the patient, signs and symptoms include sexual pseudoprecocity, menstrual irregularity, secondary amenorrhea, endometrial hyperplasia, or even endometrial carcinoma.

**Why aren't granulosa and theca cell tumors classified separately?**

A strict division between granulosa and theca cell tumors is not useful because of frequent histologic coexistence and similar endocrinologic effects.

**What is the gross appearance of these tumors?**

Vary in size, tend to be yellow or gray in color, and have a smooth lobulated surface

**What are Call-Exner bodies?**

Arrangement of granulosa cells in small clusters around a central cavity; present in granulosa- stromal cell tumors

**What is the metastasis/ recurrence pattern seen in these tumors?**

Usually stage I at diagnosis, but may recur 5 to 30 years later.
Hematogenous spread to lungs, liver, or brain is also possible and may occur years after the initial diagnosis.

**What factors should be taken into account when planning treatment of granulosa- stromal cell tumors?**

Age of patient, desire to preserve fertility, and extent of disease determined by surgical staging

**What is the treatment if fertility is not an issue?**

TAH/BSO
Primary therapy with chemotherapy and radiation reserved for recurrent or metastatic disease

**What is the treatment if fertility preservation is desired?**

For stage Ia disease, unilateral salpingo-oophorectomy followed by a dilatation and curettage of the uterus because of the possibility of coexistent endometrial carcinoma

| | |
|---|---|
| **What is the prognosis following treatment?** | Granulosa tumors have a prolonged natural history with possibility of late recurrence.<br>Ten-year survival is about 90%; drops to a rate of approximately 75% after 20 years. |

## SERTOLI-LEYDIG CELL TUMORS

| | |
|---|---|
| **How common is this malignancy and in what age-group does it usually occur?** | Quite rare (0.2% of all ovarian cancers)<br>Occur most frequently in the third and fourth decades of life |
| **What are the signs and symptoms?** | Virilization secondary to androgen production is seen in about 85% of cases. Signs of virilization include acne, hirsutism, breast atrophy, oligomenorrhea or amenorrhea, receding hairline, and a deepening of the voice. |
| **What laboratory abnormalities may be associated with Sertoli-Leydig tumors?** | Plasma testosterone and androstenedione levels may be elevated.<br>Rarely, these tumors may produce estrogen (gynandroblastomas) and may thus cause signs and symptoms typical of granulosa-theca cell tumors. |
| **What is the treatment?** | Because bilateral lesions are rare (< 1%), the usual treatment is unilateral salpingo-oophorectomy with evaluation of the contralateral ovary. |
| **What is the prognosis following treatment?** | Five-year survival rate is about 70% to 90%, and recurrences are uncommon. |

## TUMORS METASTATIC TO THE OVARY

| | |
|---|---|
| **What percentage of ovarian tumors are metastases from distant primaries?** | Approximately 5% |
| **What primary tumors tend to metastasize to the ovaries?** | Tumors of the female genital tract, breast, or gastrointestinal (GI) tract<br>About 25% of women who die of metastatic breast cancer have evidence of ovarian involvement (usually bilateral) at autopsy. |

**What is a Krukenberg tumor?**

Cells characterized by a mucin-filled "signet ring" histologic appearance that have metastasized to the ovary, usually from the GI tract

The primary tumor most frequently originates from the stomach, and less commonly, from the colon, biliary tract, or the breast.

These tumors tend to occur bilaterally and usually present at an advanced stage of the primary disease. Most patients die of their primary tumor within a year.

**What other malignancies tend to involve the ovaries?**

Leukemias and lymphomas; involvement tends to be bilateral.

**What hematologic malignancies most commonly involve the ovaries?**

Burkitt's lymphoma: most common

Advanced-stage Hodgkin disease: About 5% of patients have some involvement of the ovaries.

**What is the treatment of metastatic tumors to the ovaries?**

Therapy consists of treating the primary disease.

# 40

# Endometrial Carcinoma

| | |
|---|---|
| **What is endometrial carcinoma?** | An adenocarcinoma involving the lining of the uterus |
| **What is the incidence of endometrial cancer in the United States?** | The most common malignancy of the female genital tract in the United States<br>Approximately 36,000 new cases and 5900 deaths occur each year. |
| **What is a possible cause of endometrial cancer?** | Exact cause is unknown; however, a positive correlation exists between exposure to unopposed estrogen and development of endometrial cancer. |
| **What are examples of hyperestrogenic states associated with development of endometrial cancer?** | Estrogen replacement therapy, obesity, anovulatory cycles (polycystic ovary disease), and estrogen-secreting tumors (such as granulosa-theca cell tumors) |
| **What factors tend to be protective against endometrial cancer?** | States of decreased estrogen or increased progestin levels (e.g., oral contraceptives) |
| **What is the typical profile of a patient with endometrial carcinoma?** | Patients tend to be obese, postmenopausal women of low parity. |
| **What are the signs and symptoms of endometrial carcinoma?** | Postmenopausal bleeding, perimenopausal intermenstrual bleeding, or premenopausal abnormal uterine bleeding, particularly in the presence of anovulation. |
| **How is endometrial carcinoma diagnosed?** | All patients presenting with the previously mentioned signs and symptoms should undergo an endometrial biopsy.<br>Because of a 10% false-negative rate, a negative endometrial biopsy in a |

symptomatic patient should be followed by fractional curettage under anesthesia.

**Describe the current staging system for endometrial carcinoma.**

Endometrial carcinoma is surgically staged (as recommended by the International Federation of Gynecologists and Obstetricians).

**Stage I: tumor limited to the uterine corpus**
  Ia–limited to the endometrium
  Ib–invasion of less than half of the myometrium
  Ic–invasion of greater than half of the myometrium

**Stage II: cervical involvement**
  IIa–endocervical glandular involvement only
  IIb–cervical stromal invasion

**Stage III: local spread**
  IIIa–invasion of the serosa, adnexa, or both, with or without positive peritoneal cytology
  IIIb–vaginal metastasis
  IIIc–metastasis to pelvic nodes, para-aortic nodes, or both

**Stage IV: distant spread**
  IVa–invasion of bladder/bowel mucosa
  IVb–distant metastasis, including intra-abdominal or inguinal nodes

**How does this cancer spread?**

Direct extension is the most common route.
Can also spread via the following routes:
  Transtubal dissemination, leading to widespread peritoneal metastasis
  Lymphatic spread to pelvic and para-aortic nodes
  Hematogenous spread (usually to lungs)

**What tumor features represent important prognostic factors?**

**Advanced tumor grade and increased depth of myometrial invasion** are associated with increased risk of hematogenous and lymphatic spread, local vault recurrence, adnexal metastasis, and positive peritoneal cytology.

| | |
|---|---|
| **What are the histologic subtypes of endometrial carcinoma?** | Approximately 90% are endometrioid. Remaining 10% to 15% consist of papillary serous, adenosquamous, clear cell, malignant mixed mesodermal tumors, sarcomas, undifferentiated and, rarely, squamous cell carcinomas. The uncommon subtypes are associated with a poorer prognosis. |
| **How does the presence or absence of hormone receptors affect survival?** | Presence of estrogen receptors (ER) and progesterone receptors (PR) is associated with increased survival, even in patients with lymph node metastasis. |
| **What is endometrial hyperplasia and what is its relationship to endometrial cancer?** | All endometrial hyperplasia was once thought to represent the benign end of a continuum of morphologic severity eventually resulting in carcinoma in situ, but this concept has been recently challenged. Endometrial hyperplasia with atypia is thought to be premalignant. |
| **What are the risks of progression to carcinoma for endometrial hyperplasia and hyperplasia with atypia?** | Endometrial hyperplasia: approximately 1.5% <br> Endometrial hyperplasia with atypia: approximately 25% |
| **What is the treatment of stage I endometrial cancer?** | Total abdominal hysterectomy and bilateral salpingo-oophorectomy (TAH-BSO) <br> Some authorities treat microscopic cervical involvement (unofficially designated as stage II occult disease) in the same manner as stage I disease. |
| **What is the treatment of stage II disease?** | Two options: <br> 1. TAH-BSO with bilateral pelvic lymphadenectomy <br> 2. Combined preoperative radiation (external pelvic irradiation and intracavitary radium or cesium), followed in 6 weeks by surgery. |
| **What risks are associated with the second option?** | Ten percent risk of associated severe gastrointestinal/urologic complications |

**What is the treatment of stage III disease?**

Treatment is individualized and is aimed at surgical eradication of all macroscopic tumor, including any enlarged pelvic or para-aortic nodes, to improve the prognosis.

**What is the treatment of stage IV disease?**

Management, because patients with stage IV disease respond poorly to treatment

Treatment is individualized and usually involves surgery (palliative), radiation therapy, and progestins. Pelvic exenteration may be considered if disease extension is limited to bladder or rectum.

**What are the 5-year survival rates for each stage of endometrial carcinoma?**

Stage I: 70% to 95%
Stage II: 60% to 85%
Stage III: 40%
Stage IV: < 10%

# 41

# Gestational
# Trophoblastic Disease

**What is trophoblast?**

The extraembryonic ectoderm surrounding the blastocyst

**What is gestational trophoblastic disease (GTD)?**

Tumors originating from trophoblastic tissue
These tumors may spread either locally or distantly metastasize.

**What are the four main types of GTD?**

The four types represent a continuum:
1. Hydatidiform mole
   Complete—swelling of the chorionic villi
   Partial—cystic changes in the placenta, fetus present
2. Invasive hydatidiform mole
3. Gestational choriocarcinoma
4. Placental site trophoblastic tumor

**How are these types differentiated?**

On the basis of histopathologic and cytogenetic findings
However, the clinical features are more important in determining prognosis.

**What are the tumor markers for GTD?**

With the exception of placental site trophoblastic tumor, which is marked by human placental lactogen (HPL), the primary tumor marker is human chorionic gonadotropin (hCG).

**In general, what is the diagnostic evaluation for all forms of GTD?**

Complete history and physical examination
Ultrasound
Measurement of serum hCG level
Hepatic, renal, and thyroid function tests

**What is the diagnostic evaluation for metastatic disease?**

Chest x-ray
Ultrasound or computed tomography scan of the abdomen and pelvis

Measurement of the hCG level in
    cerebrospinal fluid (hCG levels are
    elevated in central nervous system
    metastatic disease)
Angiography of selected pelvic organs

**When should a diagnostic
evaluation for metastatic
disease occur?**

If hCG levels either plateau or continue
to rise

**List the common
metastatic sites of GTD
and their relative
incidence.**

Lung: 80%
Vagina: 30%
Pelvis: 20%
Brain: 10%
Liver: 10%
Bowel, kidney, spleen: < 5%
Other: 10%

**How is GTD staged?**

Stage I: limited to the uterus
Stage II: extends outside the uterus,
    limited to the genital structures
Stage III: extends to the lungs
Stage IV: all other metastatic sites

**What factors indicate a
good prognosis?**

Less than 4 months since the pregnancy
hCG level < 40,000 mIU/ml
No liver or brain metastasis
No prior chemotherapy

**What factors indicate a
poor prognosis?**

More than 4 months since the
    pregnancy
hCG level > 40,000 mIU/ml
Evidence of liver or brain metastasis
History of prior chemotherapy
Following a term pregnancy

**What is the overall cure
rate for GTD?**

Ninety-two percent

**What are the cure rates
for each stage of GTD?**

Stage I: 100%
Stage II: 88%
Stage III: 90%
Stage IV: 40%

**What is the cure rate for
low-risk disease (good
prognosis)?**

Ninety-seven percent

**What is the cure rate for high-risk disease (poor prognosis)?**

Sixty-four percent

**What is the effect of GTD on subsequent pregnancies?**

Patients with complete molar pregnancy have no increased risk of antenatal or intrapartum complications in later pregnancies.

Partial mole: Available data are limited but reassuring.

Choriocarcinoma: with successful treatment with chemotherapy, no increased risk of complications in later pregnancies

The frequency of congenital anomalies is not increased despite the teratogenic and mutagenic potential of the chemotherapeutic agents.

Risk of molar pregnancy in subsequent pregnancies:

Patients with molar disease are at an increased risk of developing molar pregnancy in later conceptions. The incidence is 0.6%–2.0%.

After two episodes of GTD, the risk of repeat disease rises to 28%.

## HYDATIDIFORM MOLE

**What are the two types of hydatidiform mole and how are they differentiated?**

Complete and partial
Differentiated based on cytogenetics, histopathology, and gross appearance

**What is the incidence of hydatidiform mole?**

In North America and Europe, the rate is 1 in 125 live births (1 in 1500 pregnancies)
Incidence is increased by 7- to 10-fold in Asian countries.

**What percentage of patients will develop malignant sequelae?**

Approximately 20%

**Do these tumors metastasize?**

No, unless persistent disease develops

**What are the risk factors?**

Maternal age:
  Increased risk in women over age 35
  Risk is five times greater in women over age 40.
  Risk may be increased in teenagers.
Previous molar pregnancy: Women with a previous mole have 10 times the risk of having a subsequent mole, regardless of partner.
Paternal age: increased risk if father is over age 45

**What are the cytogenetic features of a hydatidiform mole?**

Maternal genome regulates the growth and development of the embryonic tissue, while the paternal component regulates tissue proliferation.
In general, a haploid normal sperm fertilizes an ovum; the sperm then duplicates its own chromosomes, producing a 46XX karyotype. Maternal chromosomes may be either inactive or absent.
46XY complete moles result from fertilization of an empty ovum by two separate sperm, one contributing the X, the other the Y.

**Table 41–1.**

|  | Complete | Partial |
|---|---|---|
| Fetal or embryonic tissue | Absent | Present |
| Hydatidiform swelling of villi | Diffuse | Focal |
| Trophoblastic hyperplasia | Diffuse | Focal |
| Trophoblastic stromal inclusions | Absent | Present |
| Karyotype | (90%) 46XX | (66%) 69XXY |
|  | (10%) 46XY | 69XYY |
|  |  | (33%) diploid |
| % of total hydatidiform moles | 95% | 5% |
| % that develop to persistent disease | 20% | 5% |

**What are the signs and symptoms?**

Pregnancy-induced hypertension in the first half of pregnancy is virtually diagnostic of a mole.
Hyperthyroidism is secondary to the high level of hCG, which behaves like TSH.

**What is invasive hydatidiform mole?**

Features are those of hydatidiform mole, but edematous chorionic villi persist with invasion into the myometrium and continue to produce hCG. Rarely metastasize

**Table 41–2.**

|                                      | Complete | Partial |
|--------------------------------------|----------|---------|
| Vaginal bleeding                     | 97       | 73      |
| Excessive uterine size               | 51       | 4       |
| Prominent ovarian theca lutein cysts | 50       | 0       |
| B-hCG > 100,000                      | 50       | 6       |
| Pre-eclampsia                        | 27       | 3       |
| Hyperemesis                          | 26       | 0       |
| Hyperthyroidism                      | 7        | 0       |
| Trophoblastic emboli                 | 2        | 0       |

**What is the treatment of hydatidiform mole?**

The preferred method of treatment is evacuation of the uterus by suction and curettage.
Hysterectomy is an alternative in selected patients.

**What is the follow-up for hydatidiform mole?**

Weekly measurement of serum hCG levels until levels are normal for 6 consecutive months. If levels plateau or rise during the 6-month interval, patient should be evaluated for metastasis. Virtually all episodes of malignant sequelae occur within 6 months of evacuation.
Patient **MUST** use effective contraception for the entire interval of hormonal follow-up.

**What is the treatment of invasive hydatidiform mole?**

First-line therapy is methotrexate (MTX). Since MTX is secreted by the kidney, urine creatinine levels must be normal before each treatment. Patients whose levels of hCG plateau or rise during therapy should be switched to alternative therapy.
Alternative therapy: actinomycin-D or etoposide
Early hysterectomy shortens the duration and amount of chemotherapy needed to produce remission.

Failure of alternative therapy or the appearance of new metastasis mandates the use of multiagent chemotherapy.

**What is the follow-up for invasive hydatidiform mole?**

Same as the follow-up for hydatidiform mole

## GESTATIONAL CHORIOCARCINOMA

**What is choriocarcinoma?**

Malignant form of trophoblastic disease, generally referred to as gestational trophoblastic neoplasm and always preceded by a pregnancy

Characterized by proliferation of cytotrophoblasts and syncytiotrophoblasts, but in contrast to invasive hydatidiform mole, no villi are present

**What percentage of patients develop metastatic disease?**

Approximately 50%

**What is the incidence of gestational choriocarcinoma?**

Rare, but can follow any type of pregnancy:
   Forty percent follow hydatidiform moles
   Thirty percent follow spontaneous abortions
   Twenty-four percent follow term deliveries

Difficult to assess exact incidence of choriocarcinoma because of its rarity and the difficulty in distinguishing between an invasive mole and nonmetastatic choriocarcinoma.

In North America and Europe, the rate is 1 in 20,000 to 1 in 40,000 pregnancies.

Slightly higher risk in Asia

**What are the risk factors for choriocarcinoma?**

History of hydatidiform mole
   Two percent to nineteen percent of women with a molar pregnancy will develop choriocarcinoma.

Approximately 50% of patients with choriocarcinoma have a history of a mole; the other 50% have had either a spontaneous abortion or a term delivery.

Maternal Age
  Increased risk after the age of 35
  Women over age 40 have a 5% to 15% greater risk than younger women.

ABO blood group incompatibility: More cases than statistically expected occur in women with blood type A.

Oral contraceptive pill (OCP) use: Long-term OCP use has been associated with an increased risk.

**What are the features and histologic findings?**

No chorionic villi
Cytotrophoblasts and syncytiotrophoblasts

**What are the signs and symptoms?**

Same as those for hydatidiform mole

**What is the treatment of choriocarcinoma?**

**Low risk** (good prognosis)
  MTX or actinomycin-D
  Hysterectomy in conjunction with chemotherapy
**High risk** (poor prognosis)
  Triple therapy (MTX, actinomycin-D, cyclophosphamide, vincristine)
  Hysterectomy does not appear to improve the outcome in patients with high-risk metastatic disease.
  ± Radiation therapy to brain and liver to control metastatic disease

**What is the follow-up for choriocarcinoma?**

Weekly measurements of serum hCG levels until levels are normal for 3 consecutive months
Monthly measurements of serum hCG levels until levels are normal for 12 to 24 consecutive months depending on the stage of the disease
Again, effective contraception is a **MUST.**

## PLACENTAL SITE TROPHOBLASTIC TUMOR

**What is placental site trophoblastic tumor?**

Consists primarily of intermediate trophoblasts
Usually limited to the uterus but may metastasize late in the course of disease

**What is the incidence of placental site trophoblastic tumor?**

Rarest form of GTD

**What are the risk factors?**

All are subsequent to a pregnancy; 5% of patients may have a history of a spontaneous abortion.

**What are the features and histologic findings?**

Histologically composed of only one cell type (intermediate trophoblast)
Can follow any type of pregnancy

**What features of placental site trophoblastic tumor differentiate it from other GTDs?**

Differs from choriocarcinoma primarily because of absence of syncytioblasts and cytotrophoblasts
Unlike other forms of GTD, hCG production is variable or may be absent and does not correlate with the extent of the disease. Measurement of HPL may be more reliable than hCG.

**What are the signs and symptoms?**

One-third of patients present with amenorrhea, positive β-hCG, and uterine enlargement.
Patients may present with menometrorrhagia.

**What is the treatment of placental site trophoblastic tumor?**

Often can be treated with dilation and curettage, but if it persists, it is fairly resistant to chemotherapy. Therefore, early hysterectomy is recommended.

# 42

# Vulvar Cancer

**Vulvar cancer comprises what percentage of all malignancies of the female genital tract?**

Four percent

**What are the etiologic factors?**

A specific factor has not been identified. The relationship of vulvar cancer to vulvar intraepithelial neoplasia, human papillomavirus (HPV), multiple sexual partners, and smoking is controversial.

**In younger women with vulvar cancer, what percentage have evidence of HPV infection?**

20% to 60%

**What are the signs and symptoms?**

The usual presenting symptom is a palpable mass on the vulva. Most of the lesions occur on the labia majora, although vulvar cancer may occur anywhere on the external genitalia.
Many women present with vulvar itching.
Other presenting symptoms include bleeding and an abnormal discharge.

**How is vulvar cancer diagnosed?**

Definitive diagnosis is made by biopsy.

**How is vulvar cancer staged?**

Vulvar carcinomas are surgically staged because of the importance of evaluating the regional lymph nodes.
Stage 0: Carcinoma is situ, including Paget's disease
Stage I: Tumor confined to the vulva, < 2 cm in diameter, no suspect lymphadenopathy
Stage II: Tumor confined to the vulva, > 2 cm in diameter, no suspect lymphadenopathy

Stage III: Tumor of any diameter with
the following:
Spread to urethra, vagina, anus; and/
or
Clinically suspicious lymphadenopathy
in either groin
Stage IV: Tumor of any diameter with
any of the following:
Infiltration of the bladder or rectal or
urethral mucosa
Fixed to the bone
Distant metastases

**What are the histologic types of primary vulvar cancer and their frequency?**

Primary vulvar cancer comprises 92% of
vulvar cancers.
Squamous cell carcinoma: 85%
Melanoma: 5%
Bartholin gland carcinoma: 5%
Basal cell carcinoma: 2%
Sarcoma: 1% 2%
Lymphoma, endodermal sinus: Rare

**What percentage of vulvar cancers are metastases from other primary tumors?**

Eight percent

**What primary cancers typically metastasize to the vulva?**

Cancers of the cervix, endometrium,
kidney, and urethra

## SQUAMOUS CELL CARCINOMA

**What is the mean age of patients with squamous cell carcinoma of the vulva?**

Age 65 years

**What are the signs and symptoms?**

A mass usually located on the labia
majora. However, the labia minora,
clitoris, and perineum may be
involved. In 10% of cases, the location
of the primary lesion cannot be
determined because of the presence
of multiple lesions at the time of
presentation.
Pruritus, bleeding, or discharge

**How does squamous cell carcinoma of the vulva spread?**

By direct extension to adjacent tissues

By lymph nodes, primarily to the inguinal lymph nodes, then to the femoral lymph nodes and the external iliac lymph nodes (pelvic lymph nodes)

By circulation (hematogenous spread), primarily to the lung, liver, and bone; hematogenous spread usually occurs late in disease and is uncommon without lymphatic involvement.

**Spread to how many lymph nodes increases the risk of distant metastatic disease?**

More than three

**What is the incidence of lymphatic spread?**

Thirty percent

**What factors influence the likelihood of lymphatic spread?**

The size of the lesion and the depth of invasion

**What is the treatment of stage I disease?**

Before any treatment, the cervix, vagina, and vulva should be examined colposcopically.

Surgery:

Is the mainstay treatment: either wide local excision of the lesion or a radical vulvectomy

Wide local excision for vulvar cancer involves an incision carried down to the underlying fascia and a 1-cm negative surgical margin.

A radical vulvectomy involves excisiong both labia majora and the mons pubis to the depth of the underlying fascia.

A 1-cm negative surgical margin is predictive of excellent local control.

Wide local excision is the most appropriate treatment for lateral or posterior lesions, whereas rediotherapy may be preferred for anterior or periclitoral lesions.

Small vulvar lesions respond well to radiotherapy.

Groin lymph node dissection:
Must be considered, even in patients
suspected of having only stage I
disease
The only patients without significant
risk of lymph node metastases are
those with < 1 mm of invasion.
Recurrent disease in the undissected
groin carries a high mortality rate.
For unilateral lesions, the groin
dissection only needs to be
performed on the ipsilateral side.
If the lesion is midline, a bilateral
groin dissection should be
performed secondary to the
increased risk for contralateral
lymph node involvement.

**What is the difference between early and late stage III disease?**

Early stage III disease involves a lesion
of any size with spread to adjacent
organs. However, there is no unilateral
lymph node metastasis, as there is with
advanced stage III cancer.

**What is the treatment of stage II and early stage III disease?**

Surgery:
Radical vulvectomy and either
ipsilateral or bilateral groin
lymphadenectomy depending on
the location of the lesion
Partial resection of other involved
areas, such as the urethra, if
necessary
Radiation therapy: Preoperative radiation
therapy may decrease the size of the
primary lesion and thus allow a less
extensive surgery.

**What is the lymph node dissection that should be performed in stage II and early stage III disease if one positive lymph node is found?**

No additional treatment is needed, and a
contralateral lymph node dissection is
not necessary.

**Two or more positive nodes?**

Contralateral dissection; patient should
be considered for postoperative radiation
to the groin and pelvis.

**When is a pelvic lymph node dissection necessary?**

There is a < 10% incidence of pelvic lymph node involvement; therefore, a pelvic lymph node dissection does not need to be performed unless:

More than three positive unilateral groin nodes are found; same-side pelvic nodes should be evaluated.

There are positive bilateral groin nodes.

**What is the treatment of advanced stage III and stage IV disease?**

Radical vulvectomy and bilateral groin dissection

Postoperative radiation therapy to the pelvis and groin if more than two groin nodes are positive

Preoperative radiation with or without chemotherapy can be considered as primary treatment in very advanced lesions (in poor surgical candidates, this may be the only option).

Pelvic exenteration may be necessary if bladder or rectal mucosa is involved.

**What is the treatment of recurrent disease?**

If the primary lesion is > 4 cm, there is a significant risk for recurrence. Treatment is further surgical resection or radiotherapy if the patient was not previously radiated to maximal dosage.

Systemic recurrences (lung, bone) are treated with chemotherapy; the most commonly used agents are cisplatin, cyclophosphamide, methotrexate, bleomycin, or mitomycin C. Systemic recurrences are associated with poor prognosis.

**What are the complications from treatment?**

Radical vulvectomy and groin dissection are associated with wound infection and breakdown in 40%–50% of patients secondary to the inability adequately to mobilize healthy skin to close the defect.

Sixty to 70% of patients will have chronic leg edema.

Mortality rate from radical vulvectomy is 2%, usually as a result of a pulmonary embolism or myocardial infarction.

Seromas occur in 10%–15% of patients and can be treated by aspiration if the patient is symptomatic.

Femoral nerve injury may occur, resulting in sensory loss to the anterior thigh; often resolves spontaneously.

Chronic cellulitis occurs on the side of the lymph node dissection in approximately 10% of patients.

Rare: Femoral hernias and fistula formation

**What is the overall 5-year survival rate?**

Seventy percent

**What are the 5-year survival rates for each stage?**

Stage I: 90%
Stage II: 77%
Stage III: 50%
Stage IV: 18%

**What is the most important predictor of recurrence in squamous cell carcinoma of the vulva?**

Number of involved groin nodes

**What are the rates of recurrence based on this factor?**

Less than three positive nodes: 12% rate of recurrence to the vulva, groin, pelvis, or systemically

More than three positive nodes: 66% rate of local or systemic recurrence

**What is another predictor of recurrence in squamous cell carcinoma of the vulva?**

Location of positive lymph nodes

**What are the 2-year survival rates based on the location of the positive lymph nodes?**

Unilateral groin nodes: 70%–80%
Bilateral regional nodes: 50%
Bulky regional nodes: 30%
Pelvic nodes: 10%

## MELANOMA

**What is the incidence of primary vulvar melanomas?**

Rare

| | |
|---|---|
| **In what age-group and race do these cancers commonly occur?** | Postmenopausal white women |
| **Where on the vulva do the melanomas commonly arise?** | May arise either de novo or from a previously existing nevus<br>Occur primarily on the labia minora or the clitoris |
| **What are the signs and symptoms?** | Patients usually present with a mass, bleeding, or pruritus. |
| **What staging criteria are used for primary vulvar melanomas?** | Traditional staging for vulvar cancer does not apply, because the prognosis for melanomas depends on the depth of invasion.<br>Clark, Chung, or Breslow staging criteria are used.<br>Breslow is most commonly used for vulvar melanoma. It measures the thickness of the lesion from the surface to the deepest point of invasion. |
| **What are the Breslow stages for primary vulvar melanomas?** | Stage I: < 0.76 mm<br>Stage II: 0.76–1.50 mm<br>Stage III: 1.51–2.25 mm<br>Stage IV: 2.26–3.0 mm<br>Stage V: > 3 mm |
| **What is the treatment of lesions with < 1 mm of invasion?** | Wide local excision |
| **What is the treatment of lesions with > 1 mm of invasion?** | Radical excision and groin dissection. If the lesion is located laterally, an ipsilateral dissection is needed. If the lesion is located medially, a bilateral dissection is indicated.<br>If the groin lymph nodes are involved, there is no benefit from a pelvic lymph dissection secondary to the poor prognosis.<br>No role for radiation therapy<br>Poor results with chemotherapy or immunotherapy |

| What is the overall 5-year survival rate? | 20% to 30% |
|---|---|
| What is the 5-year survival rate for lesions with < 1 mm of invasion? | One hundred percent |

## BARTHOLIN GLAND CARCINOMA

| Where are the Bartholin glands located? | In the labia majora |
|---|---|
| What is the most commonly occurring type of cancer of the Bartholin glands? | Multiple histologic types occur because of the various cell types that comprise a gland; the most commonly occurring type is adenocarcinoma. |
| What is the treatment? | Wide local excision of the primary tumor or a hemivulvectomy with ipsilateral groin lymph node dissection. If the ipsilateral groin nodes are positive, the patient may benefit from a contralateral lymph node dissection and pelvic radiation therapy. |
| What is the overall 5-year survival rate? | Similar to that for a primary squamous cell carcinoma of the vulva |

## BASAL CELL CARCINOMA

| In what age-group and race do basal cell carcinomas commonly occur? | Primarily postmenopausal white women |
|---|---|
| Where are these cancers commonly located? | On the labia majora |
| What is the treatment? | Three percent to five percent contain a squamous cell component and should be treated as a primary squamous cell to the vulva. Primary treatment is wide local excision. |
| What is the prognosis? | Overall, good. There are too few cases to assign percentages. |

| | |
|---|---|
| **Is metastatic disease to the lymph nodes common or rare?** | Rare |
| **What is the rate of local recurrence?** | Twenty percent |

## VULVAR SARCOMA

| | |
|---|---|
| **What are the most common histologic subtypes of vulvar sarcoma?** | Multiple; the most common are leiomyosarcoma and rhabdomyosarcoma. |
| **Where does leiomyosarcoma commonly occur and what is the most common presentation?** | In the labia majora and usually presents as a large, painful lesion |
| **What is the treatment of vulvar leiomyosarcoma?** | Wide local excision because lymph node involvement is rare |
| **What is the overall 5-year survival rate for vulvar leiomyosarcoma?** | Thirty percent |
| **Rhabdomyosarcoma is the most common vulvar sarcoma of what age-group?** | Children |
| **In what percentage of vulvar rhabdomyosarcomas is the pelvis involved?** | Twenty percent |
| **What is the treatment of vulvar rhabdomyosarcomas?** | Similar to that for rhabdomyosarcoma in other pelvic organs (see Chap. 44) Involves a combination of surgical resection, chemotherapy, and radiation therapy |
| **What is the overall 5-year survival rate for vulvar rhabdomyosarcoma?** | 20% to 30% |

# 43

## Fallopian Tube Carcinoma

**Primary fallopian tube carcinoma comprises what percentage of all primary cancers of the female genital tract?**

0.3%

**Fallopian tube carcinoma is similar to what other female genital tract cancer?**

Epithelial ovarian carcinomas; diagnosis, treatment, and prognosis are therefore similar.

**What primary cancers commonly metastasize to the fallopian tubes?**

Ovarian, uterine, breast, and gastrointestinal tract

**In what age-group does fallopian tube carcinoma primarily occur?**

Fifth to sixth decades of life

**What are the signs and symptoms?**

Classic triad of symptoms occurs in 15% of patients:
    Profuse, watery vaginal discharge
    Pelvic pain
    Pelvic mass
Fifty percent of patients present with vaginal bleeding or vaginal discharge.
Sixty percent of patients have a pelvic mass at the time of presentation.
Ten percent of patients have abnormal cells detected on a routine Papanicolaou smear.

**How is fallopian tube carcinoma staged?**

Staging is based on that used for ovarian carcinoma.
Stage I: Confined to the fallopian tubes, with or without malignant ascites
Stage II: Extends beyond the fallopian tubes but confined to the pelvic organs, with or without malignant ascites

Stage III: Confined to the abdominal
cavity
Stage IV: Distant metastases

**What are the histologic
types of fallopian tube
carcinoma and their
frequency?**

Epithelial serous: > 90%
Sarcoma: Rare

## EPITHELIAL SEROUS CARCINOMA OF THE FALLOPIAN TUBES

**What are the signs and
symptoms?**

Classic triad of pelvic pain, pelvic mass,
and a watery discharge

**What is the percentage of
patients who present at
each stage?**

Stage I: 20%–25%
Stage II: 20%–25%
Stage III: 40%–50%
Stage IV: 5%

**What is the treatment?**

Overall, identical to that for ovarian
carcinomas
The mainstay of treatment is exploratory
laparotomy to resect the bulk of the
tumor and adequately stage the
disease. Adequate staging includes
lymph node evaluation, biopsies of
suspect areas, and cytologic evaluation
of the peritoneal fluid.
The chemotherapeutic regimens are
similar to those for ovarian cancer and
include platinum-based agents,
cyclophosphamide, and doxorubicin.

**What is the overall 5-year
survival rate?**

Forty percent

**What is the 5-year survival
rate for each stage?**

Stage I: 65%
Stage II: 50%–60%
Stages III–IV: 10%–20%

## SARCOMA OF THE FALLOPIAN TUBES

**What is the most common
sarcoma of the fallopian
tubes?**

Primary mixed müllerian mesodermal
tumor (MMMT)

**Is MMMT common or rare?**

Very rare

**What is the common stage at presentation?**

Advanced stage III–IV disease

**Treatment?**

Attempted resection of disease as described previously, with adjuvant chemotherapy. Radiation therapy has limited usefulness.

**What is the overall 5-year survival rate?**

Zero percent

# 44

# Vaginal Cancer

| | |
|---|---|
| **Primary vaginal cancer comprises what percentage of all malignancies of the female genital tract?** | 1% to 2% |
| **What percentage of vaginal cancers are metastases from other primary cancer?** | 80% to 90% |
| **What cancers *usually* metastasize to the vagina?** | Cervical or vulvar |
| **What other cancers can metastasize to the vagina?** | Uterine, gestational neoplasms, and (by direct extension) rectal and bladder |
| **What are the signs and symptoms?** | Fifty percent to seventy-five percent of patients present with painless vaginal bleeding, either postcoital or postmenopausal. Vaginal discharge is common. Five percent present with pelvic pain. Five percent to ten percent of patients are asymptomatic. |
| **How is vaginal cancer diagnosed?** | Diagnosis is often difficult if the lesion is small or endophytic or if the lesion is covered by the blades of the speculum. The speculum should be manipulated so that the anterior and posterior vaginal walls are well visualized. Definitive diagnosis: Biopsy |
| **What findings are suspect for vaginal cancer?** | An abnormal Papanicolaou smear and normal cervical colposcopy |
| **How is vaginal cancer staged?** | Clinically staged (similar to cervical cancer) based on physical examination, cystoscopy, proctoscopy, and chest radiography: Stage 0: Carcinoma in situ Stage I: Limited to vaginal mucosa |

Stage II: Submucosal tissue involvement but no extension to the pelvic sidewall

Stage III: Extension to the pelvic sidewall

Stage IV: Extension beyond the pelvis or involvement of the bladder or rectal mucosa

    IVa: Extension to adjacent organs

    IVb: Spread to distant organs

**What are the histologic types of primary vaginal cancer and their frequencies?**

Squamous cell carcinoma: 84%
Adenocarcinoma: 9%
Sarcoma: 3%
Melanoma: 2%
Miscellaneous (e.g., lymphoma, small cell): 2%

## SQUAMOUS CELL CARCINOMA

**What is the mean age of patients with squamous cell carcinoma?**

Age 50–60 years

**Where is squamous cell carcinoma usually located?**

Upper posterior wall of the vagina

**From what metastatic cancers is squamous cell carcinoma of the vagina difficult to differentiate?**

Metastases from the cervix or vulva

**Is squamous cell carcinoma associated with human papillomavirus?**

Yes

**What percentage of patients have a history of severe cervical dysplasia or cervical cancer?**

Thirty percent
May be secondary to the treatment for cervical cancer, especially if previously treated with radiation therapy.
If diagnosed more than 5 years after the cervical cancer, it is most likely a second primary lesion.

**What percentage of patients present at each stage?**

Stage I: 25%
Stage II: 34%
Stage III: 25%
Stage IV: 16%

**How does squamous cell carcinoma spread?**

Direct spread or invasion
Lymphatic spread, primarily to the inguinal and the pelvic lymph nodes
Hematogenous spread

**What is the treatment of squamous cell carcinoma?**

Overall, radiation is preferred.
Surgical treatment is indicated in a few circumstances:
  Stage I disease in the upper vagina
  In young patients, to preserve ovarian function
  Patients with advanced local disease may undergo pelvic exenteration.
  Radiation failures

**What are the treatment options for carcinoma in situ?**

Surgical excision to rule out invasive cancer
Laser ablation
Interstitial radiation
Radioactive implants placed in the vagina to provide local radiation dose to the affected area
Topical chemotherapy with 5-fluorouracil

**What are the treatment options for stage I disease?**

Radical hysterectomy with pelvic lymphadenectomy and partial vaginectomy
Interstitial radiation

**What are the treatment options for stages II, III, and IV disease?**

External and interstitial radiation

**What are the complications from treatment?**

Complications occur in 10%–15% of patients and include radiation cystitis, fistula formation, vaginal stenosis, and proctitis.

**What is the overall 5-year survival rate?**

Forty-two percent

**What are the 5-year survival rates for each stage?**

Stage I: 70%
Stage II: 46%
Stage III: 30%–40%
Stage IV: 10%–15%

## ADENOCARCINOMA

**What is the frequency of primary adenocarcinoma of the vagina?**

Rare

**In what age-group does this cancer primarily occur?**

Except for clear cell adenocarcinoma, primarily in postmenopausal women
Most clear cell adenocarcinomas occur in women 17–20 years of age.

**What is the relationship between diethylstilbestrol (DES) exposure and clear cell adenocarcinomas?**

Sixty-five percent of women with clear cell adenocarcinoma have documented evidence of DES exposure.
Ten percent have exposure to an "unknown" drug.
Twenty-five percent were not exposed to DES.

**What is the estimated risk of clear cell carcinoma in DES-exposed women?**

One in 1000

**Where are adenocarcinomas primarily located?**

In the exocervix or the upper third of the vagina

**At what stage do most patients present?**

Seventy percent present with stage I disease.

**What is the treatment?**

Similar to that for squamous cell carcinoma
Stage I disease: Surgery is the primary treatment.
Advanced stages: Radiation therapy is the primary treatment.

**What is 5-year overall survival rate?**

Seventy-eight percent

**What are the 5-year survival rates for each stage?**

Stage I: 87%
Stage II: 76%
Stage III: 30%

## EMBRYONAL RHABDOMYOSARCOMA

**What are the two types of embryonal rhabdomyosarcoma?**

Solid and cystic.
The cystic form is referred to as sarcoma botryoides, and is the most common vaginal tumor in infants and children.

**In what age-group do most embryonal rhabdomyosarcomas commonly occur?**

Ninety percent occur in children younger than 5 years of age.

**Where in women of reproductive age are embryonal rhabdomyosarcomas primarily located?**

The cervix

**Where in postmenopausal women are embryonal rhabdomyosarcomas primarily located?**

The uterus

**At what stage do most patients present with embryonal rhabdomyosarcoma?**

Usually at an advanced stage

**What is the treatment?**

Previously treated with exenteration, which was ineffective and associated with a high complication rate
Currently, treatment involves a combination of surgical resection, chemotherapy, and radiation therapy.

**What is the overall 5-year survival rate?**

20% to 30%

## MELANOMA

**What is the mean age of patients with melanoma?**

Age 60 years

**In what race do melanomas almost always occur?**

White

**What are the signs and symptoms?**

Most patients present with vaginal bleeding, discharge, or a mass.

**Where are melanomas primarily located?**

Most commonly arise in the distal vagina and may or may not be pigmented.

**At what stage do most patients with melanoma present?**

Melanoma is too rare to assign percentages.

**What is the treatment?**

Surgery has been the primary treatment, including radical exenteration, although local control is difficult to achieve with surgery alone.
Radiation therapy may be helpful in selected patients.

**What is the overall 5-year survival rate?**

Less than 10%

# 45

# General Gynecologic Oncology

## RADIATION THERAPY

**What is radiation therapy?**

Use of x-rays and gamma rays to treat cancer

**How does radiation therapy kill cancer cells?**

Cells are sensitive to the effects of radiation during the G2 phase of mitosis. The radiation kills cells by breaking DNA strands, either directly or by producing free radicals.

**What is the relationship between tumor size and depth and the dose of radiation required to cause cell death?**

As a tumor increases in size and depth, an increasing dose of radiation needs to be applied to cause cell death.

**How is radiation therapy administered?**

External beam: X-ray beam therapy in which electromagnetic energy is directed to the target tissue from an "external" source

Brachytherapy: Gamma-ray therapy in which the source is placed into the patient's body

In interstitial therapy, the source (e.g., cesium needles) is placed directly into the area of the tumor.

In intracavitary therapy, the source is placed indirectly in the area of the tumor (e.g., vaginal colpostats and uterine tandems).

Radioisotopes: Radiation therapy in which a radioisotope in solution (e.g., gold in solution) is placed in the peritoneal cavity to deliver radiation directly to the surface of the tumor

| | |
|---|---|
| **What is the inverse square law?** | The dose of radiation delivered to the tissue is the inverse square of the distance from the source to the tissues. |
| **What is the conventional unit of radiation used in radiation oncology?** | Centigray (cGy) One cGy is equal to 1 rad. |
| **What are the dosage limitations for normal tissues?** | Ovary: 1000 cGy Kidney: 2500 cGY Liver: 5000 cGY Intestine: 6000 cGY Bladder: 6500 cGY |
| **What are the complications?** | Both tumor cells and normal cells absorb radiation; surrounding tissues also undergo cell damage. Acute complications: Nausea and diarrhea secondary to mucosal damage leading to mucosal irritation and sloughing; "sun burn" secondary to radiation absorption by the skin Chronic complications: Radiation causes microvascular damage and fibrosis, leading to poor tissue oxygenation and repair. Genitourinary tract: Fistulas between the bladder and surrounding organs, ureteral strictures, hemorrhagic cystitis Gastrointestinal tract: Fistulas and strictures that may require surgical resection and repair Vaginal stenosis, fistula tract formation Ovarian failure with subsequent anovulation; hormone replacement should be considered in premenopausal women. |

## CHEMOTHERAPY

| | |
|---|---|
| **What is chemotherapy?** | Use of drugs that exert a cytotoxic effect on cells |
| **What are cycle-specific drugs?** | Act only during a specific phase of cell division and therefore depend on cellular proliferation |

**What are cycle-nonspecific drugs?**

Act during all phases and therefore depend less on cellular proliferation

**What are the mechanisms of cytotoxicity of chemotherapeutic agents? Give examples of drugs for each mechanism.**

DNA synthesis inhibitors [e.g., 5-fluorouracil (5-FU), methotrexate, bleomycin]

Mitotic inhibitors (e.g., vincristine, vinblastine, taxol)

Alkylating agents [e.g., ifosfamide, cyclophosphamide, doxorubicin (Adriamycin), cisplatin, carboplatin]

**How are dosages calculated?**

Most dosages are determined in clinical trials. Dosages are then individualized to the patient based on renal and hepatic function, body surface area, and side effects such as myelosuppression, nephrotoxicity, and neurotoxicity.

**What is the mechanism of action of 5-FU?**

Interferes with DNA synthesis by disrupting the DNA chain. It is a DNA synthesis inhibitor and cycle specific, and acts during the G2 phase of the cell cycle.

**When is 5-FU used?**

Primarily to treat cervical cancer and for vulvar and vaginal dysplasia

**How is 5-FU excreted?**

Renal

**What are its toxicities?**

Myelosuppression, nausea, vomiting, alopecia

**What is the mechanism of action of methotrexate?**

Interferes with DNA synthesis by interfering with folate reduction. It is a DNA synthesis inhibitor and cycle-specific, and acts during the G2 phase of the cell cycle.

**When is methotrexate used?**

Primarily to treat gestational trophoblastic disease

**How is it excreted?**

Renal

**What are its toxicities?**

Myelosuppression, mucositis, liver and kidney damage, alopecia

| | |
|---|---|
| **What is the mechanism of action of bleomycin?** | Bleomycin is an antibiotic that forms free radicals that cause breaks in the DNA strand during mitosis. It is a DNA synthesis inhibitor and cycle-specific, and acts during the G2 phase of the cell cycle. |
| **When is bleomycin used?** | To treat squamous cell carcinoma of the vagina and vulva and ovarian germ cell tumors |
| **How is it excreted?** | Renal |
| **What are its toxicities?** | Interstitial pneumonitis, alopecia, and pulmonary fibrosis<br>Total dose must be limited to 400 mg secondary to an increased risk of pulmonary fibrosis.<br>Patients should be followed by chest x-ray and diffusion capacity of carbon monoxide. |
| **What is the mechanism of action of vincristine?** | Vincristine interferes with microtubule function during mitosis. It is a mitotic inhibitor and cycle-specific. |
| **When is vincristine used?** | To treat gestational trophoblastic disease and ovarian germ cell tumors |
| **How is it excreted?** | Renal |
| **What are its toxicities?** | Myelosuppression, neurotoxicity, alopecia |
| **What is the mechanism of action of vinblastine?** | Interferes with spindle formation during mitosis. It is a mitotic inhibitor and cycle-specific. |
| **When is vinblastine used?** | For the same conditions as vincristine |
| **How is it excreted?** | Renal |
| **What are its toxicities?** | Nausea, vomiting, myelosuppression, stomatitis, alopecia, and neurotoxicity |
| **What is the mechanism of action of Taxol?** | It is an alkaloid derived from the yew tree and acts by interfering with spindle cell function during mitosis. It is a mitotic inhibitor and cycle-specific. |

| | |
|---|---|
| **When is Taxol used?** | Primarily to treat ovarian cancer, but also used as second-line therapy for uterine and cervical carcinomas |
| **How is it excreted?** | Hepatic |
| **What are its toxicities?** | Myelosuppression, allergic reactions including anaphylaxis with cardiopulmonary collapse, seizures, nausea, vomiting, alopecia, neurotoxicity |
| **What is the mechanism of action of ifosfamide?** | Interferes with DNA linkage. It is an alkylating agent and cycle-nonspecific. |
| **When is ifosfamide used?** | To treat cervical and ovarian cancers, all sarcomas |
| **How is it excreted?** | Renal |
| **What are its toxicities? ?** | Myelosuppression, nausea, vomiting, alopecia, hemorrhagic cystitis, nephrotoxicity |
| **What is the mechanism of action of cyclophosphamide?** | Interferes with DNA linkage. It is an alkylating agent and cycle-nonspecific. |
| **When is cyclophosphamide used?** | Used primarily to treat ovarian and endometrial carcinoma |
| **How is it excreted?** | Renal |
| **What are its toxicities?** | Myelosuppression, nausea, vomiting, alopecia, hemorrhagic cystitis |
| **What is the mechanism of action of doxorubicin?** | Doxorubicin is an antibiotic that interferes with DNA and RNA synthesis by forming free radicals. It is an alkylating agent and cycle-nonspecific. |
| **When is doxorubicin used?** | To treat uterine and ovarian cancer |
| **How is it excreted?** | Hepatic |
| **What are its toxicities?** | Myelosuppression, nausea, vomiting, cardiomyopathy<br>Cardiomyopathy is dose-related; usually begins with 500 mg/m$^2$ |

| | |
|---|---|
| **What is the mechanism of action of carboplatin?** | Carboplatin cross-links DNA. It is an alkylating agent and cycle-nonspecific. |
| **When is carboplatin used?** | To treat ovarian carcinoma |
| **How is it excreted?** | Renal |
| **What are its toxicities?** | Thrombocytopenia, nausea, vomiting, nephropathy, peripheral neuropathy |
| **What is the mechanism of action of cisplatin?** | Cross-links DNA; it is an alkylating agent and cycle-nonspecific. |
| **When is cisplatin used?** | To treat ovarian carcinoma and cervical cancer |
| **How is it excreted?** | Renal |
| **What are its toxicities?** | Decreased white blood cell count, ototoxicity, nephrotoxicity, peripheral neuropathy |

## SURGICAL PROCEDURES

| | |
|---|---|
| **What is a type I hysterectomy?** | Surgical removal of the uterine corpus and cervix |
| **What is a type II hysterectomy?** | Surgical removal of the uterine corpus, cervix, and medial half of the cardinal ligaments |
| **What is a type III hysterectomy?** | Surgical removal of the uterine corpus, cervix, cardinal ligaments, uterosacral ligaments, and upper third of the vagina with pelvic lymph node dissection. Also known as a radical hysterectomy. |
| **What is a type IV hysterectomy?** | Type III hysterectomy with removal of periureteral tissues and three-fourths of the vagina |
| **What is a type V hysterectomy?** | Type IV hysterectomy with removal of the distal ureters and bladder; similar to an anterior exenteration |

**What is an anterior exenteration?**

Removal of the uterine corpus, cervix, bladder, and vagina

**What is a posterior exenteration?**

Removal of the uterine corpus, cervix, rectum, and vagina

**What is a total pelvic exenteration?**

Removal of the uterine corpus, cervix, bladder, rectum, and vagina

# 46

# Urinary Incontinence

## INTRODUCTION

**What is urinary incontinence?**

The objective, involuntary loss of urine; presents a social and/or hygienic problem for the patient
Note: Urinary incontinence is a symptom, not a diagnosis, and therefore requires careful, thorough evaluation.

**How common is it?**

Reports among women less than 65 years of age range from 15% to 30%. In patients older than 65 years, the estimated prevalence is 30%.

## ETIOLOGIES

**What are some causes of urinary incontinence (especially in elderly patients)?**

Anatomic abnormalities
Urinary infection
Drugs
General atrophy
Neurologic impairment

**What is the most common form of urinary incontinence among women?**

Stress incontinence (SUI) occurs during periods of increased intra-abdominal pressure (e.g., coughing, sneezing, exercise).

**What is the pathophysiology of SUI?**

In general, there is loss of anatomic support of the urethra, bladder, and/or urethrovesical junction, which allows the proximal urethra to be located outside the abdominal pressure zone. Thus, any increase in intra-abdominal pressure is transmitted to the bladder without a simultaneous rise in urethral pressure, so urine is involuntarily lost.

**What factors contribute to the development of stress incontinence?**

Denervation injuries from labor, childbirth, or pelvic surgeries
Previous bladder surgeries
Advanced age
Hypoestrogenism

**What is intrinsic urethral sphincter deficiency?**

Specific type of SUI, which may or may not coexist with an anatomic abnormality of the urethra
Usually results from previous bladder surgery or severe denervation injury
Urethra is rigid ("pipe stem")

**How is the condition diagnosed?**

Urodynamic evaluation

**What is the treatment?**

Pubovesical sling or collagen injections

**What is urge incontinence?**

Involuntary loss of urine associated with an abrupt and strong desire to void
Also known as **detrusor instability** because of overactivity of the detrusor muscle
In the presence of detrusor overactivity and a neurologic lesion (e.g., Parkinson's disease), the term **detrusor hyperreflexia** is commonly used.

**How does the detrusor muscle normally serve to maintain urinary continence?**

Normal micturition is under voluntary and involuntary control. The detrusor muscle is the smooth muscle wall of the bladder and normally contracts reflexively after voluntary relaxation of the pelvic floor and urethral musculature.

**What is mixed urinary incontinence?**

Urinary incontinence due to both detrusor instability and genuine stress incontinence

**What are some other causes of urinary incontinence?**

Urethral diverticulum
Congenital abnormalities (e.g., ectopic ureter)
Urinary fistula
Bladder cancer

| **What drugs can cause incontinence?** | Diuretics:<br>Methyldopa<br>Prazosin<br>Antihistamines:<br>Phenothiazines<br>Diazepam |
|---|---|
| **What is overflow incontinence?** | Results from underactivity of the detrusor muscle, most commonly from a neurogenic (e.g., diabetic) or postoperative bladder<br>Bladder fails to empty adequately, resulting in a large postvoid residual (PVR), usually > 300 ml<br>Leakage can thus be precipitated by small increases in intra-abdominal pressure because the bladder is always full. |

## EVALUATION

| **What are the pertinent questions to ask when taking the patient's history?** | "Do you leak when coughing, sneezing, laughing, or with exercise?" (suggests SUI)<br>"Do you leak before you reach the toilet with a strong urge to void?" (suggests urge incontinence)<br>"How many voids per day?" (frequency suggests infection or overflow)<br>"Nocturia or incontinence with intercourse?" (suggests urge incontinence)<br>"Do you wear pads? How disabling is the problem?"<br>"How often do you have leaking?"<br>"History of UTIs?"<br>"Painful urination?" (suggests obstruction, cancer, infection)<br>"Hematuria?" (suggests cancer, infection)<br>"Difficulty initiating voiding?" (suggests obstruction, loss of bladder support, neurologic impairment)<br>"Straining with urination?" (suggests obstruction)<br>"Feeling of incomplete emptying?" (suggests obstruction, loss of bladder support)<br>Note: Some patients may benefit from keeping a voiding diary. |
|---|---|

**What should be looked for on physical examination?**

Atrophy
Vaginal infection
Urethral diverticulum
Cystocele
Descent of bladder

**What is the Q-tip test?**

A Q-tip lubricated with viscous lidocaine is placed in the urethra at the urethrovesical junction.
To check for hypermobility of the urethra (a condition often associated with stress incontinence), have the patient Valsalva. If the Q-tip deviates more than about 30°, the test is positive.

**What tests can be performed in the office to assess urinary incontinence?**

Urinalysis with culture should always be performed.
Urine cytology for women with unexplained hematuria

**What are office cystometrics?**

After the patient empties her bladder, postvoid residual is checked.
A sterile catheter is then placed in the bladder, which is filled with increments of 50 to 100 cc sterile water.
Patient is asked to relay her first filling sensation, first urge to void, and maximum bladder capacity.

**What does a detrusor contraction look like?**

A rise in the meniscus of fluid in the catheter suggests a detrusor contraction.

**What is a stress test?**

After maximal filling, the patient is asked to cough.
If she **immediately** leaks urine, the test is positive.
If leakage occurs several seconds after provocation, the patient may have a component of detrusor instability.
It is essential to check in both the supine and the standing position.

**Who should be referred for more sophisticated urodynamic testing?**

Approximately 10% to 15% of patients will require multichannel urodynamic testing for diagnosis. Such studies might be useful for patients with:
  Mixed urge and stress symptoms
  Prior bladder surgeries

Suggestive history, but negative office
evaluation
Also used to rule out intrinsic sphincter
deficiency, which may predict surgical
failure

**What are the benefits of
cystoscopy?**

Can diagnose fistulae, foreign bodies,
tumors, or aberrant ureters

**What is the purpose of
multichannel urodynamic
tests?**

Specialized catheters simultaneously
record urethral, vesical, and intra-
abdominal pressures, and precisely
diagnose detrusor instability and/or
stress incontinence.

## TREATMENT

**What are the treatment
options for urinary
incontinence?**

Behavioral modification
Pharmacologic treatment
Surgical management

**What are some behavioral
techniques used to treat
urinary incontinence?**

Encouraging patient to avoid excess fluid
and/or caffeine intake
Regularly scheduled voiding
Biofeedback techniques
Clean, intermittent self-catheterization
Vaginal pessaries, if pelvic organ
prolapse is also present

**What are some
pharmacologic agents used
to treat urinary
incontinence?**

Antispasmodics (e.g., oxybutynin)
Tricyclic antidepressants (e.g.,
imipramine)
α-adrenergic agents (e.g.,
phenylpropanolamine)

**Is hormone replacement
recommended?**

In postmenopausal women, estrogen
replacement (topical or oral) is
recommended to treat stress or urge
incontinence.

**What is the Burch
procedure?**

Abdominal retropubic urethropexy
operation
Uses suture to suspend the paravaginal
fascia (which supports/surrounds the
urethra) to the abdominal side of the
pubic bone
Point of attachment is Cooper's
ligament, better known as the
iliopectineal line
Success rate is 75% to 90%

**What is the Marshall-Marchetti-Krantz procedure?**

Abdominal retropubic urethropexy operation
Uses suture to suspend the paravaginal fascia to the abdominal side of the pubic bone
Point of attachment is the cartilage in the symphysis pubis
Success rate is 75% to 90%

**What complication is associated with the MMK procedure?**

Osteitis pubis, a painful inflammatory condition (occurs in up to 5% of patients)

**What complications are associated with the Burch procedure?**

An enterocele (occurs in 7% to 15% of patients)

**What is a Pereyra procedure?**

Type of vaginal suspension for SUI

**What is the advantage of a Pereyra procedure?**

Vaginal approach

**What is the disadvantage of this procedure?**

Potential bladder injury and smaller objective cure rate (40%–70%)

**What is a suburethral sling procedure?**

Reserved for patients at most risk for operative failure (those with intrinsic sphincter deficiency, severe obesity, prior surgical failures, or a scarred, fibrotic urethra)
Restores continence by elevating the urethrovesical junction and mechanically compressing the urethra against the pubic symphysis
Autologous graft material, usually a thin strip of rectus fascia, is tunneled under the urethra and sewn to the abdominal wall

**What are the possible complications of a suburethral sling procedure?**

Postoperative voiding dysfunction, especially urinary retention

**What are some other surgical techniques?**

Periurethral collagen injections
Insertion of an artificial urinary sphincter

# Index

Page numbers in *italics* represent figures; page numbers with a *t* indicate tables.

Agranulocytosis, 377
AIDS. *See* Acquired immunodeficiency
  syndrome (AIDS); Human
  immunodeficiency virus (HIV)
Alcohol
  during pregnancy, 41
  teratogenicity and/or adverse effects of,
    176
Alpha-fetoprotein (AFP), definition of, 3
Amenorrhea, 351–358
  axes in, 352–353
  evaluation of patient, 353–356
  postpill, 299
  primary, 351, 356
  secondary, 351, 356, 357
  specific disorders, 356–358
  types of, 351
Aminoglycosides, teratogenicity and/or
  adverse effects of, 176
Amniocentesis, 3, 109
Amnioinfusion, 63
  in intrapartum management of post-
    term pregnancy, 128
Amniotic fluid, 3, 183
  volume of, in assessing intrauterine
    growth restriction (IUGR), 107
Ampicillin in treating bacterial vaginosis,
    243
Anatomy, female, 18–32
Androgen excess
  signs and symptoms indicative of, 297
  tests for, 341
Androgen insensitivity syndrome, 316–
  317
Android pelvis, 19
Anemia
  in pregnancy, 14
  defining, 112
    etiologic factors of, 112
    iron deficiency, 112–113
  relationship between folate deficiency
    in pregnancy and megaloblastic,
    114
Angiography during pregnancy, 224
Angiotensin-converting enzyme
  inhibitors, teratogenicity and/or
  adverse effects of, 178
Anovulatory cycles, differentiation
  between ovulatory cycles and, 325
Anovulatory dysfunction, management of,
  300
Antepartum testing, 126–127

Anthropoid pelvis, 19
Antibiotics. *See also specific antibiotic*
  for premature rupture of membranes,
    102
  teratogenicity and/or adverse effects of,
    176
  for tuberculosis, 159–160
Anticonvulsant medication for
  preeclampsia, 140
Antihistamines, teratogenicity and/or
  adverse effects of, 176
Antihypertensive medication for
  preeclampsia, 140–141
Apgar score, 3
Appendicitis, effects of pregnancy related
  to, 16
Arcuate line, 18
Artificial rupture of membranes (AROM)
  as controversial, 56
Asherman syndrome, 347–348
Aspirin, teratogenicity and/or adverse
  effects of, 177
Assisted reproductive technologies, 348–
  350
Assisted vaginal delivery
  goals of, 48
  steps in, 48–49
Asthma, 149–152
  diagnosis of, 149
  effect of pregnancy on, 149–150
  etiologic factors of, 149
  incidence of, 149
  management of, 150
  pathophysiology of, 149
  symptoms of, 149
  treatment of, 150–152
Asymptomatic bacteriuria, 161–162
  complications of, 162
  diagnosis of, 161–162
  incidence of, 161
  treatment of, 162
Auscultation in monitoring labor, 45

Backache during pregnancy, 42
Bacterial cystitis, 236
Bacterial infections
  diagnosis of, 217–218
  group B streptococcus, 216–219
    fetal effects of, 216–217
    incidence of, 216
    signs and symptoms of, 216
  *Listeria monocytogenes,* 219–220